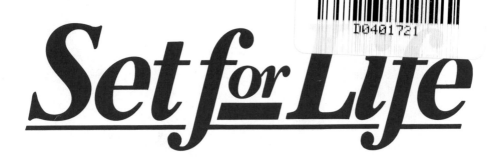

Set for Life

Eat More...
Weigh Less...
Feel Terrific!

Featuring More Than
350 Lowfat Recipes ...

Jane P. Merrill • Karen M. Sunderland

Foreword by Dennis Remington M.D.

Copyright © 1988, 1995 by
Sunrise Publishers
P.O. Box 112112
Salt Lake City, UT 84147
Phone (801) 595-8155

Library of Congress Catalog Card No.: 88-92562

ISBN 0-9621168-3-1

Sixth Printing, Revised 1995

Published in the United States of America

Contents

The Authors

Jane P. Merrill is a professional health and weight control counselor. She has taught the Setpoint principles both as an independent consultant and as an owner and operator of three health and weight control centers. Jane and her husband Jay have six children and twenty-three grandchildren.

Jane finds much personal fulfillment in teaching the *Setpoint* lifestyle. She sees the principles proven daily in the lives of clients and their families as lifestyle changes occur. For the past twenty years Jane has taught cooking and nutrition classes based upon simple, practical methods of food preparation. She believes people are getting back to eating *real food*, and that they need help in streamlining menu planning and food preparation. She believes in eating well without spending all day in the kitchen. In *Set For Life* she shares secrets and recipes that will make this possible for every family who wants to enjoy better health and weight control. Everyone is delighted to learn that they too, can: Eat More - Weigh Less - Feel Terrific!

The second half of this mother-daughter team is Jane's oldest daughter, *Karen M. Sunderland*. She has a bachelor's degree in home economics with an emphasis in nutrition.

College training was just the beginning of Karen's interest in nutrition. Karen and Merrill Sunderland are the parents of 6 children. As their family grew, Karen realized the importance of diet to a child's physical and mental development. She has undertaken a specialized, intense study in pre-natal, infant and child nutrition, and attends every available Nutrition Seminar dealing with this subject. In addition, she applies what she learns in her own home with her young family.

Foreword

Reduced-calorie dieting does not help with long-term weight control; it only makes you fatter. Besides that, dieting causes fatigue, weakness, depression, irritability, excessive hunger, headaches, and a wide range of other unpleasant symptoms.

In addition to these problems, it is clear that cutting calories over the long term is also dangerous. Researchers evaluated a large group of people for twelve years. They found that those women who died of strokes ate 361 calories per day less than the women who lived! In spite of eating considerably fewer calories, the people in this group who died were actually heavier on the average than those in the healthy group. The conclusion from the study was that these people could have reduced their risk of dying by 40 percent simply by increasing their potassium intake by the equivalent of one serving of fresh fruits or vegetables per day. (Khaw K-T. Barrett-Connor E. "Dietary Potassium and stroke-associated mortality: a 12 year prospective population study." *N Engl J Med* 1987; 316:235-40) A number of other population studies have shown the same results — those who died prematurely ate less food, on the average, than those who lived.

Eating adequate amounts of good, nutritious, low-fat, high-complex-carbohydrate food is very important for good health. The idea that you could eat plenty of food and still lose weight was first presented in a book I coauthored, *How to Lower Your Fat Thermostat* (Vitality House International, 1983). With this program, not only *can* you eat plenty, you *must* eat plenty of food to be effective in lowering the fat thermostat (Setpoint) for permanent weight control. The type of food we recommend for weight control is very similar to that recommended by the American Heart Association, the American Diabetes Association, and the American Cancer Society.

It is now clear from a scientific viewpoint what foods we should be eating and that we should eat adequate amounts. However, to actually eat this way is not always easy. In this book, Jane and Karen offer many helpful guidelines in changing your attitudes and lifestyle. The principles that they teach are very much in harmony with my own beliefs. By following their suggestions, you should not only lose weight naturally and comfortably, but you should also feel better and greatly reduce your risks of developing serious diseases.

Dennis W. Remington, M.D.
Bariatric (weight control) Physician

Preface

Once every dozen years or so a new book comes into the marketplace that is destined to have a major impact in the lives of its readers. We believe *SET FOR LIFE* is just such a book. While there are hundreds of cookbooks on the market, few of them combine the results of extensive experience in health and weight-control counseling with proven recipes that complement the total program. These recipes provide delicious alternatives to the typically drab fare being offered to persons struggling with health and weight problems.

The concepts contained within these pages have been taught to thousands of people over the past several years; the results have been outstanding. Those who follow these simple principles look and feel better than they have in years. Success has been accomplished with careful attention to attitude, moderate exercise, and eating patterns.

This is not a diet book. It does not prescribe a diet. Rather, it teaches a lean, healthy way of life and includes more than 350 tasty recipes for foods which enhance that lifestyle.

Our message is simple:

Eat More - Weigh Less - Feel Terrific.

That's what this book is all about.

Introduction

As I discovered the *Setpoint* principles, I was reminded of a story in the Old Testament. Naaman, a mighty Syrian captain, suffered from leprosy. A servant suggested that the Israelite prophet Elisha could heal him. Accordingly, Naaman traveled to Samaria to see Elisha. Elisha sent a messenger to Naaman, telling him to bathe seven times in the River Jordan and he would be cleansed.

Naaman was so angry at the simplicity of the cure that he refused to comply. He had his own ideas on how he should be healed. His servants contended that if Elisha had asked Naaman to perform some great feat in order to be cleansed, he would have readily obeyed. Therefore, why not obey the simple request and be made clean? Seeing the logic, Naaman finally followed the instructions and was healed.

In like manner, the *Setpoint Lifestyle* is rather simple in concept and application. This does not take away from its effectiveness, however, but rather enhances it. Truths are simple, and because they are, we tend to look elsewhere for our answers.

In light of recent research, there is little doubt that the program outlined in this book is one of the most effective health and weight-management programs in existence. It *is* built on simple truths, but don't be fooled by its simplicity; anything worthwhile requires effort. Your success will be assured if you make the effort to follow each step as outlined.

Unlike Naaman, who received no reasons for his instruction, this book contains many good reasons as to why these principles work so effectively. It includes a step-by-step plan, plus more than 350 tasty recipes to make this lifestyle change as easy as possible. These recipes provide good everyday eating your whole family will enjoy.

As I counsel people with health and weight problems, they repeatedly ask: "What can I eat that tastes good? I want to fix something that my family likes; I don't want to fix two meals." I began to share these recipes with clients and friends, and their responses were similar: "My husband said he could eat that dish three times a week. Even our three-year-old enjoyed it. It was so simple, yet so good!" Sometimes they brought me recipes to help others share in their good eating, and some are included.

Since many people aren't into cooking these days because of busy lifestyles, most of the recipes in this book are simple and not too involved. They call for ordinary ingredients you can find in almost any grocery store. Menu planning becomes surprisingly easy by following the simple guidelines. Don't wait to make the exciting discovery of how you, too, can:

Eat More - Weigh Less - Feel Terrific!

Acknowledgments

We gratefully acknowledge the assistance and inspiration of many people. A very special thanks to our dear husbands, Jay and Merrill. They never wavered in their patience, support and encouragement. To our children: Debra and Steve Parks; Julie and Rick Dooley; Alan and Debbie, Dale and Debbie, and Junius Merrill; Heidi, David, Shaun, Marc and Lisa Sunderland, we say thank you for helping us in so many different ways. You have all been totally supportive.

Dona Jo Osterhout has rendered countless hours of service. We also thank Vall Gene Mills, Janis Hardy, Lane Godfrey, Debbie Hunt, Rose Kreiger, Joan Parr, Annjean Scholer, Kathie Maughan, Dana Thornock, Florence Johnson, Cindy Holiman, R.D. and others who have contributed recipes, assistance, and encouragement whose names cannot be included here.

Debbie T. Merrill gave invaluable help in computations and proofreading. Dale Merrill gave freely of his time and talents in the tedious final editing. Many others helped too.

The beautiful pictures add so much to our book. Thanks to Brett Kennedy and his outstanding team for their extraordinary work of art. Working with them was an education!

Art Director — Brett Kennedy
Photographer — Steve Bunderson
Food Stylists — Melanie Shumway & Jill Turner
Typesetting — Accu-Type Typographers, Paula Conway
Cover Design — Dan Ishii

We acknowledge the great contribution made by Dr. Dennis Remington (M.D.), Dr. Garth Fisher (Ph.D.), and Dr. Edward Parent (Ph.D.). Their book, *How to Lower Your Fat Thermostat*, introduced an entirely new approach to weight management that is sweeping the country. *Set For Life* does not attempt to duplicate the sound research and documentation of these bariatric (weight-control) specialists. Instead, it helps you implement their ideas and avoid the greatest con game of all—dieting.

CHAPTER 1

Eat More — Weigh Less

If you want to lose weight or if you've already lost weight and are struggling to keep it off, you'll be delighted to learn that living the *Setpoint* lifestyle provides the simple, permanent solution to your problem. Dieters know that losing weight is only half the battle — keeping it off is the real war. Who wants to stay on a restrictive diet forever?

If you really want to *eat more, weigh less, and feel terrific,* keep reading. Don't just skim a page or two. Invest an hour in yourself and read every word of the first five chapters so that you thoroughly understand how you can be lean and healthy naturally. Then follow the simple guidelines step by step to achieve success. The rules are the same whether you want to lose weight, gain weight, maintain your ideal weight, or simply improve your health.

Best of all, no more mealtime dilemma. Packed between the covers of this book are hundreds of quick, delicious family recipes. They're "real food", not "diet" food. As you get lean, you and your family will get healthy—a winning combination!

Starvation Is Not The Answer

SET FOR LIFE is a lifestyle of abundance, not starvation. It is the normal, natural diet your body needs to achieve good health and weight control. Instead of starving your body into abnormally disposing of the excess fat, you eat and exercise yourself into a condition of good health and a normal weight. This naturally high-fiber diet is packed with the nutrients your body needs to be healthy and strong. It is low in cholesterol, fats, and sugars; high in whole grains, vegetables, and fruits. And as you eat these complex carbohydrates, you are much more likely to feel satisfied before you overeat.

SET FOR LIFE is the ideal family plan for good health and weight control; one you can live for the rest of your life — anytime, anywhere. This lifestyle has been successful for people of all ages; for those in top physical condition, and for those who can barely get from the house to the car. It is ideal for pregnant women and nursing mothers. Men as well as women love it because it is common-sense eating, not starvation.

Living this *Setpoint* lifestyle induces an internal feeling of calmness and tranquility. You will feel satisfied and content, knowing that your body is finally functioning as it should and that you're getting lean and healthy in the process.

Band-Aids: Do They Cover or Cure?

The problem with dieting is that it treats the symptoms related to weight problems. *SET FOR LIFE* treats the underlying cause. People have become avid consumers of band-aid approaches to weight control—diet pills, diet shots, diet drinks, and diet foods. For years the prescription for losing weight has been to simply decrease food intake—quit eating. After all, it's logical to think that if you consume fewer calories, you'll automatically lose weight.

This prescription sounds great and looks good on paper, but the results have been disappointing. About 95 percent of those persons who adhere to a diet plan will regain their weight plus some additional pounds within two years. Going without or eating less food doesn't lower weight in the long run, *unless you follow it with a positive lifestyle change.*

Dieting can actually cause the body to retain fat. Why? Because our bodies have been genetically programmed against starvation or restrictive eating. Historically, the greatest single threat to human existence—greater than wars, disease, or plague—has been famine. More people have died from starvation than from any other cause. As a result, our bodies have developed an elaborate protective defense and have become intricately tuned to overcoming the threat of famine. The body cannot tell the difference between starvation and restrictive dieting, but it does know when it isn't getting enough food and nutrients to keep going.

Don't Fight Your Body

When you diet, you are fighting your body. You're forcing it to go without adequate food (nutrients), something it is not designed to do. Your body immediately feels threatened and goes to work to keep you from starving. First, your appetite increases and you are always hungry. In fact, you may become obsessed with food and think about it all the time. Your favorite reading material becomes your cookbook. Next, your metabolic rate decreases and you have no energy. You just want to sit quietly or take a nap. You may also have poor mental endurance and be unable to think clearly. You are nervous, irritable or depressed. These symptoms of starvation have been experienced by most dieters.

Strange Things Happen When You Diet

You do need food to fuel your body, even if you don't feel hungry. Those who suffer from anorexia are never hungry, but they are actually starving. Like many dieters, they suffer from an artificial suppression of hunger. Sooner or later, a binge is inevitable. A binge is one way the body can force you to eat, preventing the starvation it senses.

Dieting raises the *Setpoint*. It goes higher with each diet you try. After successive diets, your metabolism is so confused that it stays suppressed, even after you quit dieting. That's why you can eat a little and gain a lot.

What Is The Setpoint?

Think of the *Setpoint* as the fat level of the body which is determined by a weight-regulating mechanism in the brain. The *Setpoint* is the weight that the body naturally gravitates toward under a normal pattern of eating, drinking, and exercising. The *Setpoint* is the weight at which you stabilize when you make no special effort to gain or lose — the "set" amount of weight at which the body feels comfortable and naturally tends to maintain.

The *Setpoint* can be raised and lowered because it is governed by how effectively the body burns or stores fat for energy. The weight-regulating mechanism controls body weight by increasing or decreasing the appetite as needed to control this *Setpoint* weight and to protect the body from a deficiency of nutrients. It can also trigger systems in the body to "waste" excess energy if you overeat or "conserve" energy if you under-eat. This weight-regulating mechanism works tirelessly to protect your *Setpoint* weight.

Lower Your Setpoint!

How do you lower your *Setpoint*? Eat regular wholesome meals, exercise daily, and live positively! With this balance, the overweight body begins to feel uncomfortable and senses a need to change. As your body adjusts to being fueled and exercised regularly, it will begin to burn more calories. Burning more calories raises your metabolic rate and causes your metabolism to reset at a higher level. (A simplified explanation of the metabolic rate is the number of calories the body burns each day to keep you going.) In this way the body seeks to rid itself of excess fat so it can accommodate your new lifestyle. As you raise your metabolic rate your *Setpoint* lowers naturally!

If you've been a yo-yo dieter and are making the switch to this *Setpoint* lifestyle, it may take a while for your body to readjust and raise your low metabolic rate. You may even have a temporary gain as your body adjusts to normal eating again, but don't panic! Be assured that as you follow the guidelines as outlined, you will soon begin to look and feel terrific as you shed those unwanted inches and pounds naturally.

When you work *with* your body, it is given a sense of security. Your body no longer needs the fat for survival protection because you are meeting its nutritional needs. With a high *Setpoint*, the body stores fat readily and carefully guards its fat stores. With a low *Setpoint*, the body burns fat readily and stores fat slowly.

Don't Be Impatient!

Most people who begin living the *Setpoint* lifestyle start to look and feel better right away. For a few, however, the process will be slower, and they must be patient. The body seems to take care of first things first! If your body is nutritionally deficient due to poor eating habits, extreme stress, ill health, anorexia, restrictive dieting, or for any other reason, health must be reestablished first.

If you are using all your daily food intake to provide the necessary energy just to get you through the day, there may be little or none left to repair and rebuild the body and to burn excess fat. All these activities take energy, and food is the fuel which provides that energy. Your body deserves the best high grade fuel available (wholesome foods), so be selective about what you eat. Would you put low-grade fuel in a new Mercedes?

Help Yourself

Most people benefit from taking a good whole-food concentrate or food supplement to help support the body's own healing activity so that it can regenerate more quickly. (Regeneration means strengthening the body so that it can heal itself.) As you begin to meet your body's nutritional needs you will probably go through a natural cleansing and healing as this regeneration process takes place.

When the body is completely nourished with good food, it feels secure. The appetite decreases and you automatically stop thinking about food all the time. Once you achieve a normal healthy body by following the *Setpoint* guidelines, your weight begins to regulate naturally.

Balance Brings Success

Good nutrition must be coupled with regular exercise and positive living. They are an unbeatable combination, and their combined strength or synergism forms a powerful triangle that assures success.

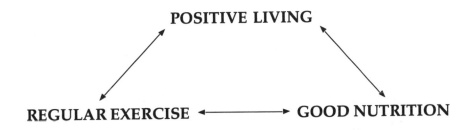

POSITIVE LIVING

REGULAR EXERCISE ⟷ GOOD NUTRITION

The importance of balance was forcefully brought to my attention while writing this book. I found myself feeling out of control while under the stress of trying to meet a deadline. Many workdays were eighteen hours long, filled with early and late hours of writing and a full schedule of clients to counsel. Additionally, I had homemaking responsibilities. Could I hold up under the pressure? I didn't have time to collapse or become ill.

I discovered that it could be done by keeping my life in balance every day. To accomplish it I blocked out the only hour of uninterrupted time available — early in the morning. It became "the hour a day that changed my life" and worked so well that it has become an integral part of my life. This hour brings harmony as well as balance into my life and more than compensates for the missed sleep.

Morning devotions are first: reading, giving thanks, and planning. This provides a positive foundation for the day. At least thirty minutes of brisk walking or cycling comes next. This helps to relieve stress, increase vitality, and maintain control. I plan simple family menus, taking into consideration my time, the season of the year, and what foods are readily available. I rarely skip meals and try to be selective (without being fanatical) about what goes in my mouth because food is fuel, and I want lots of go-power.

Maintaining balance in my life helped me achieve my goal, and it will help you achieve yours. Nothing is better for the body than good wholesome food, regular exercise plus adequate rest, and positive living. This harmonious balance brings success. Let's see how each helps build a leaner, more healthy and active you.

CHAPTER 2

You Can

Set For Life offers a positive lifestyle change, one that will work for you. The light at the end of the tunnel is not an oncoming train. It is the light of hope. You *can* be successful. *This* is the way!

Have the vision to see, the faith to believe,
and the courage to do.

Take Control of Your Life

Good things start to happen when you take control of your life, and that control lies within you. As you seek for balance you will learn to control your mind as well as your body. This balance helps to develop a sense of purpose and direction which is very energizing. Whenever you put yourself whole-heartedly into something worthwhile, energy flows. You will succeed with *Set For Life* because you have purpose and direction — which gives energy — which leads to success!

Feeling out of control causes emotional and mental stress. Stress can tear health down faster than almost any other cause. Living the *Setpoint* lifestyle makes you less vulnerable to stress. As you incorporate the balance of adequate rest, regular exercise, proper diet, and positive living into your life, you'll feel in control again!

Make a Lifestyle Change

Temporary changes are what diets are all about. This is *not* a diet. It is a lifestyle change — a comfortable, workable, lifestyle change. At first, it may seem a little frightening because it takes commitment, time, thought, and planning. But soon everything will become second nature — from the way you buy your food to the way you prepare and eat it. Be patiently consistent, and you'll become lean and healthy — naturally.

There are other benefits, too. In addition to losing fat and keeping it off, your mental and physical health will improve. You will have an increase in energy and strength and will find it easier to be more active. You can work and play longer and harder without getting tired. Your endurance will increase, and you will begin to get by on less sleep. It feels so good to be lean, fit, and in harmony with your body. You are then free to think about other things as you'll no longer need to worry about your health and your weight.

YOU Must Decide

You are the one who must decide to change your lifestyle — to incorporate positive living, moderate exercise, and wholesome foods into your daily life. Change is difficult to achieve, because we all cling to our own comfortable habits — good or bad. It's only through change that you can improve your life, and the only one you can change is yourself!

Unfortunately, we are all victims of "hurry sickness." We want excess weight off yesterday, and we want someone else to do it for us. We want to be lean and healthy right now, but it just doesn't work that way. Good health and weight control take time and consistent effort. You may go forward two steps and slide back one for a while, but that is how positive physical and mental changes are made. Anything worthwhile is worth working for. You will succeed as you realize that success doesn't come from luck. Success comes from work and consistent effort.

Start Now

Don't wait until you are "in the mood" or until you "feel like it" to start; you may wait forever. Just start — regardless of how you feel. Action often comes before motivation. You will get "in the mood" *after* you get started and can see your progress. I wasn't "in the mood" when I started exercising, and I didn't begin to enjoy it until several months later. You may not "feel like" giving up fast foods, diet pop, candy bars and chips; just do it, and you'll begin to like the way you look and feel. Remember, if you cheat, you are cheating yourself.

As you develop this "willpower," also develop some "won't" power. Say "I won't" to those negative things or people that would thwart your progress. You must be strong-willed and firm about your commitment. Successful people seem to have the habit of doing things failures don't like to do. They don't like doing them either, necessarily, but realize that the results are worth the effort.

Be Happy!

As you awaken each morning, consciously determine that you are going to be happy and have a good day. Be positive about every challenge that life offers you. Don't let a negative thought enter your mind, and don't listen and accept negative comments from others. Push them away, and replace them with positive, uplifting ambitions and goals. Happiness comes from within. *Decide* to be happy, positive, and successful and you will be. You possess the inherent power to control your thoughts, desires and actions. You will have an increased feeling of self-disipline as you realize that *you can succeed*. Change "I can" to "*I will*," and your success is assured.

Commit to Twenty-One Days

Give yourself twenty-one days of true, all-out commitment and dedication to this way of life. At that time, you will *know* you are going in the right direction by the way you feel. You will begin to look and act younger than you have for years. In fact, these changes will come about so naturally that you may take them for granted and forget how the "old you" looked and felt.

To help measure your progress, take time right now to write down how you really feel about yourself. Don't be too critical, but do be honest! Next, get on a scale. Weigh yourself, and write it down. Take your measurements, and write them down. Now put the scales and measuring tape away and forget about them.

Use the Power of the Mind

No changes will occur that don't happen mentally first. You need a change on the inside to help you become lean and healthy on the outside. Psychologists tell us that the picturing power of the mind is one of our strongest motivations for success. We can use it to achieve whatever we want in life. Your mental image should reflect what you want instead of what you don't want. This takes mental discipline and practice.

During the day, visualize your excess fat cells as little round balls which are being gobbled up by Pac-Man, or any other image you feel comfortable with. The more he gobbles, the leaner and healthier you become. Also, program your subconscious to raise your metabolic rate so you will burn more fat all day.

Focus On The "New You"

Find a picture of yourself taken at a time when you liked the way you looked. If you don't have one, cut the head off one of your photos and paste it on a photograph of a lean, healthy body from a magazine or catalog. Put this picture in a conspicuous place, and take a long look at the "new you" each evening as you get ready for bed. Say to yourself: "That's the way I am going to look."

When you get into bed, relax and feel good about yourself. You are on the way to the "new you." As you fall asleep, keep repeating this phrase: "Every day, in every way, I'm getting leaner and leaner and leaner." Say it at least seven times each day, and wonderful things will begin to happen. Your positive affirmations and the mental visualization of your ideal body will register in your subconscious mind. You'll be surprised how your subconscious will instruct every part of your body to help you accomplish your goal. Your eating habits will improve, your willpower will increase, your *Setpoint* will begin to lower, and everything will work together to help you reach your desired goal. The power of the mind is limitless and can accomplish wonders. Let it work for you!

Talk Back to Those Inner Voices

If you start slipping, talk back to those inner voices that tell you failure is inevitable, If you find yourself saying, "Every time I've lost weight before, I've always regained it," come back with: *"This time will be different. I can and will succeed. I am not on a diet. I'm just changing my eating habits, my lifestyle, and my attitude!"*

Don't say: "I knew I couldn't do it. I ate all that rich gooey dessert." Instead, say: *"I made a mistake and ate too much of the wrong thing. If I stop overeating now, I haven't lost much ground. Tomorrow will be better!"*

Don't rationalize by saying: "Others eat as much as I do and stay thin. There must be something wrong with my metabolism." Simply say: *"I may have a sluggish metabolism, but that will change as I eat fewer fats and sugars and increase my activity. I am losing fat, and I feel better."*

Don't make excuses: "Everyone in my family is overweight. I guess it's in my genes." Take heart and say: *"My genes may make it more difficult, but not impossible."*

Don't be unduly hard on yourself: "I ate way too much last night." Be positive: *"I went on a binge because I haven't been eating enough of the right foods. I learned a good lesson. Besides, I made some wise choices too. I'll get back in balance to-day.''*

When you are tempted, give yourself a pep talk: *''It's not going to taste that good, and it won't be worth the way I'll feel after I eat it. I don't need it. I'll eat this whole wheat bread or fresh fruit instead. It's delicious and makes me lean and healthy. There are so many good things to eat which help me reach my goal. Why bother with the junky stuff?''*

As you begin to eliminate the poor food choices from your diet, replace them with good wholesome foods so that you won't feel deprived. Replacing, not just eliminating poor choices, helps overcome the mental addiction we have to many foods. This mental addiction often triggers psychological hunger. Train yourself to eat only when physically hungry; not when you are psychologically hungry from boredom, depression, loneliness, anger, or nerves.

If you make mistakes, don't degrade yourself. Merely correct them and move on. Tell yourself: *''That wasn't like me. I'll do it right the next time.''* Be your own best friend. Lift yourself up, and be happy that you are you! Never give up. There are no failures unless you fail to keep trying. Finish what you begin!

You WILL Be Successful

No formula for success will work unless you do; nothing worthwhile can be accomplished without effort.

First, decide what you want to achieve. Make sure your goals are realistic and practical for you. Write them down so you'll remember them. Set short-term goals that you can see materialize *today!* Set weekly goals, monthly goals, and lifetime goals. Review them often; pat yourself on the back as you achieve them. Be your own best friend.

Second, give your goals priority — put them high on your list of dos. They must be important to you. You will find time in each day for those things which you feel are important, no matter how busy you are. Make *you* a priority. You can best serve the needs of those around you — your family, loved ones, and friends — by first giving necessary attention to your own needs. You must feel good about you!

Happiness is victory over self. It brings an inner peace and feelings of well-being and self-worth. You were born to succeed. Don't put the responsibility for your success on anyone else. Remember, *''If it is to be, it is up to me!''* After you do all you can do, God will help you realize your righteous goals and ambitions.

CHAPTER 3

Feel Terrific

Many people begin feeling middle-aged long before they are. They consider those nagging aches and pains an inevitable aspect of aging. The truth is, these aches and pains are usually the result of inactivity. Proper exercise is the best preventive medicine. Exercise gives energy and improves general health. It tones up the muscles and improves elimination, digestion, and cardiovascular fitness. It also relieves stress. Moderate daily exercise helps to keep all body cells and tissues full of oxygen and in the peak of their efficiency. Thus the aging and degenerative processes can actually be slowed by a program of regular exercise plus wholesome foods.

The Fountain of Youth

The body is designed to be active. The more it's used, the better it works. No matter when in life you start to exercise, improvements occur. It's almost never too late to start. Many people who are middle-aged and older who begin to exercise regularly testify that exercise is their Fountain of Youth. They look and feel ten to twenty years younger than before they started. Exercise gives vitality and a sense of purpose and well-being. It helps you stay committed to eating right and it can lower your *Setpoint*. Start today and prove it to yourself!

Break the Inactivity Cycle

Obesity in children is a growing problem (no pun intended). Dr. Susan Finn, a clinical professor at the College of Medicine at Ohio State University, says that the major factors contributing to child obesity are a diet high in fats and sugars and too little activity. Dr. Finn recommends limiting children's unnecessary sedentary activities such as television viewing, while encouraging regular daily exercise.[1] If this is true for children, could it not also be true for adults?

Inactivity starts a cycle that makes becoming active difficult. The less active you are, the less energy you have. With less energy, you have less desire to move. The less you move, the less you are able to move. Pretty soon you have neither the desire nor the ability to be active. You *can* break this cycle and quickly turn it around by following the guidelines in this chapter. *Do it!* It will change your life.

Be Lean and Healthy

Good food choices alone won't do it. Exercise and junk food won't do it. It's regular exercise in combination with wholesome foods that make this lifestyle work most effectively. The body has great difficulty storing fat when you exercise regularly and eat right. The body seems to sense that an active person needs to be lean, and willingly lowers the Setpoint to get rid of the excess fat. It may take from three months to three years or longer to get lean and healthy, depending on where you are when you start and how strictly you live the program. The key is to be consistent and persistent as you work at what you want.

Be aware that any abrupt change in lifestyle that combines richer foods and lots of sitting can raise your *Setpoint*. This could be a vacation, a new job, retirement to a small apartment, or some other change. If you must sit most of the time, you must consciously work at being active the rest of the day. A brisk walk during work breaks or at noon plus morning or evening exercise will make a big difference in how you look and feel. Be extremely careful to avoid fats and sugars at this time.

Exercise Regularly

Exercise cannot be hit-and-miss if it is going to be effective. Studies show that most people who lose weight are unable to keep the weight off without a change in lifestyle that includes regular exercise. When you reach your desired goal, you can usually maintain that fitness level by exercising three days a week or every other day. Set an upper weight limit for yourself and never exceed it. If your weight and inches do begin to creep up, exercise more often and for longer periods of time as you decrease your fat and sugar intake. You'll quickly get back into shape. It's much easier to "keep it off" than it is to "take it off" later!

I Don't Have Time

You will rarely *have time* for exercise. You must *make time*. If you are too busy now to make time for good health and weight control, you may eventually have to make time for illness. You can always find time for the things you really want to do. Make exercise a top priority by scheduling a *regular time* each day for a fat-burning workout; even 25 to 30 minutes every single day will make a difference. Consistency brings results.

Early-morning exercise is ideal. Then you are done for the day and nothing can come along to interfere. You will find that your resolve to exercise tends to weaken in the afternoon and evening, so get it in early if possible. The important thing, however, is not what time of day you exercise, but that you do it regularly. You must be strong-willed and firm about this commitment to be successful.

Easy Does It!

Many people start an exercise program thinking that if a little is good, a lot is better. They overdo and consequently suffer from stiff muscles, sore feet, bad knees, or some other ailment that quickly ends their good intentions. Please *don't overdo*. Begin exercising slowly, 10 to 20 minutes per day if you are able. Increase gradually by adding five minutes per week or every two weeks, depending on your fitness level. Don't try and speed up the increase. Too many people develop foot and knee problems when they do. Use moderation, and every part of your body will gradually strengthen to meet the need.

As you exercise, your fitness level will increase rapidly. By the second week you will probably be walking farther and faster or exercising harder, just to keep your heart rate up; yet you won't feel any more stress than you did the week before. Why? Your heart and lungs have already grown stronger. You are using oxygen more efficiently, increasing the flow of nourishment to the body, and decreasing blood pressure. This lessens the load on the heart, helping prevent stroke and heart disease. The more you exercise, the better you feel; the better you feel, the more you are able to exercise. Exercise reverses that vicious cycle of inactivity.

Inch Loss Denotes Fat Loss

Regular exercise helps decrease fat as it increases the resting metabolic rate. Moderate exercise increases this metabolic rate and keeps it high for hours after you stop. The real value of exercise, then, is not only from the calories burned while exercising but, more importantly, the additional fuel your body burns for hours after exercise because of this raised metabolic rate. It is difficult for the body to store fat if you exercise regularly and eat wholesome foods.

As you begin to exercise, you may find that you are losing inches faster than pounds. Your clothes start fitting better as your body burns fat and builds muscle, but you see no reduction on the scale. Don't be frustrated. This phenomenon is due to the fact that muscle is denser and heavier than fat. Fat floats—muscle sinks. Pound for pound, fat has more volume than muscle. Just remember that *an inch loss denotes a fat loss*. Once you build your lean body mass, the scale weight should drop at a faster rate. Lean body mass (LBM) is muscle, bones, organs, and body fluids. In other words, LBM is your body without the fat!

Muscle Curves—Fat Hangs

Exercise helps build muscle. This makes a more efficient fat-burning body because fat burns in the muscles for energy. Fat in the body has a necessary function, but an excess can be very detrimental. You want to lose excess fat. Muscle curves—fat hangs. Muscle is attractive—fat is not.

Many who diet become littler fat people because when they diet, they often burn muscle, not the fat. They think they must either be fat and have a nice full face or be thin and have a drawn face with wrinkles. *Set For Life* is a fat-loss program. Now you can be lean and also have a firm, younger-looking face because you will be losing fat. Muscle conforms to the skeletal body shape and is both masculine and appealing on a man, and beautiful and feminine on a woman. Muscle gives the strength, endurance, and stamina needed to be truly healthy.

Burn Fat!

Interestingly enough, we cannot *diet* fat off the body. Fat must burn in the muscles for fuel. Our goal, then, should be to make our body an efficient fat-burner and to thus lower the Setpoint. Let's evaluate exercise against that criteria.

The Body Has Two Sources of Fuel: Glucose or Blood Sugar, and Fat

Glucose or blood sugar is the fuel that gives large quantities of energy for short periods of time. It is our "fight or flight fuel," our "stop and go fuel!" Burning sugar is easy. If our fuel need is of a short duration, glucose or blood sugar will suffice. With our modern lifestyle, sugar is the fuel we use most often as we vacuum the house, mow the lawn, go to the supermarket, and so on. Even most farm work falls into this category. Sports, such as golf and tennis, are lots of fun, but they are not very effective for burning fat. When you start and stop frequently during an activity, or if you work out at a high intestity but for a short period, the body primarily burns sugar.

Fat is our second source of fuel — our efficient endurance fuel, the one we carry on our body. Since fat is very concentrated, the process of converting it to energy or fuel for the body is more complex. To be most successful in burning fat, choose a fat-burning exercise — one that uses your large muscles for at least 25 to 30 minutes without stopping. As this non-stop exercise combines with deep breathing, fat burning increases as the body calls on its higher octane endurance fuel — fat. You must *keep moving* to be an efficient fat burner.

Oxygen Is Vital

The burning of fuel in the body requires the same ingredient any burning requires — oxygen! Burning fat requires more oxygen than burning sugar. If the body doesn't have enough oxygen, it cannot burn fat efficiently. Thus, a fat-burning exercise must be aerobic which means *with oxygen*. If you overexert to the point that the cells do not have sufficient oxygen, the exercise becomes anaerobic and the fat-burning stops. You are above the aerobic threshold if the cells require more oxygen than the heart can supply. Breathe in deeply during exercise, using both your mouth and nose if necessary. Breathe out through your mouth.

Regular deep breathing can do much to improve your health so make a conscious effort to breathe deeply, even when you are not exercising. Deep breathing provides a rich supply of oxygen to the cells, which is vital to all body functions. Its value in good health and weight control has long been underestimated. Oxygen is truly the "breath of life."

Enjoy An Energy High

Exercise at a moderate intensity, and pay attention to your breathing rate. *Heavy breathing is normal as you exercise*, but be sure you are able to talk at the same time. Take the *"walk-talk test"*: Are you able to talk while you walk, jog, or exercise without being *totally* winded? If you can't, slow down. If you start to feel faint or if you're not perspiring, stop exercising immediately! Find a cool place, drink liquids, and rest until you feel better.

How do you feel when you get through exercising? Are you exhausted, shaky, or hungry, especially for sweets? If so, you were probably burning sugar. I learned this lesson the hard way several years ago. Anxious to get in shape one winter, I began jumping on my new mini-trampoline. After a few days, I decided I was in terrific shape and jumped hard for a full hour. When I quit, I was bushed—totally wiped out for the remainder of that day and for the next day, too. In fact, I couldn't face any kind of exercise for a week. I did myself more harm than good as I definitely burned sugar, and not the fat I was trying to lose.

A fat-burning exercise should leave you with an energy high, not a feeling of total exhaustion. You may want to sit down for a few minutes, but you should feel invigorated—as if you could get up and do it again. Pay attention to your breathing rate during exercise and how you feel afterwards to assure that you are burning fat and are not exceeding your aerobic threshold.

Check your Pulse

Another indicator of aerobic intensity is your heart rate. During exercise your heart rate can be checked by taking the pulse on the inside of your wrist just below your thumb or on either side of the Adam's apple in the neck. Place the tips of your index and middle finger over the region of the artery, and press down lightly. Stop exercising, and count your pulse for ten seconds. Don't wait to take your pulse or take more than a ten-second count because the pulse rate drops very quickly once exercise is slowed or stopped.

If you wish to convert your exercise pulse rate to a one minute heart rate, multiply the number you counted in ten seconds by six. For example, 20 beats (in 10 seconds) x 6 = 120 beats per minute.

Table 1

	10-SECOND HEART RATE		ONE-MINUTE HEART RATE	
	Beats in 10 Seconds		Beats in 1 Minute	
Age	70 percent of maximum heart rate	80 percent of maximum heart rate	70 percent of maximum heart rate	80 percent of maximum heart rate
20	23	27	138	162
30	22	25	132	150
40	21	24	126	144
50	20	23	120	138
60	19	21	114	126
70	17	20	102	120

Your Target Heart Rate

For cardiovascular fitness and efficient fat loss, you should exercise between 70 and 80 percent of your maximum heart rate. Your target heart rate zone may be estimated from the table above or derived from a simple formula. Subtract your age from 220 and multiply the result by .70 and .80.

Remember, however, that heart rates are only guidelines. They are averages for healthy individuals. If you are on a heart-slowing medication, you may not be able to get your heart rate up to the target heart rate. Use the "walk-talk test" as a measure of exercise intensity. Always pay attention to your breathing rate and how you feel. Check with your personal physician if you have questions regarding your health and ability to engage in moderate exercise.

What Type of Exercise is Best?

A *nonstop* rhythmic exercise such as walking, jogging, bicycling, low-impact aerobics that keep you on your feet, or rebounding on a mini-trampoline are excellent fat-burning exercises. These exercises use the largest muscle mass. This makes them the most effective because you'll burn more fat as you fuel those large working muscles. Choose exercises that are fun for you — those that you *could and would do continuously for a long, uninterrupted period of time.* This factor is critical for your success! Sit-ups, leg lifts, and even weight lifting promote muscle strength and toning but are not very effective for burning fat because they are all stop-and-go exercises.

Don't confuse work with exercise. Housework, yard work, tending children, or on-your-feet jobs help keep you moving and are certainly beneficial, but this stop-and-go activity simply does not put the body in a full fat-burning mode. You still need 30 to 60 minutes of daily aerobic exercise to burn fat and to condition your heart and lungs. Once you start to exercise, don't stop! *You must keep moving to burn fat efficiently!*

Join An Exercise Class

Exercise classes are a popular way to get in shape and stay in shape. They are a lot of fun and group support can keep you motivated. If your goal is to burn fat, be selective. Choose a low-impact aerobics class which keeps you moving on your feet for a *minimum* of 30 to 40 minutes; a class that follows the fat-burning rules as outlined in this chapter.

THE PERFECT EXERCISE

Walking has long been called the perfect exercise. The growing consensus among experts is that walking is the best and safest exercise for people of any age. Except for a disability that specifically prevents walking, people in almost any condition, age, or state of health can walk. The American Heart Association says that walking briskly is one of the simplest and best forms of exercise.

Walking feels good *while* you are doing it, *not just when you stop*! It's as natural as breathing! It has the lowest dropout rate of any form of activity, particularly if you have a compatible walking partner. If you are looking for fitness without sacrifice, walk! Walking outdoors gives the added therapeutic benefit of fresh air and sunshine.

If You Can Walk...

You can walk anywhere without special equipment other than good shoes. Walk out your front door for five to ten minutes; turn around and walk back home. Walk slowly for the first three to five minutes to warm up your muscles. This warm-up is especially important as you get older. After warming up, don't stroll. Pick up your pace until you are walking rapidly, with a goal to work up to at least three to four miles in an hour.

Brisk walking is the key to success. Many people don't walk fast enough or long enough to really burn fat effectively and then wonder why they aren't making progress. As your body condition improves, you must exercise harder or longer to really get results. Get your heart rate into your target zone and keep it there for 25 to 30 minutes, with a goal to work up to 45 to 60 minutes daily.

Listen To Your Body

Learn to listen to your body as you compete with yourself—walk a little farther and a little faster each day, but never to the point of stress. An inexpensive sports watch with a chronograph (stop watch feature) helps track your progress. As your fitness level increases you may want to alternate jogging and walking to keep your heart rate up. As you finish, slow down to a leisurely walk for the last three to five minutes to let your body functions slow back down to normal. This cool-down is important.

Use affirmations as you walk. Here are a few suggestions to get you started: With every step, tell your body, "Fat burn, fat burn, fat burn all day" and "Every day in every way, I'm getting leaner, and leaner, and leaner." If you have trouble keeping up your speed, tell yourself, "Faster, faster, faster." As you deep breathe in and out, think: "Life's pure energy in, stress and tension out." Let your mind help your body get lean and healthy. Believe it, and you will soon achieve it!

Walk With Style!

Practice good posture as you walk or jog. Stand up straight with your shoulders back, head level, and stomach tucked in. Hold your arms slightly away from the body with a ninety-degree bend at the elbow. Swing your arms naturally with your hands held about waist high. This posture builds a natural momentum and also helps eliminate the swollen hands many walkers complain about.

To increase walking speed, lengthen your stride. Tilt your weight slightly to the back. To help propel you forward, use lots of arm movement. Notice how your arms swing to counter-balance your feet. When your right foot swings forward, your left arm swings with it. Keep your arms bent at a ninety-degree angle and let them swing from the shoulder blades, forward across your body to about the center of your chest. You'll be surprised at how fast and effortlessly you can walk. Don't forget to breathe deeply! If you prefer to jog, take shorter steps. Make it a low, smooth, rolling jog. To avoid injury, land on the bottom, not on the ball or front part of your foot.

Good Shoes Are a Must!

I've become a fanatic about the importance of wearing *good shoes*. Too many people have foot and knee problems when they try to walk or jog in the wrong shoes. Get running or walking shoes, not aerobic, court, or any other type. Buy the best and the most comfortable shoes you can afford to support and cushion your feet. Good shoes are worth the investment. You will cover hundreds of miles in those shoes so select them carefully and replace them before they get too worn. If possible, have two different brands of shoes to alternate daily. Changing shoes changes the pressure points and rests the feet. Altering the weight and type of absorbent socks also helps reduce foot fatigue.

Protect Your Body

In cold or windy weather, dress in several layers of light clothing to increase insulation. It's easy to peel off a layer if you become too warm. A windbreaker is a good investment, but any zippered jacket or sweatshirt allows you to adjust the heat of your body. Protect your hands with gloves, and use ear muffs or a warm hat to cover your ears. A towel or scarf around your neck prevents the cold from creeping in. If you keep your head, ears, and neck warm, you will rarely get chilled.

In hot weather, wear light-colored clothing to reflect the heat of the sun. Choose loose-fitting clothes which breathe. If needed, wear a hat to guard against heat stroke.

Avoid outdoor exercise when there is heavy smog or air pollution. These conditions are hazardous to your health. Stay upwind or away from busy roads to avoid the carbon monoxide from cars. Always exercise in the cleanest air available.

Don't Take Chances

Have a walking companion if possible — spouse, friend, or dog. Walk facing traffic so that you know what's coming. Choose a safe route and alter it occasionally. Stay away from dark or deserted places. Avoid anyone or any place that makes you feel uneasy. If necessary, scream for help and run!

Anyone who walks knows about dogs; they can be a real problem. Avoid them if possible. My favorite route takes me past big dogs and little dogs. At first they barked and chased me. I soon discovered that dogs are a lot like people; they like to be acknowledged and receive a kind word. I wasn't overly friendly, just cordial. A simple "Good morning, how are you today?" began to change their attitude. After a week or two, they decided I was a friend and they could ignore me. Be advised that this approach doesn't always work; dogs can be dangerous.

Bicycling Is Fun!

Cycling, indoors or out, is another great way to get in shape. It is a "non-weight-bearing" exercise. This makes it particularly good for the overweight person, those with artificial knees or hips, or a bad back.

Bicycling outdoors is a good fat-burning exercise if you have an area where you can ride nonstop for an extended period on a fairly level surface to keep pedaling constant. Indoor cycling is a good winter or year-round exercise. A number of excellent exercise bikes are now available. If you have a disability, those bikes with body-contoured seats and full back support may be the most comfortable and easiest to use. Try several bikes before you purchase one. Learn to adjust the tension or the speed until your heart rate reaches your target zone.

Drink Water

Drink plenty of good, pure water before, during (if needed), and after exercise. Drink more if you perspire heavily and certainly in warm weather. Even in cool weather the body needs water to increase endurance and promote overall good health. Studies show that drinking adequate water causes a measurable increase in endurance. Muscle cramps and fatigue are often caused by dehydration as well as a lack of oxygen.

Nature's Tranquilizer

We live in a stressful world. Exercise is an excellent natural remedy for stress. It helps you feel refreshed and energized by reducing anxiety, tension, and depression. Just getting away from your problems for an hour of daily exercise is most beneficial. You have time to think and will return home with a more positive perspective and a greater sense of well-being. It helps you stay in control of your life.

You'll also develop a calmer, more relaxed attitude toward daily pressures because of the endorphine release from exercise. Endorphines are small morphine-like chemicals that are secreted in the brain as a result of endurance exercise. Endorphines are nature's tranquilizer! Exercise makes you feel soooo good—but you must experience this feeling yourself to know what I mean!

Exercise Can Be Addictive

You may have met someone with an exercise addiction. These individuals have such a powerful commitment to exercise that it takes priority over their work, their family, and their entire lives. They seem to use exercise as an escape and often live in a state of chronic fatigue and inferior health. They become self-centered and totally preoccupied with fitness, diet, and body image. Living the *Setpoint* lifestyle is the ideal deterrent to this addiction because of the daily balance it provides.

Get Adequate Rest

Nothing takes the place of adequate rest. Getting to bed early can be difficult, but do it whenever you can. The hour or two just before bedtime is often wasted with television, aimless reading, or winding down after a busy day. Get in the habit of heading for bed before 10 p.m. whenever possible. Seven to eight hours of sleep each night is essential for most people, although you may find you need less as your fitness improves.

A quiet bedroom helps you relax. You may need to use the masking effect of a fan, soothing music, or some other steady background sound to help drown out disturbing noises.

If you've built up a sleep deficit that has sapped your energy, take the time to catch up. Once you're back to your norm, don't let yourself get run down. Learn to rest before you get too tired. A short nap or a few minutes of total relaxation when needed helps prevent fatigue and keeps you in control.

Feel Terrific . . .

Exercise gives a higher quality life. It is the Fountain of Youth we all search for. Exercise is a critical factor in lowering the *Setpoint* and in improving body circulation. These factors are vital to good health and weight control.

Cultivating good health habits is a lifelong pursuit that requires consistent effort. This responsibility is yours and yours alone. Take charge of your life. The rewards are worth the effort!

EXERCISE GUIDELINES

1. **Exercise three to six days a week.**

2. **Exercise 30 to 60 minutes.**

3. **Choose an aerobic exercise that uses a large muscle mass.**

4. **Work at a moderate pace—not too fast, not too slow.**

5. **Breathe deeply.**

6. **Drink water before, during (if needed), and after exercise.**

CHAPTER 4

You Are What You Eat

Good Nutrition Is Common Sense

We are not into "health food". We *are* into healthy food. Good nutrition includes healthy food and good common-sense eating based on three balanced meals each day. These meals are naturally high in nutrients and fiber from complex carbohydrates (whole grains, vegetables and fruits). They are low in cholesterol, fats, and refined carbohydrates (sugar and white flour) and lower than the norm in sodium. They are similar to the foods recommended by the American Heart Association, the American Diabetes Association, and the American Cancer Society.

You soon develop an awareness of good wholesome foods and the wisdom of eating a wide variety of them. You do not have to weigh or measure your food, use exchanges, or count calories. What freedom! You will not be hungry, so you won't be thinking about food all day. You eat when you *are* hungry, so you avoid guilt eating. Best of all, you will develop a healthy attitude toward food. Your tastes will change as you *eat to live, not live to eat!*

How Much Can I Eat?

"Dieters" are accustomed to being told exactly what and how much to eat. The *Setpoint* lifestyle is not a diet. It simply gives realistic guidelines and allows you to make the choices. You're probably wondering: How much can I eat? The answer is: How much do you need? Some days you will have higher energy requirements than on other days, so it's not wise to give specific amounts. The amounts given in this book are suggestions only. Allowing your body to dictate its own needs is the beauty of this lifestyle. You will be happy to learn that *what you eat* is much more important than *how much you eat!* Give the body the nutrients it requires, and the appetite will begin to regulate itself. You will find yourself naturally cutting back as you begin to get in harmony with your own eating drives.

Don't Be A Breakfast Skipper

Don't be a breakfast skipper. I know...you're not hungry in the morning — but you will be later. Food is fuel, and you can't run on empty very long. By 10 a.m. you'll have the blahs and will be looking for some quick energy from fats, sugars, or caffeine such as doughnuts, hot chocolate, or a cola drink. You'll probably end the day feeling unsatisfied, even after a good dinner as your body tries to catch up on the needed nutrients it missed earlier in the day. This explains the old failure-oriented diet routine: skip breakfast, have a light lunch, and then eat out of control all evening.

For Long-Term Energy

Do eat breakfast! It needn't be elaborate, just nourishing. A nutritious breakfast can eliminate that mid-morning slump that gets many people into trouble. It also does marvelous things for your energy and your weight. Don't worry if you get hunger pangs before lunchtime for a few days. When you're used to eating only one or two meals a day, your body learns to cope with this limited food supply by manifesting an artificial suppression of hunger. When you begin eating breakfast, you may actually feel hungrier during the day than you did when you were skipping meals. These hunger pangs are simply your body signaling for more of the nutrients and high energy foods it needs to maintain good health and weight control. Continue eating a nutritious breakfast and this extreme hunger response will disappear in a few days as your body adjusts to regular eating. Keep in mind that eating refined carbohydrates (sweets and white flour products) will make you feel hungry within a short time because of their effect on your blood sugar levels. In contrast, a whole grain breakfast gives high, long-lasting energy. Your appetite may increase as your metabolism speeds up and you develop more fat-burning muscle. Don't be afraid to eat. Just enjoy the phenomenon of eating more and weighing less!

Skipping Meals Can Make You Fat

Eat regularly. Meal skipping activates the starvation defense we discussed earlier, and statistics show that meal skippers are fatter than regular eaters. Skipping meals forces the body to store fat for survival and lowers the metabolic rate (calorie burning), leaving you with a "fat metabolism."

Eating three *Setpoint* meals each day, plus nutritious snacks between meals, helps raise your metabolic rate. You begin to burn more calories naturally, and this helps to create a "lean metabolism." That's why you can eat more and weigh less.

Sweets make you feel hungry so avoiding them will automatically cut your appetite for sweets. Your tastes will change and you'll begin to look forward to eating wholesome, high energy foods. Eat until you feel comfortable and satisfied. Feeling completely satisfied helps relax the *Setpoint* so that it comes down willingly with regular moderate exercise.

Eat Before You Get Too Hungry

Eat something every four to five hours, even if you don't feel hungry. In fact, it's better to eat something, even if it's a poor food choice, than to skip a meal. Choose the best of whatever is available. Eat just enough to last until you can get some wholesome food — and don't feel guilty! Learn to plan ahead so that having to settle for less than the best is a rare occurrence.

You may need a booster meal mid-afternoon, particularly if you will be eating a late dinner or if you had a very light lunch. Regular eating helps prevent the binges that often result from going too long without proper foods. It also helps to keep your energy high; food is fuel. Snack on vegetables if you aren't hungry, and vegetables, grains, beans, and fruits if you are hungry.

Forewarned is Forearmed

If you do skip a meal or fast for one or two meals, your next meal should be well balanced. Be sure it includes a wide variety of fresh and raw vegetables plus whole grains. Eat slowly and drink at least two glasses of water along with the meal. Avoid the natural tendency to eat high-fat, high-sugar foods at this time. Surprisingly, you may feel hungry again in just two or three hours as your body tries to catch up on the nutrients it missed earlier. If this happens, don't feel guilty — just eat again. A bowl of Grape-Nuts, Shredded Wheat, or some other whole-grain cereal topped with a little fruit and milk usually satisfies this hunger. Another option is a piece of whole wheat toast or a lowfat whole grain sandwich. Whole grains can be very satisfying, and they help you resist the sweet treats you may otherwise indulge in. If you must have a treat, eat it *after* a full meal, never on an empty stomach.

But That's My Favorite!

We are all deeply attached to certain foods that we like and those that are familiar to us. They may represent the comfort and security of home or our life as a child. Unfortunately, they are often high in fats and sugars, especially the foods we crave and consider our favorites. These foods may always be tempting because food addiction is partly emotional. You may be eating for reasons other than physical hunger—comfort, pleasure, anger, boredom, stress, fatigue, and the like. Nearly all overeating is motivated at least in part by emotional factors.

Begin now to incorporate more wholesome foods into your meals. Your tastes will change as you bypass some of the old high-fat, high-sugar favorites. If you do eat these favorites, you may notice a drain on your energy, a change in your disposition, and an increase in your weight. Eating fats and sugars can quickly raise your Setpoint, especially when combined with a sedentary lifestyle.

Plan Ahead

Don't wait until you are hungry to start thinking about the next meal. The first line of defense against meal skipping or eating the wrong foods is having the right foods readily available. Keep a variety of wholesome foods prepared. Menu planning will help assure your success. The guidelines in Chapter Five make menu planning easy for you to implement.

WHAT CAN I EAT? COMPLEX CARBOHYDRATES

Generally speaking, the more food we eat in its natural state, *as it is grown*, the healthier it will be for us. For good health and weight control, eat more whole grains, fresh vegetables, and fruits. These complex carbohydrates should make up 65 to 80 percent of your total daily food intake. They are the only major category of foods that has never been linked to any long-term health risk. These foods are naturally low in calories and price and high in nutrition and fiber, which makes them a very good buy any time.

Whole grains are always a bargain, and you can now afford to buy more fresh vegetables and fruits as you purchase less of the expensive foods—such as meat, cheese, pop, snacks, and prepared foods. Shop the outside perimeter of the grocery store and avoid the center aisles that are full of expensive convenience foods. Your grocery bill will drop dramatically; your medical bills should, too!

Complex carbohydrates promote regular elimination which is vital for good health and fat loss. In a short time you should notice a positive change in your bowel habits. As you naturally increase the bulk of fiber in your diet and decrease the refined carbohydrates (sugar and white flour products — the real culprits of constipation), you will have an increase in favorable intestinal bacteria. You may experience a short period (a week or two) of gas and occasional feelings of fullness, but these are just temporary as your body cleanses itself and adjusts to more wholesome foods.

The Staff of Life

Whole grains form the cornerstone of good health and weight control. They make you feel satisfied and provide endurance. As you begin living this lifestyle, eating whole grains will often make the difference between success and failure. Use them as a crutch at first, and they will help you pass up the tempting sugars and fats. When used regularly, they act as a *natural appetite suppressant* and help eliminate binges and the desire for empty-calorie foods, more commonly known as junk foods.

Good whole grain bread is usually less than 20 percent fat. Eat it every day for high energy and satiety. Carry some in your purse or car so you'll have the right food available if you get hungry. "Fatigue makes cowards of us all." It's when we get overly tired and hungry that we weaken and reach for the wrong foods — usually fats and sugars. Use whole grains to help you plan ahead and prepare for these emergencies.

EAT WITH THE SEASONS

Spring

Vegetables and fruits are nature's finest carbohydrates. They are at their best when fresh-picked so try growing your own for the ultimate in good eating! After a long, cold winter the body needs a change from heavy foods. Fresh greens, asparagus, and other tender vegetables, berries, and early fruits are all a natural spring tonic. These vegetables and fruits supply the vitamins and minerals needed to make us feel vibrant and alive.

Summer

We seem to handle hot weather better when we aren't eating lots of fats and heavy foods. It's refreshing to eat more melons and other fresh fruits during the summer. Vegetables offer a wide variety, such as peas and potatoes, cucumbers, green beans, the cabbage family, and tomatoes. For high energy, fill up on these and bypass the heavy meats. Corn on the cob hits the spot in late summer, and yes, you can eat it! Just skip the butter.

Fall and Winter

With the chill of fall and the cold of winter, the desire for melons and other fruit will lessen. We look forward to the dense, sweet vegetables — potatoes, carrots, squash, yams, and the like. Legumes (dried beans, lentils and peas) made into stews and soups taste extra good at this time of year. Those who regularly eat these types of soups usually lose weight faster because these foods are high in nutrients, low in fat, and are very satisfying.

There are still a variety of fruits to enjoy in fall and winter such as apples, pears, and plums. Citrus fruits are at their prime about holiday time, just when other fruits lose their best flavor and nutrition.

Make a conscious effort to eat those foods that are in season. When you learn to eat this way, you get a wide variety of foods and nutrients naturally. Imagine being able to eat all these wholesome foods and still get lean and healthy!

Use Lowfat Dairy Products, Lean Meat, and Eggs in Moderation

Choose lowfat dairy products: 1% or skim milk, lowfat cheese and cottage cheese, nonfat yogurt, buttermilk, and evaporated skim milk. Most cheese is high in cholesterol and fat.

Fish and poultry are good meat choices. Remove the skin from poultry because fat clings to it. Red meat is the single largest source of fat in the American diet according to Dr. Hans Diehl.[3] Limit red meat to two or three servings per week. Choose lean cuts and trim away any visible fat. Even extra-lean ground beef is high in fat. Venison and elk are better red meat choices because they are naturally lean. Use red meat as a condiment or seasoning for vegetables and whole grains; make a little bit go a long way. A good assortment of beef recipes following these guidelines are included in this book.

Eggs are a good food, but use them in moderation. They are an excellent source of protein and are easy to prepare. In comparison — an ounce of most hard cheeses has more fat than an egg yolk, and fat is considered a bigger culprit than dietary cholesterol when it comes to heart disease.

Bacon, ham, wieners, fresh pork, cold cuts, and lamb are all high in fat and should be avoided or eaten *very* sparingly. Thinly sliced turkey ham may occasionally provide the desired flavor on a whole grain sandwich piled high with vegetables.

FATS ARE FATTENING—IT'S AS SIMPLE AS THAT!

Most people love fat. It is one of America's most popular nutrients. It tastes good and requires little chewing. Fats pack a lot of fat calories into a very few bites—cheesecake, chocolate, ice cream, salad dressings, and gravy are good examples. If it slides, don't eat it! These calorie-dense high-fat high-sugar foods can quickly raise the *Setpoint* and make you fat.

Eat Fat and Get Fat!

A high percentage of all fat calories eaten are reportedly converted to body fat, yet you can eat ample complex carbohydrates without a weight gain. Remember, not all calories are created equal! There are nine calories in one gram of fat compared to four calories in a gram of protein, sugar, or starch. Alcohol has seven calories per gram. Much of the fat we consume is combined with sugar in empty-calorie foods. In other words, we gain little nutritional value from the calories—just fat!

Fat in the diet is essential, but don't worry about not getting enough. Fats are hidden in almost all foods, including vegetables, fruits, and whole grains. It is almost impossible to get too little fat if you eat a wide variety of wholesome foods.

The natural foods highest in fat are avocados, olives, coconut, raw nuts and seeds, and soybeans. They are much better choices than refined fats—such as shortening, mayonnaise, and salad dressing—but use them in moderation as you lower your fat consumption and your Setpoint.

Drastically Reduce Fat Intake!

The body finds it very easy to take the fats from the following foods and put them right into storage...on the hips and abdomen.

Butter	Mayonnaise	Red meats
Margarine	Salad dressings	Poultry skin
Shortening	Peanut butter	Tuna in oil
Lard	Cheesecake	Cold cuts
Oils	Whole milk products	Roasted nuts

Cheese	Gravy and sauces	Roasted seeds
Sour cream	Chips	Hot dogs
Ice cream	Fried foods	Ham
Coconut	Chocolate	Pastries

Fats can be hazardous to your health. Eaten in excess, fats make you fat; they make you tired, and they can make you sick. They make your mind and your body sluggish by slowing circulation and by reducing the oxygen-carrying capacity of the red blood cells. Fats are being linked to many health problems, including heart disease, high cholesterol, some types of cancer, diabetes, high blood pressure, and obesity, to name a few. Drastically reducing your fat intake can make a big difference in a very short time in how you look and feel.

A diet high in whole grains, vegetables and fruits, and low in fats and sugars, can help *reverse* the effects of cholesterol buildup, high triglycerides, and other health problems. Diet changes can and will make a difference in avoiding heart problems and many other degenerative diseases. If you want to feel better, start eating better. There is a direct relationship between how you feel and what you eat.

Eat Lean — Get Lean

Because fats cram a lot of calories into just one bite, making small changes in your food choices can make big differences in how you look and feel. The following suggestions will help you get started.

Use nonfat dressings for salads and spreads. They're tasting better all the time. A skiff of butter or spread can taste as good as a tablespoon or two, once you've adjusted to the change. Fat free cream cheese, lowfat cottage cheese, applesauce or fruit spread are other good alternatives. You'll soon find your favorites. Even "lite" margarines, spreads, and salad dressings are high in fat, but are better choices than the regular products.

Cook without oil as much as possible. Bake or broil instead of frying in fat. Use quality nonstick or stainless steel pans. Wipe the bottom of the pan with a stick of butter or margarine if needed. Use limited amounts of nonstick cooking spray.

You can reduce the amount of fat in recipes by one-third to one-half without making much change in the taste and texture of the finished product. To do this, reduce the flour, etc. or add additional liquid such as milk, water, applesauce, pureed white beans, etc. to equal the amount of decreased fat. This may take a little experimentation so make only one change at a time. If that works well, then change something else next time.

Defat Broth Before Using

When stewing a chicken, making soup, cooking broth from bones, or making gravy from pan drippings, *always* defat the broth before using. Pour the hot broth into a specially designed fat skimmer cup. The fat will rise to the top and you can pour off fat-free broth through the spout that attaches at the bottom. These cups are worth the investment. You can also chill the broth and skim off all fat as it hardens. Additionally, an ice cube added to gravy stock hardens the fat so it can be removed.

THE REFINED CARBOHYDRATES— SUGARS AND WHITE FLOUR

We would all be much healthier and happier if refined carbohydrates — sugar and white flour — never entered our mouths again. Unfortunately, they probably will; it's too hard to keep them out. But the quantity you do eat will continue to decline as your tastes change. Until your *Setpoint* moves down to the desired level, you should avoid refined carbohydrates. They are empty-calorie foods *that make you hungry and make you fat!*

Sugar has many names. Learn to read food labels and keep to an absolute minimum those foods that contain sugar, brown sugar, corn syrup, dextrose, fructose, sucrose, honey, molasses, sorghum or any artificial sweeteners. When cooking, you can decrease sugar in most recipes by a fourth to a third; the taste is almost the same.

Sugars' Vicious Cycle

Sugars upset the balance in the body. When you are eating sugars, you rely on them as your energy source. The more sugar you eat, the more rapidly the body burns sugar. Your appetite may rage out of control. You are hungry all the time as blood sugar rises, then drops. The accompanying mood swings make you feel as if you are on a roller coaster. They give a quick pick-up that soon drops you down lower than when you started out. One sweet leads to another and another until sweets are almost all you want to eat — and the vicious cycle continues. As the body goes through this cycle again and again, it becomes better and better at using sugar for energy and much less efficient at using fat. Artificial sweeteners seem to affect the body in much the same way and should also be avoided.

No... Chocolate Is Not a Complex Carbohydrate!

Eating chocolate puts inches on your hips and abdomen faster than you can imagine! It is very addictive and makes you feel hungry, even when you are not. Cut back on chocolate or better yet, cut it out. You will start looking and feeling better within a very short time. Regular meals of good wholesome foods will fortify you nutritionally so that you gradually lose the craving for chocolate.

Sweets are Addictive

Giving up sweets may not be easy. Many people have a sugar addiction, even though they may not be aware of it. The easiest way to get over this addiction may be to go "cold turkey" — give up all sweets except for fruit and foods sweetened with fruit. Clean the sweets out of the kitchen, desk drawers, and the car, and avoid purchasing them at the store. Don't tempt yourself. Out of sight, out of mind!

As you give up sweets, you may experience some withdrawal symptoms — minor headaches, uneasiness, and a feeling that "something is missing" in your life. Eat more fresh fruit and more whole grains during this time to help you bypass the sweets. Within three or four days you should start to feel better and will notice a new calmness and a feeling of body control. Your appetite for sweets will drop markedly. You'll be hungry for real food and can stop eating when you are full. You will be amazed at the power sweets have had over you.

Know Yourself!

It may be easier to plan a moderate dessert once or twice a week than to try to abstain completely and then feel guilty when you overindulge or binge. Most dieters tend to think in all-or-nothing terms, where everything is either black or white. They're either completely on or totally off sweets and fats; there is no middle of the road. A workable plan must have variety and allow for occasional treats, special occasions and favorite foods. Your tastes will change and the forbidden favorites will have less appeal to you and your family as you replace them with other tasty foods that are not high in fats and sugars. Remember to eat dessert or a sweet after a full meal — never on an empty stomach. This helps prevent the blood sugar highs and lows we just discussed.

When you do prepare desserts for your family occasionally, fix those that are lower in sugar and fat and higher in complex carbohydrates. For example, instead of a cookie filled with sugars, white flour, chocolate chips, and oil, make one with whole wheat flour, oatmeal, raisins, or unsweetened carob chips and a reduced amount of sugar and fat. Try the Raisin Bars and other tasty recipes in Chapter Ten. They are much better choices than most traditional desserts.

If sweets continue to be a real problem, you may want to read *Back to Health*, an excellent book which deals with infection from the yeast Candida albicans. It is written by Dr. Dennis Remington, a noted medical doctor who specializes in weight control and related problems.[4]

What's Wrong With White Flour?

White flour is so refined that the body handles it in much the same way as it does sugar. White flour does not have the nutritional value or the satiety of whole grains. If whole grains aren't your favorite, keep trying them. Your tastes will gradually change.

A FEW MORE GUIDELINES

Decrease Salt

Gradually decrease salt in all your recipes until you have cut it at least in half; you won't miss it because your tastes will change. Try Morton's Lite Salt and use salt-free spices and herbs for seasoning foods. Soy sauce, bouillon cubes, and MSG (monosodium glutamate) are all high in salt. Use them sparingly in place of salt or avoid them.

Many foods you buy have added salt. Rinsing such foods as canned vegetables, tuna, and cottage cheese with water reduces the salt content quite dramatically.[5]

Drink Up!

Drink six or more glasses of water every day. Start the day with a large glass of the *purest drinking water available*. Drink at least one glassful with each light meal and two glasses with your main meal. Adequate water intake is vital to your success. Taking a swallow each time you pass the drinking fountain just isn't enough. Keep a full glass of water on your desk or countertop and empty it several times a day. Put a slice of fresh lemon or lime in the water if you need a little flavor.

Water naturally suppresses the appetite for soft drinks and also helps to relieve constipation. If you feel tired or hungry, drink water! You may just be thirsty. Drinking plenty of water will greatly increase endurance. If you are retaining water, drink! Drinking water helps relieve fluid retention. It stimulates the kidneys and helps rid the body of waste and bacteria that can cause disease. The overweight person needs more water to help regulate all body functions, especially during fat loss. For good health, drink plenty of pure water—at least six 8-ounce glasses and not over 20 glasses daily.

Be Wary of Beverages

Decrease or eliminate alcohol, tea, coffee, and *all drinks* containing caffeine. Caffeine is addictive, so you may want to cut back gradually. If you are accustomed to drinking large quantities of cola drinks or coffee each day, drink one less each day, or every three days, or even one less each week, and you will soon break the caffeine habit. If you prefer to go "cold turkey" and give up all caffeine at once, the withdrawal symptoms will be similar to those described under sugar addiction, so be prepared!

Decrease or avoid all soft drinks, diet pop, and punch; and limit your juice intake. They all tend to increase the appetite for sweets and are often high in empty calories. Artificial sweeteners feed the craving for sweets and stimulate the appetite without satisfying it, so avoid them also. *The Bitter Truth About Artificial Sweeteners*[3], by Dr. Dennis Remington, M.D. and Barbara Higa, R.D. cites extensive evidence indicating that artificial sweeteners promote weight gain, create a "fat metabolism", and contribute to various degenerative diseases.

Fresh vegetable and fruit juices have their place and can be therapeutic, but don't use juice as a regular meal replacement. Low-sodium V-8 or tomato juice are good if you want an occasional juice. Part of the satiety of food is in the smelling, chewing, tasting and swallowing. You miss this satiety when you drink beverages.

In Review...

Food is fuel. For high energy, good health, and weight control, eat regular meals which include whole grains, fresh vegetables, and fruits. Make meat the exception, not the rule. As you eat less meat, eat more vegetable sources of protein, particularly whole grains and legumes. Decrease or omit the empty-calorie "junk foods." This will happen naturally as you cut down on fats and sugars. The fats and sugars make your mind and your body sluggish in addition to making you fat.

Use Common Sense

Please... don't read this book and decide to change everything all at once. Gradual changes are easier to adapt to and are much more likely to be permanent. Drastic changes can cause resentment and even promote a craving for favorite foods you may now view as forbidden. Serve a "forbidden favorite" dish occasionally if you choose, but balance that meal by adding some high energy food choices too. Remember, there are no forbidden foods in the *Setpoint* Lifestyle. What you eat is *your* choice!

As you strive to improve family eating habits, don't make an issue of food. The "this is good for you and you're going to eat it!" type of thing won't work. And don't throw out those foods you may now feel are "unhealthy" such as white flour, sugar, and so on. Use them up as you make a gradual transition into eating whole grains, more vegetables, and less sweets and fats. As tastes change, you'll find yourself eating less and less of the low energy choices. Choose new recipes from this book that include some of your own food preferences.

Good health and permanent weight control require permanent change. Don't make this a temporary diet. Make it a lifestyle you can live for the rest of your life! If you eat a variety of good, nutritious foods most of the time, an occasional doughnut or hot dog won't hurt you too much. On the other hand, if most of what you eat is high in fats and sugars, a few vegetables and an occasional dish of oatmeal probably won't do much to make you lean and healthy. Learn to make tradeoffs. If you're going to eat out or have a dinner higher in fat, choose foods low in fat for the rest of your meals that day.

Good eating should become a regular habit but need not exclude less nutritious foods all of the time — unless you have a sticky Setpoint or a serious health problem. Make an honest evaluation of your eating habits to see which areas need improvement. For top performance, eat smart. Don't make food an issue — just get into good nutrition. Regular balanced meals which are low in fats and sugars and high in whole grains, fresh vegetables, and fruits, will give you the winning edge in good health and weight control as you . . . Eat more . . . weigh less . . . and feel terrific!

CHAPTER 5

Get Ready...Get Set...

SET FOR LIFE is a simple, common-sense lifestyle. If what you're doing isn't simple and common-sense, it probably isn't *Setpoint!* This lifestyle should not be a nutritional or physical stress to anyone. You shouldn't be hungry or experience pain from exercise if you follow the guidelines correctly. With conscientious effort you should average a one- to two-pound fat loss per week. Men and some women may lose a little faster.

Many people must strictly adhere to the Setpoint guidelines in order to lower their Setpoint; some do not. This may not seem fair if you are one of the first group, but we all have individual differences! Once your Setpoint moves down to the desired level, continue strict adherence to the whole program until your Setpoint is firmly set. This may take several weeks or even months. At that time, you should be able to use more flexibility in food choices and exercise. Although you may have to work diligently to lower your Setpoint initially, the good news is that it isn't hard to keep it down once it's firmly set.

Set For Life is a wonderful program to help rebuild health. However, if you are not feeling up to par, it's wise to start with a good medical and dental checkup. Get your doctor's cooperation. Low-grade infections such as yeast (Candida), periodontal gum disease, an infected tooth, or other problems such as anemia, can slow your progress.

Remember to take your weight and measurements before you begin. Do not weigh or measure again until you have lived these principles for twenty-one days. Weighing daily can cause mental stress. You will be improving your lean body mass and losing fat. Changes will occur, regardless of what the scales may show at first. Believe in the program and don't get in a hurry! Live the *Setpoint Lifestyle* and success will come slowly, naturally, and permanently as you eat more... weigh less... and feel terrific!

Dr. Garth Fisher, a well-known exercise physiologist who specializes in fitness, exercise, and weight control, says the success of this lifestyle lies in the simplicity of these words:

Don't diet! Exercise regularly! Cut fats and sugars!

These basic principles were explained in Chapters One through Four. Read these chapters before you begin living *The Setpoint Lifestyle* so that you thoroughly understand the complete program. The guidelines are summarized here.

THE SETPOINT LIFESTYLE — A Lifetime Plan

1. **Live Positively!**

2. **Exercise 30 to 60 minutes five to six days a week. Get adequate rest.**

3. **Eat three meals daily plus wholesome snacks when hungry.**
   Eat regularly. Don't starve! Don't stuff! Listen to your body.
   The amounts listed below are suggestions only. If this is more or less food than you need, cut back or add in each category. The key is to use variety and retain a balance.

4. **Eat more whole grains, legumes, vegetables, and fresh fruits.**
   Whole grains: Four or more servings per day.
   Eat a variety of whole grains daily such as wheat, oats, brown rice, and millet. Use in breads, cereals, pasta, tortillas, side dishes.

   Beans, Peas, Lentils: Eat at least two to four cups of these legumes each week. Increase amounts when not eating meat. Eat beans often but use smaller portions at first. This helps eliminate gastrointestinal problems. Add bean soup or a side dish of beans to any meal.

   Vegetables: Four or more servings per day (two to four cups minimum). Enjoy a wide variety of fresh and frozen vegetables. Include green and deep yellow vegetables, potatoes, yams, etc.

   Fresh Fruits: Two to four servings daily. Use fresh in-season fruits when available; unsweetened frozen or "lite" canned fruits occasionally; dried fruit sparingly. Dried fruits are calorically dense.

5. **DRASTICALLY DECREASE FATS!**
   Fats such as butter, margarine, salad dressing, mayonnaise, cheese, sour cream, whole milk, oil, roasted nuts, chips, peanut butter, red meats, fried foods, and ice cream.

6. **Use lean meat, eggs, and lowfat dairy products in moderation.**
   Lean meat: Two to four ounces daily if desired. Limit red meat to two or three servings per week and use more as a condiment or seasoning for vegetables and whole grains. Fish and skinned poultry are preferred.

   Lowfat dairy products: Two servings daily. Increase for children and teens and pregnant or nursing mothers.

   Eggs are a good source of protein. Eat in moderation.

7. Limit or avoid sugars, artificial sweeteners, and white flour products.

8. Avoid or limit soft drinks, diet pop, punch, coffee, tea, caffeine drinks, and alcohol. Limit juice intake.

9. Use salt sparingly.

10. Drink eight or more 8-ounce glasses of water daily.

Keep your total daily food intake within these levels:

Complex Carbohydrates	65-80%	Fats	10-20%
Refined Carbohydrates	0-very low	Protein	10-15%

A QUICK START — THE TWENTY-ONE DAY PLAN

This Plan Requires Commitment, Self-Discipline, and Work!

This Quick Start is not for everyone—just those impatient few who want to lose fat quickly and are physically and mentally prepared to do so. If your Setpoint is sticky, this often helps it lower more readily.

For greatest success be very strict. Follow this Quick Start for 21 Days only and then return to the Lifetime Plan on the preceding page. Repeat when needed. Use common sense and don't stress your body.

Follow the Setpoint Lifestyle on page 37 with these changes:

1. Exercise Daily or Twice Daily. This is a must! Get adequate rest.

2. Eat more vegetables of all kinds. Include lowfat vegetable soups. Continue to eat whole grains, beans, lentils, and fresh fruit every day, but put the emphasis on vegetables, both raw and cooked.

3. Drastically Decrease FATS to 10% of daily calories.

4. Eat two to four ounces of lowfat fish or poultry daily if desired. Avoid all red meats except as a condiment or seasoning.

5. Avoid sugars, white flour products, artificial sweeteners, and all drinks except water. Drink 8 to 10 8-ounce glasses of water daily.

6. Eat often—regular meals plus wholesome snacks when hungry. Don't Starve! Don't Stuff! Listen to Your Body!

MENU PLANNING

Does the thought of planning meals for more than a day at a time frustrate you? Planning ahead saves you time and money and makes it easier to eat a wide variety of foods. Simplify this task and make it more enjoyable by using the following guide. In just one evening you can plan menus for the next month. See Chapter 12 for specific menu plans to help get you started.

Simplify Menu Planning

On a large empty calendar, pencil in simple menus for each day of the month. Follow the *Setpoint* guidelines. Use the recipes in this book and the information below on breakfast, lunch, and dinner menu planning. Many families don't object to having the same main dish twice in a week if there are leftovers; allow for them in your planning. For easy reference, include on your calendar the page numbers of the recipes found in this book.

You can use the same month of menus repeatedly. Who remembers what they ate last month? Since it's beneficial to eat with the seasons, you will eventually want to make a month of menus for each season: spring, summer, fall, and winter.

Daily Guide For Menu Planning

Four or more servings whole grains
Four or more servings vegetables—raw and cooked
Include green and deep yellow vegetables
Two to four fresh fruits
Beans, Peas, Lentils — 2 to 4 cups per week
Two to four ounces lean meat
Two servings lowfat dairy products
Include potatoes, beans, or brown rice daily

Count As a Serving:

1 slice bread or 1/2 bun	1 muffin, roll, pancake, or waffle
1 cup prepared cereal	1/2 cup cooked cereal, rice, or pasta
1 cup raw vegetables	1/2 cup cooked vegetables

Fresh fruit: 1 medium whole fruit (apple, orange) or 1/2 cup diced fruit.
Dairy: 1 cup milk or yogurt; 1/2 cup cottage cheese.

1/2 cup cooked dry beans, peas, or lentils counts as a serving of vegetables or as one ounce of the meat group.

What's For Breakfast?

A simple and nourishing breakfast gives energy for the whole day. It helps stabilize blood sugar, emotions, and nerves and reduces the urge to snack or overeat later on.

Whole grain cereal	1% or skim milk
Whole grain toast	Water
Fresh fruit (may be eaten as a mid-morning snack)	

Whole-Grain Cooked Cereal

When purchasing cooked cereals, select whole grain products; avoid those that have been highly refined. Cooked whole-grain cereal keeps your energy high and stays with you longer than prepared cereal. Add banana, raisins, or a little sweetener if needed. Choose any of the hot cereals in Chapter Seven:

Brown Rice Cereal	Millet Cereal
Rice 'n Apple Breakfast	Oatmeal
Cracked Wheat Cereal	Steel-Cut oats
Whole Wheat Cereal	

Whole Grain Unsweetened Prepared Cereal

Prepared cereals don't have quite the staying power of a cooked cereal, but many brands are very good. Be certain to read the labels; avoid cereals with more than three or four grams of added sweeteners per serving. Try mixing two kinds for variety. Commercial granola is usually high in fat and sugars. Try the Favorite Granola recipe found in Chapter Seven.

Use prepared whole grain cereals such as:

Shredded Wheat	Nutri-Grain cereals
Grape-Nuts	100% bran cereals
Wheat Chex	Bran Flakes

Pancakes, Waffles, Eggs, Muffins

Make pancakes, waffles, eggs, and muffins an occasional choice. Plan them for the weekend or for special occasions. Many good recipes for the following foods are found in the breakfast section:

Whole grain pancakes or waffles	Eggs and omelets
Whole grain French toast	Hashbrown potatoes
Bran or blueberry muffins	Ebelskivers

Lean Lunches

A lowfat lunch helps keep your energy high throughout the afternoon. A salad won't stay with you very long. Add a whole grain sandwich or a nourishing soup for long-term endurance. Avoid salad bars or buffets if you are tempted to eat the high-fat, high-sugar choices.

If you eat a very light lunch, you may need a snack about 4 p.m. This refuels your body so that you won't get too tired and hungry during late afternoon. It also helps prevent overeating at dinner. If you won't have time for an afternoon snack, eat a little more lunch. Always strive for balance and variety.

Plan a Setpoint Lunch Such As the Following:

Soup or salad
Sandwich, whole wheat bread or roll
Fruit (may be eaten as a mid-afternoon snack)
Water

Lunch Suggestions

Lunch and dinner menus can be interchanged if you prefer to eat your main meal at noon. Recipes for the following foods can be found in either the lunch or dinner sections of this book:

Water-based vegetable soup such as Minestrone Soup, Bean Soup, Lentil Soup, Hamburger Soup, Clam Chowder, Lentil Soup, Bean Soup, or Split Pea Soup
Chili Con Carne with cornbread and raw vegetables
Taco Salad
Marinated Vegetables
Pear Salad
Fresh Fruit Salad with yogurt
Whole grain sandwich
Chicken-Rice Spread in pita bread
Crunchy Bible Sandwich
Stuffed baked potato
Pizza with whole wheat crust and vegetable toppings

Delicious Dinners

Dinner Guide: Eat until you are comfortable and satisfied.
Don't Diet — Never Overeat!

Eat the evening meal at least four hours before bedtime
if possible.

Plan a Setpoint Meal Such as the Following:

Two to four ounces lean meat (or a vegetarian meal if desired)
Three or more vegetables
Whole grains (whole wheat bread, pasta or brown rice.)
Fresh fruit (may be eaten as an after-dinner snack)
Two glasses of water

Dinner Suggestions

Menu suggestions for a complete meal are included with all dinner recipes
found in Chapter Nine. Add bread and fruit as desired.

Roast Chicken and Vegetables
Chicken Enchilada Casserole
Chicken Pineapple Stir-Fry
Crispy Oven-Fried Chicken
Baked Fish Fillets
Juicy Salmon Loaf
Stuffed Green Peppers
Spaghetti
Easy Lasagna
Taco Sundaes
Stuffed Baked Potato

SNACKS FOR SNITCHIN'

Hungry between meals? Drink a glass of water first; you may just be
thirsty. Snack if you are truly hungry, eating just enough to hold you to the
next meal. Try these for snacks:

Whole wheat bread
Breadsticks
Rice cakes
Whole grain cereal with milk and fresh fruit or raisins
Air-popped popcorn sprinkled with herbs (avoid butter and salt)
Corn tortilla chips and salsa
Raw vegetables
Cold cooked yam or sweet potato
Fresh fruit

Unsweetened applesauce
Fresh fruit shake
Unsweetened nonfat yogurt and fresh fruit
Water-base vegetable soup
Tuna or chicken sandwich
Whole wheat pizza topped with vegetables

Buy and Cook in Quantity

Prepare enough for two meals or more as you fix lunch or dinner. Use a block of time to prepare several different staple foods such as those listed below. (These recipes are all found in this book.) Refrigerate or freeze these items in meal-size containers. With these basic foods prepared and ready, you'll be able to whip up a *Setpoint* meal in a hurry.

Cooked brown rice (an automatic rice cooker is a good investment)
Stewed and deboned chicken
Ranchero Beans
Setpoint Bread
Steamed or baked potatoes and yams
Salsa

GROCERY SHOPPING

Once you have your month of meals planned, make a shopping list of the specific ingredients you will need. Having the right kinds of food readily available helps assure your success. Below are some good staple foods you will want to keep on hand to make living the Setpoint way easy and convenient:

Chicken, whole or pieces
Water-packed tuna
Fresh lean fish
Extra lean beef
Lowfat cottage cheese
Nonfat unsweetened yogurt
1% or skim milk
Whole grain cereals, hot and cold
100% whole wheat bread
Whole wheat pocket bread
Brown rice

Sliced white turkey, cooked
Mock crab meat
Thinly sliced turkey ham
Eggs
Buttermilk
Evaporated skim milk
Parmesan cheese
Lowfat cheddar cheese
Miracle Whip Light
Reduced Calorie Mayonnaise
Fat-free salad dressings

Pinto beans, canned and dry
Cornmeal
Whole wheat spaghetti
Fresh vegetables and fruit
Spices and seasonings

Popcorn
corn tortillas
Spinach lasagna noodles
Canned tomatoes and juice
Salsa or mild taco sauce

READING LABELS

Take Time to Read Labels

Learn to read labels so you'll know what is in the foods you buy. This can be done in seconds once you know what to look for. Don't buy from the advertising label. Words such as *natural, lite, organic, low-cal* or *high-energy* can be misleading. Always read the list of ingredients and the nutritional analysis. Ingredients appear in order of abundance or weight—the most first and the least last.

1. Check serving size first. The nutritional analysis is keyed to this.
   Be realistic when comparing the listed serving size to your own serving size.

2. Check calories per serving next. If the number is high, study the list of ingredients to see where the calories are coming from—fats, sugars, or both.

3. Find the number of fat grams per serving and choose products which are low, preferably under five grams of fat per serving for a single item; a main meal may have more than 10 grams of fat.

4. Watch for regular or artificial sweeteners and avoid heavily sweetened foods. Many products contain several types of sweeteners. Artificial sweeteners include NutraSweet (aspartame), saccharin, sorbitol, and xylitol.

5. Look for 100 percent whole wheat on the label. Enriched, unbleached, or wheat flour are other ways of saying white flour.

Don't Be Fooled By Fat Percentages

Many health authorities make food recommendations in terms of fat percentage. *Percent fat by weight and fat as a percentage of calories* are not the same. Fat as a percentage of calories tells the true story.

For example, when ham is advertised as 95 percent fat free, it sounds like a good choice, but you are only told the *percent fat by weight*. The total *fat as a percentage of calories* is usually over 60 percent, making it a poor choice.

Milk is another good example. Popular 2% milk is two percent fat by weight but 38 percent fat as a total percentage of calories. One percent milk at 18 percent fat or skim milk at three percent fat are better choices.

Compute Fat as a Percentage of Calories

Follow these steps to determine fat as a percentage of calories in any given food, recipe, or meal.

1. Multiply the number of fat grams by 9 to determine the number of fat calories.
2. Divide the number of fat calories by the total number of calories.
3. Multiply the answer in number 2 by 100 to get the percentage of fat.

Let's figure the fat as a total percentage of calories in a can of chicken noodle soup:

1. 2 grams fat per serving x 9 calories per gram = 18
2. 18 divided by 70 calories per serving = .26
3. .26 multiplied by 100 = 26 percent fat

To keep daily fat intake at 20% or less of total calories, combine small amounts of higher-fat foods with plenty of lowfat grains, beans, vegetables, and fruits each day; then average your *total* daily food intake. Eating 15 to 30 grams of fat per day will keep your average under 20% fat if you eat between 1200 and 2600 calories. Count fat grams, not calories!

EATING OUT

Everyone eats out occasionally, and some eat out every day. Choose your restaurant with care — one that offers lots of good choices. The more often you eat out, the stricter you should be in both where and what you eat. Don't hesitate to say you are on a lowfat diet. Inquire as to how the dishes are prepared, and ask if they can be made with little or no fat. Always ask, don't assume you can tell from the menu.

Salad bars can sabotage your good intentions unless you know where the fats are hidden. Most salad dressings are almost 100% fat so use the no-oil dressings now available. Read the label and make sure there are 0 grams of fat per serving. Another option is to have your dressing served on the side. Dip your empty fork in the dressing, and then spear some salad. You'll get the same good taste, but only a fraction of the fat. Or choose flavorful fruits and vegetables for seasoning your salad.

Baked potato bars offer a wide range of toppings. Water-base soup, cottage cheese, mushrooms or chili are all good. Avoid butter, sour cream, cream soups, gravy, and cheese.

Be careful at a buffet or smorgasbord. It is easy to overeat because you want to taste a little of everything. Look the buffet over before you start. Determine to avoid the sweets and the high-fat foods. When you are full, stop eating. Don't feel obligated to clean up your plate.

Eating Out Guide

Yes	No
Appetizers	
V-8 or tomato juice	Cocktails
Unsweetened fruit juices	Sweetened juices
Seafood cocktail	Cream soups and chowders
Water-base soups	Vegetables in oil marinade
Fresh vegetables	
Fresh fruits	
Salads and Salad Dressings	
Green salads	Potato and macaroni salads
Fresh fruits	Fruit with whipped cream dressing
Carrot salad, drained	Gelatin salads
Coleslaw, drained	Pasta in oil marinade
No-oil or low-fat dressings	Regular salad dressings
Lemon juice	Mayonnaise
	Sour cream
	Cheese
	Nuts, seeds, croutons
	Bacon bits
	Cold cuts
Breads	
100% whole wheat bread	White bread
Rye Bread	Dinner rolls

Yes	No
Cornbread (one piece)	Biscuits and muffins
Bran muffins	Danish and sweet rolls
Breadsticks (a few)	Coffee cake
Crackers (a few)	

Vegetables

Baked, stewed, steamed, or broiled without fat	Scalloped, au gratin, fat fried, sauteed, or creamed

Meats and Eggs

Fish, chicken, turkey	Meats which are fried,
Lean red meat occasionally	grilled, sauteed, breaded,
Roasted, baked, broiled or	or served with gravy or
boiled without added fat	sauces
Eggs: boiled, poached, or scrambled without added fat	

Miscellaneous

Beans, all kinds	
Steamed rice	
Pasta without high-fat sauces	

Desserts

Fresh fruits	All high-sugar, high-fat desserts

Beverages

Water	Alcoholic beverages
Lowfat milk	Soft drinks, regular and
Buttermilk	diet
	Chocolate milk and cocoa
	Coffee and tea
	Milk shakes

Eating Out Meal Suggestions:

Breakfast:

Oatmeal or a prepared bran or whole grain cereal
Banana
Lowfat milk

Lunch:

Turkey sandwich on whole grain bread. Ask for cottage cheese, yogurt, mustard or horseradish as a spread
Salad or water-base vegetable soup
Fresh fruit
Large bowl of vegetable soup or chili
Whole grain roll or occasional small piece of cornbread

Main meal:

Baked fish, turkey or teriyaki chicken
Baked potato (try pouring your vegetables over potato)
Vegetables (cooked and raw)
Whole grain roll or bread
Fresh fruit

One counselor used to tell her clients: "If friends think you are not eating sweets or drinking alcohol because you are 'on a diet,' they may pester you to sample this 'wonderful pie' or 'have just one drink.' Some people find it helps to say, 'I've discovered that I'm allergic to sugar (or alcohol), it gives me a terrible headache.' It seems that many people will try to tempt you away from your good food choices, but when it comes to your health, they have a little more respect!"

IDEAS FOR ENTERTAINING

Entertaining need not undermine your *Setpoint* lifestyle. All of the recipes in this book produce wonderful dishes you'll proudly serve to any guest. Here are a few suggestions:

Light Refreshments

Cinnamon rolls with hot apple cider
Fresh fruits and vegetables with dips
Salsa with tortilla chips
Layered Tostada Party Dip with tortilla chips
Lavender Fruit Ice
Layered Fruit Parfait

Light Meal

Marinated Vegetables with Danish "Birdseed" Rolls
Salad Bar with whole grain rolls
Minestrone Soup with German Dark Rye Bread
Clam Chowder with pan rolls

Dinner

Menu suggestions are given with each dinner recipe in Chapter Nine. Add bread and a dessert if desired.

Soup buffet with a variety of breads
Chili with cornbread
Chicken Divan
Hamburger Stroganoff
Baked Potato Bar
Swedish Hot Dish
Taco Sundaes

"LEAN" Suggestions

- Don't Diet!
- Eat three satisfying, well-balanced meals daily.
- Eat Setpoint snacks if hungry.
- Eat regularly and don't skip meals.
- Don't count calories, measure foods, or use exchanges.
- Eat before you get too hungry.
- Eat slowly. Enjoy your food without feeling guilty.
- Don't pass up the bread—just bypass the butter.
- Leave food on your plate if you've had enough.
- Never eat sweets on an empty stomach.
- Put thoughts of dieting completely out of your mind.
- Ignore that nagging voice that says "if you eat less, you'll lose faster."
- Eat only when physically hungry, not when psychologically hungry from food advertisements, boredom, depression, loneliness, anger, or nerves.
- Drink six to eight glasses of water each day.
- Don't wear loose-fitting clothes any time. You'll have a natural tendency to grow into them.
- Know that *you will* be successful, and GO for it!

Go!

Everything you've read in this book thus far has been geared to getting you ready. All the principles have been thoroughly explained and then summarized. You're ready, you're set . . .

Go...and you'll be *SET FOR LIFE*!

It will be the best thing you've ever done for yourself and for your family. Turn the page to discover more than 350 wonderful Setpoint recipes for foods that will dramatically improve the way you look and feel. Start now to...

Eat More - Weigh Less - Feel Terrific!

NUTRITION INFORMATION

All recipes have been nutritionally analyzed as follows to help assure success in achieving good health and weight control.

CAL — Calories
% FAT — Percent of calories from fat
P — Grams of protein
F — Grams of fat
C — Grams of carbohydrate
Na — Milligrams of sodium

Optional ingredients are omitted from the nutritional analysis. When options appear in the ingredients in a recipe, such as molasses or honey, the first one mentioned is used in the analysis. The first serving size listed is also used.

RCU — REFINED CARBOHYDRATE UNIT

1 RCU = 6 grams of sugar, honey, molasses, etc.
12 grams of white flour
24 grams of raisins, dates, dried fruit
48 grams of fruit juice concentrate

0 to 2 Refined Carbohydrate Units (RCUs) per day are within recommended limits.

FAT UNITS

1 FU = 6 grams of refined fat such as oil or margarine
8 grams of naturally occurring fat such as meat, milk, eggs, nuts and seeds, avocados, and so on.

2 to 5 Fat Units (FUs) per day are within recommended limits.

Keep fat intake between 15 to 30 grams of fat daily. Increase fat intake up to 45 or more fat grams daily if pregnant, nursing, or very active; keep fats between 10 to 20% of total calories.
For babies age 2 and under—see pages 294-296.

For further information on these principles of weight control see: "How to Lower Your Fat Thermostat" and "The Neuropsychology of Weight Control."[6] "Eat & Be Lean," an informative book by Dana and Chris Thornock, gives additional insight and strong reinforcement to this Setpoint lifestyle.[21]

CHAPTER 6

Breads—Rolls—Muffins

There's nothing like fragrant, fresh-from-the-oven bread and rolls. They fill the home with an unforgettable aroma and will create never-to-be-forgotten memories for your family.

Making good whole wheat bread is an art made easy with the right equipment. An electric grain mill and a heavy-duty electric bread mixer are worth the investment. To bake without these marvelous appliances, once you've used them, would be like returning to a scrub board to do the wash. Bread and rolls are prepared quickly and effortlessly, so there's no need to spend countless hours in the kitchen. In fact, it is so easy that you'll almost feel guilty when your friends praise your work. These appliances soon pay for themselves—not just in money saved, but in good eating and good health.

To make breadmaking easy and enjoyable, develop a routine and make it exactly the same way each time. As it becomes a habit, breadmaking will get easier and faster. Before long you will be able to whip up a delicious batch of bread and have it raising in the oven in just 15 minutes. Making a good loaf of homemade bread is a very satisfying experience.

The bread recipes in this book have all been streamlined for quick and easy preparation. Beginners and professionals alike will appreciate the simplicity of breadmaking as outlined here and the high quality finished products. While the instructions given are for use with an electric mixer, all the recipes can be made and kneaded by hand.

We've included a baker's bounty of everyone's favorites—crusty French, spicy muffins, fruit-filled quick breads, moist delicious breads for everyday eating and much more. You'll enjoy baking them, delight in eating them, and love the way they contribute to a leaner, healthier you.

All recipes marked with an asterisk* are found in this book.

BREADS

Eight secrets for making perfect whole wheat bread:

The first secret for making bread the modern way is to start with *fresh flour*. You can't make fresh bread with old, stale, prepackaged flour. Find a good health food store that will mill whole grains for you. Better yet, mill your own. When you mill your own flour, and use it immediately, you are assured of getting all the vitamins, minerals, bran, and fiber that nature intended. You reap the goodness of whole grains and none of the preservatives. (One cup wheat makes approximately 1 1/2 cups flour.)

The second secret is to use *fresh yeast*. Be sure your yeast is active before you begin making your bread, and keep it active by using liquids at the proper temperature (see below). Mix your yeast and flour before adding the liquid. If you buy yeast in bulk, store it in a covered container in the refrigerator or freezer.

The third secret is to use *comfortably warm water*. Water temperature is very important. It should be between 120 and 130 degrees — comfortably warm out of the tap as you add it to your flour/yeast mixture. Water that is too hot will kill the yeast. If your water is not warm enough, it will not fully activate the yeast. Warm water results in warm dough which keeps the yeast active and helps the dough rise properly.

The fourth secret is to let the flour, yeast, and water mixture sit, undisturbed, for 10 to 15 minutes. This process is called sponging. During this period the bread-making action begins. *Sponging* makes lighter, fluffier, more flavorful bread and cuts down on the kneading time. It is particularly important if you are kneading bread by hand. You can skip this step if you are in a hurry, but it helps assure your success.

The fifth secret is to use the *right amount of flour*. Many factors affect the amount needed, such as the moisture in the air, fineness of the flour, and the gluten content of the flour. These factors may change from day to day. One day you may need ten cups of flour for a batch of bread, the next day the same recipe will require only nine.

How do you get a perfect loaf every time? Let your bread mixer tell you how much flour to add. With the machine running, quickly add the final few cups of flour, one cup at a time. As the batter turns to dough, it clings together, creating an empty spot in the bowl. Add flour until the dough cleans the sides of the bowl and pulls against itself as it kneads. The dough should hold its shape but still be a little tacky. Follow the same guide if making bread by hand. Be very careful not to add too much flour, a common cause of heavy, dry bread.

A good breadmaker never has a failure, but instead learns to correct the inevitable, occasional mistake. If you should add too much flour, just drizzle a little warm water over the dough while it is mixing. It will soon return to the proper consistency. If you find your dough is too moist after kneading is complete, add a little white flour to ''glue'' it back together — usually one-third to one cup, depending on the batch size. Knead only until the flour blends in well, and shape dough immediately into loaves.

The sixth secret for making perfect bread is to *develop the gluten*. Gluten is the protein in wheat which gives structure and elasticity to batters and dough. Gluten is unique to wheat; other grains don't contain very much gluten, if any. That's why you can't make leavened bread out of rice or soy flour. (Be aware that all wheat is not created equal. When purchasing wheat, shop carefully for quality. High protein hard spring and winter wheat makes the best bread because it contains the highest percentage of gluten. Soft wheat, which contains less gluten, is excellent for quick breads, pastries, and pasta.)

When you add liquid to whole wheat flour and knead it thoroughly, the gluten turns into an elastic dough. If you can be successful in fully developing the gluten in bread dough, you will get a lighter, fluffier loaf of bread instead of a hard, compact loaf. With a good bread mixer, you can do this in a matter of minutes — not after a half-day of kneading, raising, and punching down dough! The kneading arm acts like a taffy puller, pulling and stretching the dough so thoroughly that it develops all of the gluten.

Knead your dough long enough to properly develop the gluten. The dough will be smooth and elastic. This kneading time will vary according to the size of the batch, the quality of the wheat used, and the quality of your bread mixer or the strength of your arms!

The seventh secret is to put a *little oil* on your hands as you mold your dough into loaves. Using flour to help you shape your dough only makes for dry, crumbly bread. Besides, it gets all over you and the floor! If the dough sticks to your countertop or work surface, put a small amount of oil on the countertop for this batch and add a little more flour next time. For convenience, keep a small squeeze bottle of oil handy.

The eighth and final secret is to *let the dough proof*. Proofing — more commonly called rising — allows the yeast to ferment, forming gases. These gases are captured by the elastic framework of the gluten. Like tiny balloons, they cause the bread to rise, making it light.

Proofing may be done at room temperature or in the oven. Room temperature proofing takes longer and is harder to control. Many people prefer this method, however, especially for free-formed loaves, such as French, round, or braids. Preheat your oven before baking when using this method.

Oven proofing is a wonderful shortcut for busy bakers. The combination of a warm oven, warm dough, and moisture creates the perfect environment for yeast to rise.

Preheat your oven to 150° while the dough is mixing. After preparing the loaves, *turn off the oven before you put in your bread*. If the dough appears a little dry on top while proofing, lightly mist it with water from a spray bottle. Dough that is too dry cannot rise properly. If desired, coat the tops with a light layer of shortening or oil after shaping to help prevent this problem.

Always set a timer and keep a close eye on rising bread. In approximately 20 to 30 minutes the dough will double in size.

When bread dough has almost doubled in bulk, test for lightness by touching it lightly near the edge of the pan. A slight indentation should remain when it is ready for baking. If the indentation remains completely, the bread is over-proofed. Your bread will be too light and may have a coarse texture or even fall. Bake immediately or reshape your loaves and allow them to rise again. Your finished product will not be quite as good once the elastic framework breaks down.

If the indentation does not remain, allow your bread to rise a few minutes more. Under-proofing makes bread heavy and compact, often with a large crack down one side. With a little practice, you'll know just when it is ready.

If your bread has proofed at room temperature, it's usually best to preheat your oven before baking. For oven proofing you do not need to preheat the oven. Leave your bread in the oven and turn the temperature to 350°. In just 30 to 35 minutes you'll have mouth-watering, fresh, crispy bread! Whole wheat bread seems to require a lower baking temperature than other types, but be careful not to overbake. Ovens vary, and your altitude will affect the baking time. After a few batches you'll learn the right time and temperature for your oven.

Tip: One proofing is sufficient if your dough has been kneaded by an efficient electric bread mixer. If kneaded by hand, let your dough *sponge* (step 4) for 15 minutes and then let it rise once in the bowl after kneading is complete until dough is almost double. This improves the quality and makes lighter bread. Knead dough down, then proceed with steps 7 and 8.

The last step is always the best: *Eat and enjoy!*

How to Shape Breads

Regular Loaves: A loaf of bread may be formed in many ways, and most bakers have their favorite. Here are two simple methods that produce good, consistent results.

1. Slightly flatten a ball of dough with your hands, and then cross-grain the dough by folding in each of the four sides, directly across from each other. Using the palms of your hands or a rolling pin, flatten the dough into a rectangle, 7 x 15 inches for a large 4 x 8 1/2-inch loaf, or 5 x 8 inches for a small 3 x 5 3/4-inch loaf. Roll up, starting at the narrow side, sealing each turn tightly with the edge of your hand. Tuck in the uneven ends, and seal the ends of the loaf into two very thin strips. Tuck the strips under the loaf, and roll the loaf back and forth to make it even. Place in a lightly greased loaf pan. If the loaf is

a bit too long for the pan, lift up the center, allowing the ends to fit, and then lay the center down. The dough will fit without remolding.

2. Hold a ball of dough in your hands and keep tucking the edges of the dough underneath, turning the ball as you go until you have a smooth turtle's back shape. Gently elongate the ends until the dough resembles a football. Seal the edges underneath with your fingers. Place in a lightly greased bread pan.

Using the right size bread pan is very important. Too much or too little dough results in a poor loaf of bread, particularly when using whole wheat. Whole wheat dough is heavier than white dough and cannot support itself in a wide pan. For best results, bake whole-grain bread in a 4 x 8 1/2-inch or narrower bread pan.

The following were calculated using 100% whole wheat bread dough.

Pan Size	Dough Weight	Cups of Dough
4 x 8 1/2″	1 1/2 pounds	3 cups
3″ x 5 3/4″	3/4 to 1 pound	1 1/2-2 cups
46 ounce juice can	1 pound	2 cups
1 quart can	1/2 pound	1 cup

Round Loaves: Form dough into a ball. Holding the dough in your hands, tuck the edges of the dough underneath, turning the dough until you have a smooth ball. Seal the underneath edges with your fingers. Place in a lightly greased 8-inch pie or cake pan and let rise until almost double.
Bake: 350° 30-35 minutes

French Loaves: Roll dough into a large rectangle, about 12 x 15-inches. Beginning at the long edge, roll up tightly. Pinch the edge to seal, and taper the ends. Place seam-side down on a lightly greased baking sheet which has been sprinkled with cornmeal, or place in a French bread pan. Using a sharp knife, make 1/4-inch deep diagonal slashes every 2 1/2 inches across the top. Brush with an egg-water mix*. Let rise until double.
Bake: 375° 25-30 minutes

Braids: Form dough into three ropes, each about 1/2-inch in diameter. Starting in the center, braid the ropes together. Pinch the ends together to seal. Turn the braid over, and braid the other half. Again pinch the ends to seal. Pull the braid slightly to lengthen, if necessary. Place on a lightly greased baking sheet or place in a bread pan to rise.
Bake: 350° 30-35 minutes

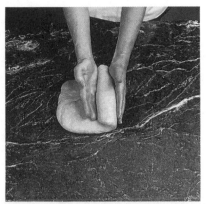

How to shape dough into loaf of bread

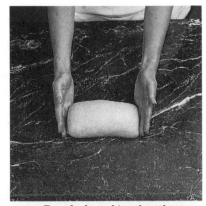

Dough shaped into bread

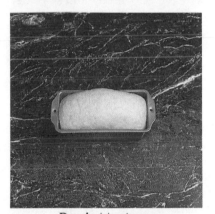

Dough rising in pan

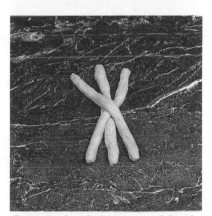

Beginning braid: three ropes of dough

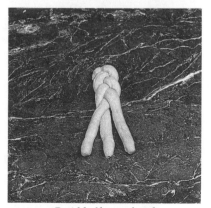

Braid half-completed

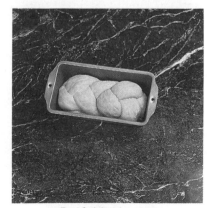

Braid rising in pan

You Can Freeze Dough

Have you found yourself stopping by a bakery for fresh bread or rolls to complement a special dinner? You won't need to once you've learned to freeze your own bread and roll dough. On a busy day, simply take the frozen bread or rolls out of the freezer. Let the dough rise and then bake. Hot breads make a welcome addition to any meal, elegant or simple, and now you can make them part of your everyday routine. Your family and friends will praise you as the best cook in the world!

Frozen Bread

Shape your bread dough as directed in the recipe. Place it on a baking sheet or in a bread pan. Freeze immediately. As soon as the dough is frozen solid, remove it from the pan and place it in a heavy plastic bag and seal. Use the dough within six to eight weeks.

To use, lightly grease bread pan with shortening. Put the frozen dough into the pan, and cover it loosely with waxed paper. Let the dough rise until double, four to six hours, depending on room temperature. If your dough dries out while rising, mist it lightly with water from a spray bottle.
Bake: 350° oven 30 to 35 minutes

Quick-Rise Method

Transfer your frozen bread dough to a lightly greased bread pan as directed. Preheat your oven to 150°. Turn off the oven. Place the frozen dough in the oven, and put a pan of hot water on the rack immediately below the dough. Let the dough rise from one to three hours. When dough is light, remove the pan of water. Turn oven to 350°, and bake 30 to 35 minutes.

Tip: If your dough should get too light, remove from the pan, reshape it, and let dough rise again until double.

Frozen Rolls

Rolls can be made from regular bread dough or any of the richer roll dough recipes. Shape as desired and place on a nonstick or lightly greased baking sheet. Freeze immediately. When frozen, cover with foil or a heavy plastic bag. If freezer space is limited, remove the rolls from the baking sheet and seal in a heavy plastic bag. Keep frozen until needed.

To use, position rolls close together but not touching on a lightly greased or non-stick baking sheet. Cover loosely with waxed paper. Let rise until very light and doubled in size, about four to five hours. The time will vary according to room temperature. If rolls appear to dry out on top, mist them lightly with water from a spray bottle while they rise.
Bake: 350° oven 18 to 20 minutes

Quick-Rise Method

Transfer frozen rolls to a lightly greased or non-stick baking sheet. Position rolls close together but not touching. Preheat your oven to 200°, and then *turn off the oven*. Place the rolls in oven, and put a pan of hot water on the rack immediately below the dough. Let rise until rolls are double in size. Mist with water from a spray bottle if rolls dry out on top while rising. Remove the pan of water from the oven. Leave rolls in oven and turn oven to 350°.

Bake: 350° 18 to 20 minutes

Reheat Breads in the Microwave

Breads and rolls may be reheated in the microwave without becoming rubbery or tough. Use 50 or 70 percent power for even reheating and to keep the bread tender. Reheat on paper toweling to absorb any moisture and prevent soggy bottoms. Do not cover breads or they will become too moist.

Bread: **15 to 30 seconds per slice**
                1 1/2 to 3 minutes per loaf
Buns and rolls: **5 to 10 seconds per roll**
                15 to 20 seconds for 4 rolls

Diastatic Malt

The dictionary says diastatic malt is "barley or other grain soaked in water and spread until it sprouts, then dried and aged. It has a sweet taste."
The purpose of sugar in breads is to feed the yeast, make the crust brown, and improve the flavor. Diastatic malt, which is widely used in Europe, does all of these things. Diabetics and hypoglycemics especially, will appreciate this inexpensive natural sweetner.

1-2 cups whole wheat
3 cups lukewarm water

Place wheat and water in a quart jar for 24 hours. Drain well and pour wheat into a plastic sprouter or leave in the bottle, turning the bottle on its side. Cover with a cloth. Rinse and drain the wheat at least twice daily until the sprout is slightly longer than the seed. This takes about 48 hours.

Place sprouted wheat on a large baking sheet. Bake at 150° until thoroughly dry, about 3 to 4 hours, or dry in a dehydrator.

Place the dried sprouted wheat in a blender and blend on high for about 30 to 45 seconds or until it is of fine meal consistency.

Store diastatic malt in a tightly closed glass jar in the refrigerator or freezer. It will keep indefinitely.

Use in any bread recipe. Eliminate or reduce the amount of sweetener in the bread. Use 1 teaspoon Diastatic Malt for each 2 loaves of bread or each 5 cups flour.

Use on cereal as a natural sweetener if desired.

Simply Perfect Setpoint Bread

This bread is a staple to enjoy every day, as it helps form the foundation of the Setpoint lifestyle. This versatile recipe enables you to make just the right-size batch for your family.

Regular Batch
14 to 16 cups whole wheat flour (10 to 12 cups whole wheat)
2 rounded tablespoons dry yeast
1/2 cup high-gluten (80%) flour* (optional)
500 mg vitamin C (optional)
6 cups warm water (120 to 130°)
1/2 cup vegetable oil
1/2 cup honey or sugar
1 1/2 tablespoons salt

Medium Batch
10 to 12 cups whole wheat flour (7 cups whole wheat)
2 tablespoons dry yeast
1/3 cup high-gluten (80%) flour* (optional)
300 mg vitamin C (optional)
4 cups warm water (120 to 130°)
1/3 cup vegetable oil
1/3 cup honey or sugar
1 tablespoon salt

Small Batch
6 to 7 cups whole wheat flour (5 cups whole wheat)
1 rounded tablespoon dry yeast
1/4 cup high-gluten (80%) flour* (optional)
250 mg vitamin C (optional)
2 cups warm water (120 to 130°)
3 tablespoons vegetable oil
3 tablespoons honey or sugar
2 scant teaspoons salt

   High-gluten flour* is a high protein (80%) flour available at most health food stores. It adds volume and improves texture in whole wheat bread. If using regular gluten flour, double the amount called for in these recipes.
   Mill whole wheat in an electric grain mill. Place 9, 6, or 3 cups fresh flour (depending on desired batch size) into mixer bowl equipped with kneading arm. Add dry yeast, gluten flour and vitamin C. Pulse to mix well. Add water, and mix for 1 minute. For lighter bread, turn off mixer, cover bowl, and let dough sponge for 10 minutes. This is very important if kneading by hand. Sponging makes lighter bread and reduces kneading time. Add oil, honey, and salt. Turn on mixer, and quickly add remaining

flour, 1 cup at a time, until dough forms a ball and cleans the sides of the bowl. The amount of flour needed may vary. Knead 7 to 10 minutes. If mixing by hand, knead at least 12 to 15 minutes or until dough is smooth and elastic.

Preheat oven to 150° during this time. Lightly oil hands. Divide dough into equal portions. Shape into loaves and place in greased bread pans. *Turn off oven.* Place bread in oven, arranging pans with space between to allow heat to circulate freely. Set a kitchen timer, and watch closely. Let rise until almost double in bulk, approximately 20 to 30 minutes. Leave bread in oven and turn heat to 350°.

Bread may also rise uncovered on countertop until double. Bake in a preheated oven 350° oven for 30 to 35 minutes. Immediately remove from pans; let cool on wire racks. For a soft crust, mist lightly with water from a spray bottle while still hot. Slice bread when cool, and store in plastic bags in freezer, not refrigerator.

Bake:		Time:		Temp:			Yield:		
Regular Batch		**30-35 min**		**350°**		5-6	4″ x 8 1/2″ loaves		
							or		
						8-9	3″ x 5 3/4″ loaves		
Medium Batch		**30-35 min**		**350°**		4	4″ x 8 1/2″ loaves		
							or		
						6-7	3″ x 5 3/4″ loaves		
Small Batch		**30-35 min**		**350°**		2	4″ x 8 1/2″ loaves		
							or		
						3-4	3″ x 5 3/4″ loaves		

Per Serving	RCU	FU	Cal	% Ft	P	F	C	Na
	0	0	88	15	3	1.5	16	119

Tip: To assist in making the transition to 100% whole wheat bread, in this and subsequent recipes you can replace a fourth to a half of the whole wheat flour with unbleached white flour. Gradually increase the ratio of whole wheat flour.

To improve bread texture:
Add 1 cup buttermilk or yogurt in place of 1 cup of the water.
Add approximately 500 milligrams of vitamin C with your flour.
Add 2 tablespoons lemon juice instead of vitamin C.
Add 2 tablespoons dry or liquid lecithin to the dough.
Replace 1 to 3 cups whole wheat flour with white flour.

Diabetics or hypoglycemics may wish to substitute a natural sweetener for the honey or sugar, such as 1/2 to 3/4 cups unsweetened applesauce per average batch. You can also use Diastatic Malt.

BREAD VARIATIONS

Use any of the basic bread doughs in this book.

Easy Rye Bread

Into 2 cups of dough knead 1 tablespoon caraway seeds and 1/2 teaspoon anise seeds. Shape into a round loaf. Place in lightly greased pie pan. Let rise until almost double.
Bake: 350° 30 min

Raisin Bread

Flatten a scant 2 cups of dough into a 5 x 12″ rectangle. Sprinkle with cinnamon and a handful of raisins. Roll up, beginning with the narrow edge. Pinch seam to seal. Place in lightly greased 3 x 5 3/4-inch loaf pan. Let rise until double.
Bake: 350° 30 min

Busy-Day Cinnamon Rolls

Roll out 3 cups dough into a 12 x 16-inch rectangle. Brush with 1 tablespoon soft butter and sprinkle with cinnamon/sugar mix made from 1 tablespoon cinnamon and 1/3 cup brown or white sugar. Sprinkle with 1/2 cup raisins. Any of the fruit fillings may be used in place of the butter, cinnamon/sugar, and raisins. Roll up tightly and pinch edges to seal. Cut roll into 15 1-inch slices using a piece of string or fishing line. Place three across and five down in a greased 9 x 13-inch baking sheet. Flatten slightly with palm of hand. Let rise until double.
Bake: 350° 16-18 min Do not overbake.

Optional: Drizzle with a light glaze made from 2 tablespoons hot water, 1 teaspoon vanilla, and 1 cup powdered sugar.

Per Serving	RCU	FU	Cal	% Ft	P	F	C	Na
	1	0	132	15	4	2	24	140

Honey-Nut Rolls

Prepare Busy-Day Cinnamon Rolls as directed above. In a small saucepan melt 2 tablespoons butter or margarine and add 1/2 cup milk or half 'n half, 1/2 cup honey, and 1 tablespoon cinnamon. Pour into a 9 x 13-inch glass baking dish or 2 9-inch pie pans. Sprinkle with 1/2 cup chopped nuts. Arrange cinnamon rolls on top of mixture in pan. Let rise until double. Bake. Invert on tray and serve warm.
Bake: 350° 18 to 20 minutes

Per Serving	RCU	FU	Cal	% Ft	P	F	C	Na
	1	1	141	23	4	4	25	149

Cinnamon Pull Aparts

Using your thumb and index finger as a pastry press, squeeze off walnut-size balls of dough. Dip in melted butter and then roll in a cinnamon/sugar mix made of 1 tablespoon cinnamon and 1/2 cup sugar. Place balls in layers in a greased bread pan or tube pan. Let rise until light.
Bake: 350° 20 to 30 min (depends on the number of layers)
Serve warm. Allow guests to pull off their own serving.

Pizza Crust

Roll out 2 to 2 1/2 cups dough on a lightly greased pizza pan using a pizza roller. Amount of dough will vary according to pan size and desired thickness of crust. Add sauce and toppings.
Makes a crisp crust when rolled thin or a chewy thick crust.
Bake: 500° 10 to 12 min for a large pizza or 5 to 7 min for a small pizza
Tip: To prevent soggy crust or to prepare for later use, prebake crust in a 500° oven for 3 to 4 minutes, just until puffed but not brown. After prebaking, spread with sauce, add desired toppings, and bake as above; or let crust cool, cover with plastic wrap, and freeze.

Bread Sticks

Roll dough into finger-thin ropes and cut into 6-inch lengths. Roll in sesame seeds. Place on a greased baking sheet.
Let raise 10 to 15 minutes.
Bake: 350° 15 to 18 min

Light Whole Wheat Bread

This is a good recipe to make if you have low-protein wheat that doesn't make light bread without some help.

11 to 12 cups whole wheat flour
2 tablespoons dry yeast
1 cup buttermilk or yogurt
4 cups hot water
1/3 cup oil
1/3 cup honey
1 tablespoon salt
1 cup unbleached white flour

In mixer bowl equipped with kneading arm, combine 6 cups whole wheat flour and dry yeast. Pour buttermilk into hot water; combined temperature should be about 125°. Add to flour mixture, and mix well for 1 minute. Turn off mixer, cover bowl, and let dough sponge for 10 minutes. Add oil, honey, and salt. Mix well. Add the 1 cup white flour and remaining whole wheat flour, 1 cup at a time, until dough forms a ball and cleans the sides of the bowl. Knead 6 to 8 minutes. Preheat oven to 150°.

Lightly oil hands. Divide dough into equal portions. Shape into loaves, and place in greased bread pans. *Turn off oven.* Place bread in oven, arranging pans to allow heat to circulate freely. Let raise until almost double in bulk, 20 to 25 minutes. Leave bread in oven; turn heat to 350°. (Bread may also rise on countertop until double. Bake in a preheated oven.) Remove from pans and let cool.

Bake: 350° 30 to 35 min
Yield: 4   4" x 8 1/2" loaves or 6   3" x 5 3/4" loaves

Per Serving	RCU	FU	Cal	% Ft	P	F	C	Na
	0	0	86	15	3	1	16	91

Potato Bread

Taste a little bit of Idaho in this moist, light bread.

10 cups whole wheat flour
1/2 cup dry potato flakes
2 tablespoons dry yeast
4 cups warm water (120 to 130°)
1/4 cup oil
1/4 cup honey
1 tablespoon salt

Mix 6 cups flour, potato flakes, and dry yeast in mixer bowl. Add hot water, and mix for 1 minute. Turn off mixer. Cover bowl, and let dough sponge for 5 minutes. Add oil, honey, and salt. Turn on mixer. Add remaining flour, 1 cup at a time, until dough forms a ball and cleans the sides of the bowl. Knead 5 to 7 minutes. Preheat oven to 150°.

Lightly oil hands. Divide dough into equal portions. Shape into loaves, and place in greased bread pans. *Turn off oven.* Place bread in oven, arranging pans to allow heat to circulate freely. Let rise until almost double in bulk, 20 to 25 minutes. (Bread may also rise on countertop until double. Bake in a preheated oven.) Leave bread in oven; turn heat to 350° and bake. Remove from pans and let cool.

Bake: 350° 30 to 35 min
Yield: 4   4″ x 8 1/2″ loaves or 6   3″ x 5 3/4″ loaves

Per Serving	RCU	FU	Cal	% Ft	P	F	C	Na
	0	0	66	16	2	1	13	87

Julienne's Wheat Seed Bread

Prepare Potato Bread to sponge stage. After sponging, add 1/4 cup sunflower seeds, 1 tablespoon sesame seeds, 1 tablespoon millet, and 1 tablespoon poppy seed. Prepare and bake as directed.

Light and Fluffy Bread

This smaller batch of bread works well with or without a bread mixer.

6 cups whole wheat flour
1/2 cup high-gluten (80%) flour* or 500 mg vitamin C
2 tablespoons dry yeast
2 cups warm water (120 to 130°)
2 tablespoons oil
2 tablespoons honey
2 eggs
2 teaspoons salt

Mix 3 cups flour, gluten flour, and yeast in mixer bowl equipped with kneading arm. Add hot water and mix for 1 minute. Turn off mixer, cover bowl, and let dough sponge for 10 minutes. Add oil, honey, eggs, and salt. Turn on mixer. Add remaining whole wheat flour, 1 cup at a time, until dough forms a ball and cleans the sides of the bowl. Knead 5 to 6 minutes. Turn off mixer, cover bowl, and let rise 20 minutes. Mix for 1 minute to knead down dough. Preheat oven to 150°.

Lightly oil hands. Divide dough into equal portions. Shape into loaves. Place in lightly greased bread pans. *Turn off oven.* Place bread in oven, and let rise until double in bulk. Leave bread in oven and heat to 350°. (Bread may also rise on countertop until double. Bake in a preheated oven.) Remove from pans and let cool.

Bake: 350° 30 to 35 min
Yield: 4   4" x 8 1/2" loaves or 6   3" x 5 3/4" loaves

Per Serving	RCU	FU	Cal	% Ft	P	F	C	Na
	0	0	45	16	2	1	8	62

Chicago Wheat Bread

Making the transition from white to whole wheat bread may be difficult for some families. This recipe makes a beautiful, light loaf that everyone will love. It comes from Debra Parks in Chicago, where the amount of flour needed varies greatly from day to day because of the high humidity. Let your mixer tell you how much flour to add.

4 cups unbleached white flour
6 to 8 cups whole wheat flour
2 tablespoons dry yeast
1/3 cup high-gluten (80%) flour* or 500 mg vitamin C powder
4 cups warm water (120 to 130°)
1/3 cup oil
1/3 cup sugar
1 tablespoon salt

Place white flour, yeast, and gluten flour in mixer bowl equipped with kneading arm. Add water and mix well. Turn off mixer; cover bowl. Let dough sponge for 15 minutes. Add oil, sugar, and salt. Turn on mixer. Add whole wheat flour, 1 cup at a time, until dough forms a ball and cleans the sides of the bowl. Knead 5 to 6 minutes. Preheat oven to 150°.

Lightly oil hands. Divide dough into equal portions. Shape into loaves, and place in greased bread pans. *Turn off oven.* Place bread in oven, arranging pans to allow heat to circulate freely. Let rise until double in bulk, 20 to 25 minutes. (Bread may also rise on countertop until double. Bake in a preheated oven.) Leave bread in oven; turn heat to 350°. Bake and remove from pans; let cool on wire racks.

Tip: This recipe is also very good using only 1 cup white flour and replacing the remainder with whole wheat flour.

Bake: 350° 30 to 35 min
Yield: 4   4" x 8 1/2" loaves or 6   3" x 5 3/4" loaves

Per Serving	RCU	FU	Cal	% Ft	P	F	C	Na
	1	0	86	15	3	1	16	87

Old-Fashioned Oatmeal Bread

This good bread makes up in a hurry.

2 cups quick-cooking rolled oats
5 to 7 cups whole wheat flour
2 tablespoons dry yeast
500 mg vitamin C powder
2 1/2 cups warm skim milk (120 to 130°)

2 tablespoons oil
1/4 cup brown sugar or molasses
2 teaspoons salt
1 egg, separated
1 tablespoon water

Mix oats, 2 cups flour, dry yeast, and vitamin C in mixer bowl equipped with kneading arm. Add warm milk, and mix well. Add oil, brown sugar, salt, and egg yolk. Mix and add remaining flour, 1 cup at a time, until mixture forms a ball and begins to clean the sides of the bowl. Dough should be a little sticky. Knead 5 to 6 minutes.

Lightly oil hands. Divide dough into two portions. Shape into loaves, and place in lightly greased pans. Mix egg white and water with a fork until foamy, and brush on loaves. Sprinkle with a little additional oatmeal. Let rise until double. Bake in a preheated 350° oven. Remove from pans, and let cool.

Bake: 350° 30 to 35 min
Yield: 2   9'' round loaves or 4   3'' x 5 3/4'' loaves

Per Serving	RCU	FU	Cal	% Ft	P	F	C	Na
	0	0	78	15	3	1	14	97

Seven-Grain Variety Bread

Enjoy the flavor and nutrition of many grains in this unique bread.

3 cups seven-grain flour
1 cup unbleached white flour
7 to 8 cups whole wheat flour
2 tablespoons dry yeast
1/4 cup dry potato flakes

5 cups warm water (120 to 130°)
1/3 cup oil
1/3 cup molasses or honey
1 tablespoon salt

Mix seven-grain flour, white flour, 2 cups whole wheat flour, yeast, and potato flakes in mixer bowl equipped with kneading arm. Add water, and mix 1 minutes. Turn off mixer, cover bowl, and let dough sponge 10 minutes. Add oil, molasses, and salt. Mix well. Add remaining flour, 1 cup at a time, until dough cleans the sides of the bowl. Knead 5 to 6 minutes.

Lightly oil hands. Divide into equal portions. Shape into loaves, and place in greased bread pans. Let rise until almost double. Bake, remove from pans and let cool.

Bake: 350° oven 30 to 35 min
Yield: 4   4'' x 8 1/2'' loaves or 6   3'' x 5 3/4'' loaves

Per Serving	RCU	FU	Cal	% Ft	P	F	C	Na
	0	0	80	16	3	1	15	87

German Dark Rye Bread

The mild rye flavor of this bread will make it a favorite.
Vall Gene Mills shares her treasured family recipe.

3 cups whole wheat flour
2 tablespoons dry yeast
1/4 cup carob powder
1 tablespoon caraway seed
2 cups warm water (120 to 130°)
2 tablespoons butter or margarine
1/3 cup molasses
2 teaspoons salt
3 to 3 1/2 cups rye flour

In mixer bowl equipped with kneading arm, combine whole wheat flour, dry yeast, carob powder, and caraway seed. In a separate bowl, combine water, butter, molasses, and salt. If necessary, warm to approximately 125°. Add to dry mixture in bowl. Mix 2 to 3 minutes. Add rye flour, 1 cup at a time, until dough cleans the sides of the bowl and forms a soft dough. Knead 3 to 4 additional minutes or until smooth.

Lightly oil hands. Divide into equal portions. Shape into loaves, and place in greased pans. Slash the tops of the loaves with a sharp knife, and lightly brush with a small amount of cooking oil. Let rise until double, 30 to 45 minutes. Bake in a preheated 350° oven. Remove from pans and cool.

Bake: 350° 30-35 min
Yield: 2 8-inch round loaves or 2 4'' x 8 1/2'' loaves

Per Serving	RCU	FU	Cal	% Ft	P	F	C	Na
	0	0	65	12	2	1	13	93

Squaw Bread

Even your fussiest little eater will like this sweet, moist bread.

1 cup rye flour
2 cups whole wheat flour
2 1/2 cups unbleached white flour
1 rounded tablespoon dry yeast
1 cup hot water
1/2 cup raisins
1 cup warm buttermilk
1/4 cup oil
1/4 cup molasses
2 scant teaspoons salt

In mixer bowl equipped with kneading arm, mix rye flour, whole wheat flour, and dry yeast. Put water and raisins in blender and pulse until finely chopped. Add buttermilk. Combined temperature of liquids should be approximately 125°. Add to flour and mix 1 minute. Add oil, molasses, and salt. Turn on mixer. Add remaining flour as needed, until mixture cleans the sides of the bowl and forms a ball. Knead 5 to 6 minutes.

Lightly oil hands. Divide into equal portions. Shape into loaves, and place in lightly greased pans. With a sharp knife, slash a large X on top of each loaf. Brush loaf tops with egg-water mix*. Let rise until double. Bake in a preheated oven.

Bake: 350° 35 min
Yield: 2   8'' or 9'' round loaves or 2   4'' x 8 1/2'' loaves

Per Serving	RCU	FU	Cal	% Ft	P	F	C	Na
	1	0	100	21	3	2	16	142

French Bread

Try these long golden loaves with their crackly-crisp crust.

3 cups whole wheat flour
2 tablespoons dry yeast
2 cups comfortably hot water (120 to 130°)
2 tablespoons oil
1 tablespoon sugar or honey
2 teaspoons salt
2 to 3 cups unbleached white flour
2 tablespoons yellow cornmeal
1 egg white
1 tablespoon water
Sesame seeds

Mix whole wheat flour and dry yeast in mixer bowl. Turn off mixer. Add hot water, oil, sugar, and salt. Mix 1 minute. Quickly add white flour, 1 cup at a time, until mixture cleans the sides of the bowl and forms a ball. Knead 3 to 4 minutes.

Lightly oil hands. Divide dough into two equal portions. Roll each into a 12 x 15-inch rectangle. Beginning at the long side, roll up tightly, pinching edges to seal. Taper ends. Place each loaf with the seam side down on a lightly greased baking sheet which has been sprinkled with cornmeal. French bread pans may also be used. Diagonally slash loaf tops every 2 1/2 inches 1/4-inch deep. Beat egg white and water with a fork until foamy. Brush tops and sides of loaves with egg-water mix. Sprinkle with sesame seeds. Let rise until double. Bake in a preheated oven.

Bake: 375° 25 to 30 min or until deep golden brown
Yield: 2 large loaves

Per Serving	RCU	FU	Cal	% Ft	P	F	C	Na
	1	0	81	13	3	1	15	120

Hard Rolls

Shape French Bread dough into small ovals. Place on cornmeal-sprinkled baking sheets. Let rise until double.
Bake: 375° 15 to 18 minutes

Braided Swiss Bread

It's as pretty to look at as it is good to eat!

1 quart warm skim milk
1/2 cup shortening
2 tablespoons honey
1 cup warm water (120° to 130°)
4 cups whole wheat flour
8 cups unbleached white flour
2 tablespoons dry yeast
1/2 cup nonfat dry milk
1/4 cup sugar
2 eggs
1 1/2 tablespoons salt

Combine warm milk, shortening, honey, and hot water. Combined temperature of liquids should be approximately 125°. In mixer bowl equipped with the kneading arm, mix whole wheat flour, 2 cups white flour, yeast, dry milk, and sugar. Add milk mixture, and mix for 1 minute. Turn off mixer, cover bowl, and let dough sponge for 10 minutes. Add eggs and salt. Mix well. Quickly add remaining flour, 1 cup at a time, until dough cleans the sides of the bowl. Knead 4 to 5 minutes. Turn off mixer, cover bowl, and let dough rise until almost double in bulk, about 20 minutes. Turn on mixer to knead dough down.

Lightly oil hands. Divide dough into 5 equal portions. Divide each portion into thirds. Roll each third into a 10 inch rope. Brade 3 ropes together to form each loaf*. Place in lightly greased bread pans. Let rise until double. Bake in preheated oven.
Bake: 375° 10 min   Reduce heat to 350° and back 20 to 22 min
Yield: 5   4" x 8 1/2" loaves

Per Serving	RCU	FU	Cal	% Ft	P	F	C	Na
	1	0	81	20	3	2	14	117

White Bread

Mary Griffin's bread has a beautiful velvety texture. It adapts easily to half-white, half-whole wheat bread.

11 to 12 cups unbleached white flour
 or 6 cups whole wheat flour and 5 to 6 cups white flour
2 tablespoons dry yeast
1 12-ounce can evaporated milk
3 cups hot water
1/4 cup oil
1/4 cup sugar
1 tablespoon salt

   Mix 7 cups flour and dry yeast in mixer bowl. Add evaporated milk and then hot water. Add oil, sugar, and salt. Mix well. With mixer running, quickly add remaining flour, 1 cup at a time, until dough just cleans the sides of the bowl. Knead 3 to 4 minutes. Do not overmix. Turn off mixer, cover bowl and let dough rise to top of bowl, about 15 to 20 minutes. Turn on mixer to knead dough down. Lightly oil hands. Divide dough into equal portions. Shape into loaves, and place in greased bread pans. Let rise until double and bake.
Bake: 350° 35 min
Yield: 4   4" x 8 1/2" loaves or 6   3" x 5 3/4" loaves

Per Serving	RCU	FU	Cal	% Ft	P	F	C	Na
	1	0	85	13	3	1	16	94

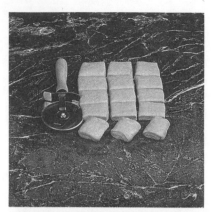

Quick Parkerhouse Rolls

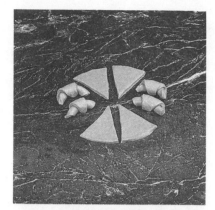

Crescent Rolls

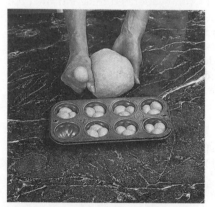

Cloverleaf Rolls

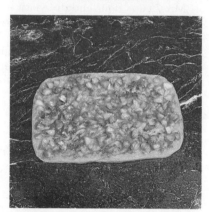

Preparing Cinnamon Rolls

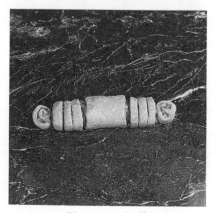

Cinnamon Rolls

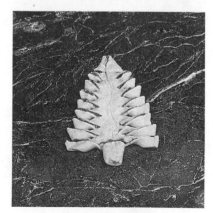

Sugar Plum Tree

ROLLS AND BUNS

Feather Roll dough is a favorite dough for most of the dinner rolls and specialty breads. Danish "Birdseed" Rolls are yummy made into parkerhouse or pan rolls. Pan rolls are delicious made from most any of the bread or scone doughs. Experiment a little and find your favorites!

Pan Rolls: Shape dough into a large, smooth ball. Using your thumb and index finger as a pastry press, squeeze off small, uniform balls of dough. Use approximately 1/4-1/3 cup dough for each dinner roll. Tuck the edges under to make smooth balls. Place rolls nearly touching in the pan. Let rise until light.
Bake: 350° 18 to 22 min

Quick Parkerhouse Rolls: On a lightly oiled countertop, roll dough into a rectangle 1/4-to 3/8-inch thick. Spread very lightly with butter if desired. Using a pizza cutter, cut the dough into 2 x 2 1/2-inch strips. Pick up each piece and stretch it slightly to thin the dough in the middle. Fold off-center so the top half overlaps the bottom just a little. Firmly press the folded edge. Place close together on a lightly greased baking sheet. Let rise until double.
Bake: 350° 18 to 20 min

Parkerhouse Rolls: On a lightly oiled countertop, roll dough to 3/8-inch thick. Cut with a biscuit cutter into rounds. Brush very lightly with melted butter if desired. Using the blunt edge of a butter knife, make a crease across each circle, just off-center. Fold so that the top half slightly overlaps the bottom. Firmly press the folded edge. Place close together on a lightly greased baking sheet. Let rise until double.
Bake: 350° 18 to 20 min

Crescent Rolls: On a lightly oiled countertop, roll dough into a circle 10 to 12 inches in diameter and 1/4-inch thick. Using a pizza cutter, cut the dough into 8 to 12 wedges. Beginning at the rounded edge, roll each piece toward the point. Place on a greased baking sheet with the point underneath. Curve slightly into a crescent shape. Let rise until double.
Bake: 350° 18-22 min

Finger Rolls: Shape approximately 1/4 cup dough into a roll about 4 inches long. Place close together in rows in a greased pan. Let rise until double.
Bake: 350° 18-22 min

Cloverleaf Rolls: Shape the dough into a large smooth ball. Using your thumb and index finger as a pastry press, squeeze off 1-inch balls of dough. Arrange 3 balls in each nonstick or lightly greased muffin cup. Let rise until double.
Bake: 350° 18-20 min

Cinnamon Rolls: On lightly oiled surface, roll approximately 3 cups of dough into a 12 x 16-inch rectangle, 1/4- to 1/3-inch thick. Spread with the desired filling* or spread with 1 tablespoon soft butter and sprinkle with a mixture of 1 tablespoon cinnamon, 1/3 cup brown or white sugar, and 1/2 cup raisins.

Roll up as for a jelly roll, starting with the long side. Seal the seam by pinching the dough together. With the seam side down, cut into 1 inch slices using fish line, heavy thread, or string. Slip the string under the roll, cross it over the top, and pull down. Place rolls cut-side up in a greased 9 x 13-inch baking pan, three across and five down, or in round cake pans. Flatten slightly with palm of hand. Let rise until very light and double in size.

Bake: 350° 18 to 20 min

Specialty Breads May be Made from Roll Dough:

Sugar Plum Tree: On a lightly oiled countertop, roll 1 to 2 cups of dough, depending on the desired size, into a triangle which is 1/4-inch thick. Transfer to a nonstick or lightly greased heavy baking sheet. Brush dough lightly with softened butter. Spoon on date filling* and spread evenly to within 1/2- inch of the edges. Gently lift the outside edges of dough and bring to the center, overlapping slightly. Seal with water, if desired. The basic tree shape should be retained. Use kitchen shears and cut about 2/3 of the way into the tree on each side. Make each branch about 1 inch wide. Twist each piece *up* to form branches. Let rise about 15 minutes. Bake and let cool. See picture page 74.

Bake: 350° 18 to 20 min or just until done
Cover with thin coat of glaze and decorate as desired.
Glaze: 1 to 2 tablespoons hot water, 1 teaspoon vanilla and 1 cup powdered sugar. To decorate use red, green, and yellow dried or candied cherries and pineapple, cut in fourths.

Fruit Braids: On a lightly oiled surface, roll dough into a 9 x 12-inch rectangle about 1/4-inch thick. Transfer to a lightly greased baking sheet. Place a 3-inch strip of raisin or apple filling* lengthwise down the center third of the rectangle. With a pizza cutter or sharp knife, cut the dough on both sides of the filling into 1/2-inch strips, cutting almost to the filling. Make the same number of strips on each side. Complete the braid by alternately laying the strips across the filling on a diagonal. Make sure the end of each strip is completely covered by the next strip. Tuck in the ends of the last strip so the filling will not leak out. Let rise only about 15 to 20 minutes.

Bake: 350° 18 to 20 min Cool and decorate if desired.

Candy Cane: Follow the instructions for Fruit Braid except roll out the dough to a narrower rectangle, approximately 6 x 12 inches. Fill the center 2 inches with any fruit filling* or use a red fruit, such as cherry pie filling*. Cut the dough into 1/4-inch-wide strips. Braid as instructed above. Gently shape into a candy cane, slightly stretching the dough to make the curve. Let rise only 15 to 20 minutes. Bake and let cool.

Bake: 350° 16 to 18 min
Cover with thin coat of glaze and decorate as desired.
Glaze: 1 to 2 tablespoons hot water, 1 teaspoon vanilla and 1 cup powdered sugar.

FRUIT FILLINGS

Date Filling

This filling is good in Sugar Plum Trees, braids, sweet rolls, and filled cookies. It's just plain good anytime!

1 1/2 cups dates, chopped (8-ounce package)
1 cup water
2 tablespoons honey
1/8 teaspoon salt
1/4 cup nuts, chopped

Combine dates, water, honey, and salt in a small saucepan. Bring to a boil. Reduce heat and simmer 5 minutes, stirring constantly. Add nuts. Cover and refrigerate until needed.

Per Serving	RCU	FU	Cal	% Ft	P	F	C	Na
	0	0	39	14	0	1	8	6

Apple Filling

This is a popular filling.

2 cups finely chopped or grated apples
1/2 cup raisins or chopped dates
2 tablespoons honey, optional
1 to 2 teaspoons cinnamon or apple pie seasoning
Pinch salt

Combine all ingredients. Use immediately. For later use, cook 1 minute to prevent the apples from turning dark. Refrigerate.

Per Serving	RCU	FU	Cal	% Ft	P	F	C	Na
	0	0	43	0	0	0	9	14

Apple-Mince Filling

This makes a festive holiday filling for braids or sweet rolls.

To above recipe add:
1 cup prepared mincemeat

Raisin Filling

This delicious filling stores well in the refrigerator or freezer. Keep some on hand through the holiday season.

1 cup raisins
1 1/2 cups water
1 teaspoon vinegar
1/8 teaspoon salt
1/4 cup honey or sugar
1/4 cup water
2 tablespoons cornstarch
1 teaspoon vanilla
2 teaspoons cinnamon
1/4 teaspoon nutmeg
1/3 cup chopped pecans

In blender, combine raisins and 1 1/2 cups water. Blend until raisins are finely chopped, about 1 minute. Transfer to a small saucepan. Add vinegar, salt, and honey. Cook 10 minutes. In a small cup, mix the 1/4 cup water and 2 tablespoons cornstarch. Add to filling. Cook until thickened. Remove from heat, and add vanilla, cinnamon, nutmeg, and pecans. Cool. Refrigerate.

Per Serving	RCU	FU	Cal	% Ft	P	F	C	Na
	0	0	23	22	0	1	3	1

Dried Fruit Filling

This filling also makes a tasty jam.

1 cup dried apricots, prunes, or other dried fruit
3/4 cup orange or pineapple juice
1 tablespoon honey (optional)

Combine all ingredients in a small saucepan. Cook until tender and thick, stirring occasionally. Cool.
Yield: 20   1 tablespoon servings

Per Serving	RCU	FU	Cal	% Ft	P	F	C	Na
	0	0	20	2	0	0	5	1

BUNS

Buns can be made from many different doughs. Basic Buns on page 82 is a favorite dough. Or use any of the regular bread doughs if you are baking bread anyway.

How To Shape Buns:

Poor Boy or Hoagie Buns: On a lightly oiled countertop, roll dough into a rectangle 1/2-inch thick. Using a pizza cutter, cut into strips 2 to 3 inches wide and 6 inches long, or any desired size. Dough may also be molded into oblong rolls. Place on a greased baking sheet, and brush with egg-water mix*. Sprinkle with sesame seeds, if desired.

Hot Dog Buns: On a lightly oiled countertop, roll dough to 5/8-inch thick. Cut into 2 x 6-inch strips. For oval buns, bend an empty 46-ounce juice can into oval and use as a dough cutter. Place dough on a greased baking sheet, and brush with egg-water mix*.

Hamburger Buns: On a lightly oiled countertop, roll dough 3/8-inch thick. Using a quart can or other large cutter, cut into large rounds. Buns may also be shaped from a 1/2-cup ball of dough. Flatten with your hand or a rolling pin. Place on a lightly greased baking sheet. Brush with egg-water mix*, and sprinkle with sesame seeds, if desired.

Let all buns rise only 12 to 20 minutes.

Bake: 350° 16 to 18 min

Egg-Water Mix

1 egg or 1 egg white, slightly beaten (use egg yolk in dough if desired)
1 tablespoon water

Mix together with a fork until foamy. Brush on tops of loaves, buns, or bread for a shiny crust.

Feather Rolls

Transform whole wheat into piping hot rolls in just 60 minutes. This favorite recipe is versatile and can be used for any dinner or sweet roll.

9 to 10 cups whole wheat flour
  or 8 cups whole wheat flour and 1 to 2 cups white flour
2 to 3 tablespoons dry yeast
1/2 cup nonfat dry milk (optional)
3 cups warm water (120 to 130°)
2/3 cup oil
1/2 cup honey or sugar
4 large eggs
4 teaspoons salt

Mix 5 cups flour, dry yeast and nonfat dry milk in large mixer bowl. Add water, oil and honey. Mix well for 1 to 2 minutes. Turn off mixer, cover bowl, and let dough sponge for 10 minutes. Add eggs and salt. Turn on mixer. Add remaining flour, 1 cup at a time, until dough begins to clean the sides of the bowl. Knead for 5 to 6 minutes. Dough should be very soft and manageable. Stiff dough produces heavy, dry rolls. If dough stiffens while mixing, drizzle a little warm water over dough as it kneads. Dough may be used immediately or covered and stored in the refrigerator for several days.

Lightly oil hands and countertop if needed. Shape immediately into rolls—see pages 75-76. Let rise until very light. Don't overbake.

Bake: 350° 18 to 20 min   **Yield: 5 dozen large rolls**

Per Serving	RCU	FU	Cal	% Ft	P	F	C	Na
	0	0	94	25	3	3	15	142

Danish "Birdseed" Rolls

These authentic Danish rolls add a special touch to any meal.
Try them once, and they'll become a family favorite.

2 cups hot water
2 cups Seed Mix (see below)
1/2 cup margarine, softened
6 to 7 cups whole wheat flour or 5 cups whole wheat flour and
  1 to 2 cups unbleached white flour
2 tablespoons dry yeast
1/2 cup nonfat dry milk
2 cups water
1/3 cup honey
3 eggs
1 tablespoon salt

Seed Mix - Makes 2 cups

3/4 cup whole wheat, coarsely cracked
3/4 cup rye, coarsely cracked
2 tablespoons flax seed
2 tablespoons sesame seed
1/4 cup sunflower seeds, slightly cracked

Coarsely crack wheat and rye separately in blender. Use high speed for about 45 to 60 seconds. Be certain no whole kernels remain. Combine all ingredients and cook as directed above.

Bring hot water to a boil. Add Seed Mix, and cook 5 to 7 minutes, stirring constantly. Remove from heat, add margarine, and set aside. Mix 3 cups flour, yeast, and dry milk in mixer bowl using kneading arm. Mix well. Add water and honey to seed mixture. (Mixture should now be comfortably warm, approximately 125°.) Add this mixture to ingredients in mixer and mix about 1 minute. Turn off mixer, cover bowl, and let dough sponge 10 minutes. Add eggs and salt. Turn on mixer. Add remainder of flour, 1 cup at a time, just until dough begins to make a ball and clean the sides of the bowl. Knead 5 to 6 minutes. Dough should be sticky but manageable.

Lightly oil hands. Shape dough into balls using about 1/4 cup dough for each. Place quite close together, but not touching, on baking sheets. Let rise until double.

Bake: 350° 18 to 22 min   **Yield: 4 to 5 dozen large rolls**

Per Serving	RCU	FU	Cal	% Ft	P	F	C	Na
	0	0	84	27	3	2	13	126

Basic Buns

You'll love this recipe. It's good for any bun you want to make.

5 to 6 cups whole wheat flour or 2 cups unbleached white flour and 3 to 4 cups whole wheat flour
2 tablespoons dry yeast
1/3 cup nonfat dry milk
2 cups warm water (120 to 130°)
1/4 cup oil
2 tablespoons honey
2 eggs
2 teaspoons salt, scant
1 egg white
1 tablespoon water
Sesame seeds (optional)

Mix 3 cups flour, yeast, and nonfat dry milk in mixer bowl. Add water, and mix well. Add oil, honey, eggs, and salt. Turn on mixer. Add remaining flour, 1 cup at a time, until dough just cleans the sides of the bowl. Dough should not be too stiff. Knead 5 to 6 minutes.

Lightly oil hands and countertop. Shape dough into hamburger, hot dog, or hoagie buns, using approximately 1/4 cup dough for each. See shaping instructions. Place on lightly greased baking sheets. Brush buns with egg-water mix. Sprinkle with sesame seeds, if desired. Let rise about 20 minutes for buns or until double for rolls.

Bake: 350° 16 to 20 min   Yield: 18 to 20 buns

Per Serving	RCU	FU	Cal	% Ft	P	F	C	Na
	0	1	148	24	6	4	23	185

Quick Cinnamon Rolls

The apple filling in these quick rolls is especially good. This recipe makes good dinner rolls too.

3 cups whole wheat flour
1 1/2 to 2 1/2 cups unbleached flour or whole wheat flour
2 tablespoons dry yeast
1 1/4 cups warm water
1/3 cup oil
1/3 cup honey or sugar
2 eggs
1 1/2 teaspoons salt

Favorite Filling
1 1/2 cups applesauce
2 apples, cored and shredded
1/2 cup raisins
1 tablespoon cinnamon

Filling #2
2 tablespoons soft butter
1/3 cup sugar
1 tablespoon cinnamon
1/2 cup raisins, optional

Glaze (optional)
2 cups powdered sugar
1/4 cup hot water
1/2 teaspoon vanilla

Mix whole wheat flour and yeast. Add water, oil, sugar, eggs and salt; mix well. Add remaining flour 1 cup at a time until dough just cleans the sides of the bowl. Do not add too much flour. Dough should be quite soft. Knead until smooth and elastic, about 6 minutes.

On lightly oiled surface roll dough into a large rectangle about 14x32 inches and a scant 1/4-inch thick. Spread evenly with applesauce, shredded apples, raisins and cinnamon. If using filling #2, spread dough with butter. Mix cinnamon and sugar and sprinkle evenly over dough. Sprinkle with raisins if desired. Or use any of the fruit fillings on page 77.

Roll up as for a jelly roll, starting with the long side. Seal the seam by pinching dough together. With seam side down, cut into 1 1/4'' slices using fish line or string. (Slide string under the roll, cross it over the top, and pull down.) Place rolls cut-side up on a nonstick baking sheet. Flatten slightly with palm of hand. Let rise until very light and double in size.

Bake: 350° 12-15 min   Yield: 24 rolls

Glaze: Mix powdered sugar, water, and vanilla. Drizzle over warm rolls if desired.

Per Serving	RCU	FU	Cal	% Ft	P	F	C	Na
Fav. Filling	1	1	145	23	4	4	24	126
Filling #2	2	1	143	29	4	5	23	136

Whole Wheat Pita Bread

Marge Miller taught me to make pita bread. Only your imagination will limit the fillings for this versatile bread.

3 to 4 cups whole wheat flour
  or 2 cups whole wheat flour and 1 to 2 cups white flour
1 tablespoon dry yeast
1 1/4 cups warm water (120 to 130°)
1/2 teaspoon salt (optional)

Mix 2 cups flour and dry yeast. Add water and salt, and mix well. Gradually add remaining flour until dough cleans the sides of the bowl. Dough should be moderately stiff. Knead 4 to 5 minutes, until dough is smooth and elastic. Do not over-knead. Form dough into 10 balls. On a floured countertop, roll each ball from the center out into a round 1/4 inch thick and 5 to 6 inches in diameter. Be certain both sides are lightly covered with flour. Place on a lightweight, nonstick baking sheet. Let rise 30 minutes or until slightly raised. Preheat oven to 500°.

Gently turn the rounds upside down just before placing in the oven. Bake on the bottom rack of the oven. The instant hot heat makes the breads puff.

Bake: 500° 5 min   Yield: 10 pita breads

Pita pockets will be hard when removed from the oven and soften as they cool. While still warm, store in plastic bags or an airtight container. Reheat in a 350° oven or in the microwave. Before filling, tear crosswise into halves.

Pita breads may be filled with virtually anything — chicken or tuna salad; taco filling, lettuce, and tomatoes; refried beans or thick chili with sprouts; stew; or leftover casserole.

Per Serving	RCU	FU	Cal	% Ft	P	F	C	Na
	0	0	142	5	6	1	30	96

Refrigerator Scones

These are tender and delicious.

1 quart buttermilk
8 to 9 cups whole wheat flour
  or 5 cups whole wheat flour and 3 to 4 cups unbleached white flour
2 tablespoons dry yeast
2 tablespoons sugar or honey
1 1/2 teaspoons salt
1 tablespoon baking powder
1/2 teaspoon soda
1/3 cup oil
2 eggs

Warm buttermilk to 125°. Combine 5 cups flour, yeast, and sugar in mixer bowl. Add buttermilk, and mix 1 minute. Turn off mixer. Add salt, baking powder, soda, oil, and eggs. Turn on mixer and add remaining flour, 1 cup at a time, until dough begins to clean the sides of the bowl. Dough should be soft.

If dough gets too stiff, drizzle a little warm water over dough as it mixes to soften.

Dough may be used immediately or covered and stored in the refrigerator for two or three weeks. Dough will continue to rise for a while in refrigerator. Knead down a few times. When ready to use, roll out room temperature dough on a lightly floured countertop. Cut into desired shape. Let rise. Cook on a nonstick griddle at 375°. Turn when brown and cook other side.

Cook: 375° until brown   Yield: 72 scones

Pan Rolls

Prepare as directed for Refrigerator Scones. Shape as desired. Let rise until light.
Bake: 375° oven 18 to 20 min

Per Serving	RCU	FU	Cal	% Ft	P	F	C	Na
	0	0	61	20	2	1	10	77

Bread Sticks

Any novice can make these tasty bread sticks.

3 to 4 cups whole wheat flour	1 1/2 cups warm water
1 tablespoon dry yeast	2 tablespoons butter or margarine
1 tablespoon sugar	Garlic salt
1 teaspoon salt	Parmesan cheese

Mix 3 cups flour, yeast, sugar, and salt. Add warm water and knead for three to five minutes. Add remaining flour as necessary to make a medium dough. If mixing by hand, cover dough and let rest for 10 minutes.

Melt butter in 9x13-inch glass baking dish in a 375° oven. Remove from oven and spread butter evenly in dish. Roll or pat dough to fit dish. Put dough into baking dish and turn once to coat with butter. Sprinkle with garlic salt and Parmesan cheese.

With pizza cutter, cut dough horizontally into nine one-inch strips, alternating directions each row to keep dough from creeping. Next, cut dough in half vertically (down the middle). Let rise only about 20 minutes. Bake in a 375° oven for 18 to 20 minutes or until golden brown.

Tip: You can double this recipe. Make one pan of breadsticks as above. Sprinkle the second pan with a mixture of 1/4 cup sugar and 1 tablespoon cinnamon to make cinnamon sticks.

Bake: 375° 18-20 min.   **Yield: 18 bread sticks**

Per Serving	RCU	FU	Cal	% Ft	P	F	C	Na
	0	0	83	17	3	2	15	135

Variation: Omit butter and add 2 tablespoons oil when adding water to the flour mixture. Mix as directed above. Lightly oil hands and countertop. Roll dough into a 7x13-inch rectangle about 1/2 inch thick. Using a pizza cutter, cut into 24 strips 1/2 inch wide and 7 inches long. Roll each strip into a 8-inch rope. Place 1/2 inch apart on nonstick baking sheet. Brush each stick with egg-water mix (see page 79), and sprinkle with sesame seeds. Let rise until almost double, 15 to 20 minutes.

Bake: 325° crisp sticks   20 to 25 min.
Bake: 350° soft sticks   12 to 15 min.   Yield: 24 bread sticks

Pretzels

Pretzels are as fun to make as they are to eat. They're best right out of the oven, but can be frozen and reheated.

1 cup whole wheat flour
1/2 cup unbleached flour
2 teaspoons baking powder
1 teaspoon sugar
1/2 teaspoon salt
2/3 cup skim milk
2 tablespoons soft butter
1 egg
Coarse salt

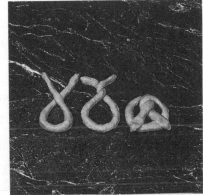

Mix flour, baking powder, sugar and salt in bowl. Add milk and soft butter. Mix with fork to make a soft dough. Knead 10 times. Divide dough in half. Roll one half of dough into rectangle 12" x 8". Cut lengthwise into eight 1-inch strips. Fold each strip in half lengthwise and pinch edges to seal. Twist each strip into pretzel shape as illustrated, tucking ends under. Place seam side down on greased baking sheet. Repeat with remaining half of dough. Beat egg in small bowl with fork. Brush pretzels with egg and sprinkle lightly with coarse salt.

Bake: 400° 16-20 min or until golden brown
Yield: 16 large pretzels
Remove with wide pancake turner and place on rack to cool.

Per Serving	RCU	FU	Cal	% Ft	P	F	C	Na
	0	0	51	30	1	2	8	129

QUICK BREADS

Microwaving Muffins

Spoon batter into a microwave muffin pan. Fill half full. Bake first at 50 percent power and then at full power according to the following schedule, or use directions given with your own microwave oven:

Quantity	50 Percent Power	Full Power
2 muffins	1 minute	30 seconds
4 muffins	2 minutes	1 to 1 1/2 minutes
6 muffins	4 1/2 minutes	1 to 1 1/2 minutes

Remove immediately from pan to prevent soggy muffins.

BRAN — Both oat bran and wheat bran make very significant contributions to overall health. The soluble fiber in oat bran helps sweep cholesterol from the veins and arteries. Wheat bran has insoluble fiber and moves rapidly through the body; a vitally important factor in good health. Use a combination of these two fibers to get maximum health benefits.

Oat bran, unprocessed wheat bran, and 100% bran cereal can all be used interchangeably in the bran muffin recipes that follow.

Oat-Bran Muffins

Mix and microwave these muffins in minutes. The batter stores well in the refrigerator.

1/2 cup hot water
1 cup 100% bran cereal
1/2 cup rolled oats
1/2 cup chopped dates or raisins
1 cup buttermilk or nonfat yogurt
1/4 cup oil or 1/2 cup applesauce

1 egg, slightly beaten
3 tablespoons sugar or honey
1 1/4 cups whole wheat flour
1 teaspoon soda
1/2 teaspoon salt

Pour hot water over cereal, oats, and dates. Let stand while mixing liquid ingredients. (If using raisins, place them in blender.) Combine raisins, buttermilk, oil, egg, and honey in blender. Pulse to mix and chop raisins. Stir liquids into bran mixture. Add mixed dry ingredients, and stir just until blended. Fill non-stick muffin pans 2/3 full.

Bake: 400° 12 to 14 min   **Yield: 18 muffins**

Per Serving	RCU	FU	Cal	% Ft	P	F	C	Na
	0	1	96	36	2	4	13	151
No oil	0	0	71	8	2	1	14	151

Refrigerator Bran Muffins

These high-fiber, melt-in-your-mouth muffins have been a family favorite for years. They complement any meal, make a good snack, and even pass for dessert! The batter stores well in an airtight container in the refrigerator for up to a month. Double the recipe to make a gallon of batter.

1 1/2 cups hot water	1/2 cup sugar or honey
3 cups 100% bran cereal	2 cups buttermilk or nonfat yogurt
1 cup chopped dates or raisins	2 1/2 cups whole wheat flour
1/3 to 1/2 cup oil or 1 cup applesauce	2 teaspoons soda
2 eggs	3/4-1 teaspoon salt

Pour hot water over cereal and dates in large bowl. Let stand while preparing other ingredients. In blender, combine oil, eggs, honey, and buttermilk. Pulse to mix well. Pour into the bran mixture, and mix together. Combine flour, soda, and salt. Add to bran mixture, mixing just long enough to blend ingredients. Do not stir batter again. Drop by tablespoonfuls into nonstick muffin pans, filling 2/3 full.

Bake: 400° 15 to 18 min   **Yield: 3 dozen muffins**

Per Serving	RCU	FU	Cal	% Ft	P	F	C	Na
	1	0	87	27	2	3	14	154
No oil	1	0	73	8	2	1	15	154

Everyone's Favorite Muffins

Try these tender, light muffins.

2 cups whole wheat flour	1 egg
1 tablespoon baking powder	1 cup skim milk
1/2 teaspoon salt	1/4 cup oil
1/4 cup honey or sugar	

Mix dry ingredients. Combine remaining ingredients in blender. Pour into dry ingredients. Stir only until combined; longer mixing makes muffins tough. Fill nonstick muffin pans 2/3 full.

Bake: 400° 12 to 15 min   **Yield: 12-15 muffins**

Per Serving	RCU	FU	Cal	% Ft	P	F	C	Na
	1	1	109	37	3	5	15	81

Half 'n Half Muffins

Substitute 1 cup unbleached white flour for 1 cup of the whole wheat flour. Prepare as directed.

Blueberry Muffins

Prepare Favorite Muffins as directed, increasing honey or sugar to 1/3-1/2 cup, depending on sweetness of berries. Fold in 1 cup blueberries just before spooning into tins.

Raisin, Nut, or Date Muffins

Prepare Favorite Muffins as directed, adding 1/3 to 1/2 cup raisins, nuts, or dates to dry ingredients.

Apple-Raisin Muffins

Orange peel gives these muffins an unusual and pleasing flavor. They are good hot or cold.

1 cup whole wheat flour
1 cup quick-cooking rolled oats
1 tablespoon baking powder
1/2 teaspoon soda
1/2 teaspoon salt
1 teaspoon cinnamon
1 teaspoon powdered orange peel
  or 1 tablespoon grated fresh orange peel
1/3 cup chopped nuts (optional)
1/4 cup sugar or honey
1 cup skim milk
1 egg
2 tablespoons oil
1 apple, cored and cut into fourths (1/2 cup)
1/3 cup raisins

Mix flour, oats, baking powder, soda, salt, cinnamon, orange peel, nuts, and sugar. In blender combine milk, egg, oil, apple, and raisins. Pulse to mix and finely chop apple and raisins. Add to dry ingredients, and stir just until moistened. Fill nonstick muffin tins 2/3 full.

Bake: 400° 12 to 14 min   Yield: 14 to 16 muffins

Tip: Decrease milk to 3/4 cup and use 1/2 cup applesauce in place of fresh apple if desired. For a change of flavor, omit orange peel and nuts and add 1/3 cup sunflower seeds.

Per Serving	RCU	FU	Cal	% Ft	P	F	C	Na
	1	1	82	28	2	3	12	183

Orange-Date Muffins

Serve these with a fresh fruit cup for a marvelous dessert.

2 cups whole wheat flour
3 tablespoons sugar
1/2 teaspoon salt
1/4 teaspoon soda
2 teaspoons baking powder
2 tablespoons grated fresh orange peel

1/2 cup chopped dates
1/4 cup chopped nuts (optional)
2 eggs
2 tablespoons oil
2/3 cup orange juice

Mix dry ingredients including orange peel, dates, and nuts. In blender combine eggs, oil, and orange juice. Pour into dry ingredients, and stir only until combined. Fill nonstick muffin pans 2/3 full.

Bake: 400° 12 to 14 min   **Yield: 12 to 15 muffins**

Per Serving	RCU	FU	Cal	% Ft	P	F	C	Na
	0	1	117	37	3	5	16	153

Banana Muffins

These muffins are moist, flavorful, and high in fiber.

1 cup whole wheat flour
1/4 teaspoon salt
1 cup bran cereal (All-Bran, Bran Buds, or 100% Bran)
1 tablespoon baking powder
2 tablespoons sugar or honey
1 egg
2 tablespoons oil
1/3 cup skim milk
2 large or 3 medium bananas

Mix dry ingredients. In blender combine egg, oil, milk, and bananas. Blend on low speed until banana is pureed. Pour into dry ingredients, and stir only until combined. Fill nonstick muffin pans 2/3 full.

Bake: 400° 12 to 14 min   **Yield: 16 muffins**

Per Serving	RCU	FU	Cal	% Ft	P	F	C	Na
	0	0	77	28	2	2	12	149

Gingerbread Muffins

Muffins make a delicious after-school snack! Bake these spicy treats in miniature muffin tins and serve instead of cookies.

1 1/4 cups whole wheat flour	1 tablespoon sugar
1/4 teaspoon salt	1/3 cup chopped nuts (optional)
3/4 teaspoon soda	1 egg
1/2 teaspoon cinnamon	1/4 cup oil
1/2 teaspoon ginger	1/3 cup light molasses
1/8 teaspoon nutmeg	1/2 cup buttermilk

Mix dry ingredients, including nuts. In blender combine egg, oil, molasses, and buttermilk. Blend on low speed until mixed. Pour into dry ingredients, and stir only until combined. Fill nonstick muffin pans 2/3 full.

Bake: 400° 12 to 14 min
8 to 10 min for miniature muffins
Yield: 12 regular muffins or 36 miniature muffins

Per Serving	RCU	FU	Cal	% Ft	P	F	C	Na
	0	0	37	43	1	2	5	47

Golden Cornbread

Here's an old favorite that complements any meal.

1 cup yellow cornmeal	1 cup skim or 1% milk
1 cup whole wheat flour or unbleached white flour	1 egg, slightly beaten
3 tablespoons sugar or honey	2-4 tablespoons oil
1/2 teaspoon salt	2 tablespoons applesauce, optional
4 teaspoons baking powder	

Mix dry ingredients. Add milk, egg, and oil. Mix only until ingredients are combined. Spread batter in a nonstick 9 x 9-inch pan; or fill nonstick muffin pans 2/3 full. Applesauce can be omitted but it keeps cornbread moist.

Bake: 400° oven Cornbread 14 to 16 min.
Muffins 12 to 14 min.
Yield: 12 to 14 muffins

Per Serving	RCU	FU	Cal	% Ft	P	F	C	Na
	0	0	103	23	3	3	17	92

Popovers

These take just minutes to make. They're best if allowed to dry out and get crispy!

1 cup unbleached white or whole wheat flour
1 cup skim milk
2 eggs
1/2 teaspoon salt
1 tablespoon oil

Put all ingredients in blender. Mix on low speed for 30 seconds. Pour into nonstick muffin pans. A few minutes before removing from oven, prick popovers with a fork to allow steam to escape. For crispy popovers, turn off oven and leave popovers in oven with door ajar for 30 minutes. Serve hot.
Bake: 450° 15 min
Reduce heat to 350° and bake 20-25 min more until firm and brown
Yield: 12 popovers

Per Serving	RCU	FU	Cal	% Ft	P	F	C	Na
	1	0	65	33	3	2	8	112

Wheat Bread (Yeast-Free)

This tasty quick bread makes crunchy toast and delicious french toast.

2 cups freshly milled whole wheat flour
1/2 cup unbleached flour
1/2 cup rolled oats (quick preferably)
2 tablespoons brown sugar
1 tablespoon baking powder
1/2 teaspoon salt
1 tablespoon grated orange peel, optional
1/3 to 1/2 cup sunflower seeds
1 egg
1 3/4 cups 1% or skim milk

Combine dry ingredients. Mix egg and milk. Add to dry ingredients and stir just until well moistened. Pour into lightly greased 4" x 8 1/2" loaf pan or 1 1/2 quart casserole.
Bake: 350° 40 to 50 min.   Yield: 1 large loaf   21 slices
Wheat-Free Bread: Use 1 1/2 cups brown rice flour and 1 1/2 cups oat flour in place of the first three ingredients. Omit sunflower seeds if desired. To make oat flour, blend rolled oats until fine.

Per Slice	RCU	FU	Cal	% Ft	P	F	C	Na
	0	0	84	25	4	2	12	132
Wheat-free	0	0	36	16	1	1	6	122

Stir n' Drop Biscuits

These biscuits are a good topping for meat pie or fruit cobbler.

2 cups unbleached white flour   2 tablespoons oil
1 tablespoon baking powder   1 egg, beaten
1/2 teaspoon salt   1 cup 1% or skim milk

Mix dry ingredients. Add oil, egg, and milk. Stir only until ingredients are combined. Drop onto a nonstick baking sheet or on top of a meat pie.
Tip: To use as a cobbler topping, add 1/4 cup sugar.
Bake: 425°   12 to 14 min.   Yield: 18 biscuits

Per Serving	RCU	FU	Cal	% Ft	P	F	C	Na
	1	0	68	28	2	2	10	126

Baking Powder Biscuits

Light and fluffy lowfat biscuits.

1 cup whole wheat flour   1 tablespoon baking powder
1 cup unbleached white flour   2 to 4 tablespoons oil
1/2 teaspoon salt   1 cup 1% or skim milk

Mix dry ingredients (all whole wheat or all white flour may be used.) Add liquid ingredients, and mix just until blended. On a lightly floured countertop, gently knead dough for 30 seconds. Pat or roll dough to 1/2-inch thick. Cut into 2-inch circles using a biscuit cutter, or cut into squares using a pizza cutter.. Place on a nonstick baking sheet.
Bake: 425°   12 to 14 min   Yield: 15 biscuits

Buttermilk Biscuits: Use buttermilk in place of milk. Decrease baking powder to 2 teaspoons and add 1/4 teaspoon soda.

Per Serving	RCU	FU	Cal	% Ft	P	F	C	Na
	0	0	75	27	2	2	12	139

Butter Dips

Julie Dooley shares this delightfully different recipe.
Butter Dips are crunchy on the bottom, tender inside, and wonderful with a hot bowl of chili
soup. They're not as rich as the name implies.

1/4 cup butter or margarine	1 tablespoon baking powder
1 cup whole wheat flour	1/2 teaspoon salt
1 cup unbleached white flour	1 cup skim milk
1 tablespoon sugar	Sesame seeds (optional)

Melt butter or margarine on a baking sheet in oven while oven preheats to 400°.
Remove pan. Mix dry ingredients. Add milk; stir until a soft dough forms. Turn out
dough onto a well-floured countertop. Roll to coat with flour. Gently knead 10 times.
Dough should be quite soft. Roll into an 8-inch square, 1/4-inch thick. Cut in half, and
cut each half into 1 x 4-inch strips. Dip each strip in the melted margarine on the baking
sheet, coating both sides. Arrange strips close together on baking sheet. Sprinkle with
sesame seeds, if desired.

Bake: 425° 12 to 15 min until golden brown   Yield: 16 pieces

Per Serving	RCU	FU	Cal	% Ft	P	F	C	Na
	1	1	82	34	2	3	12	174

Banana Nut Bread

Everyone's favorite nut bread gets even better.

2 cups whole wheat flour	1/2 cup sugar or 1/3 cup honey
1/2 teaspoon salt	1/3 cup oil
2 teaspoons baking powder	2 eggs
1 teaspoon pumpkin pie spice	1 teaspoon vanilla
1 teaspoon cinnamon	3 large ripe bananas
1/2 cup chopped walnuts or pecans	

Mix dry ingredients. In blender combine remaining ingredients. Blend on low speed
until banana is pureed. Add to dry ingredients. Mix only until combined. Pour into
greased and floured loaf pans.

Bake: 350° 40 to 50 min
Yield: 1   4'' x 8 1/2'' loaf or 2   3'' x 5 3/4'' loaves

Per Serving	RCU	FU	Cal	% Ft	P	F	C	Na
	1	1	113	44	2	6	14	91

Apple Bread

Prepare as directed for Banana Nut Bread, substituting 2 medium apples, peeled
and cored, for the bananas. Apples will chop in blender.

Zucchini Bread

You'll like the subtle blend of flavors in this good bread.

1 cup whole wheat flour
1 cup unbleached white flour
1/2 teaspoon salt
1 teaspoon baking powder
1/2 teaspoon soda
2 teaspoons cinnamon

3/4 cup sugar or 1/2 cup honey
2 eggs
1/3 cup oil
1 teaspoon vanilla
1 1/2 cups grated zucchini, drained

Mix dry ingredients. Add liquids and zucchini, and mix just until ingredients are combined. Pour into lightly greased loaf pans.
Bake: 325° 45 to 55 min
Yield: 1   4" x 8 1/2" loaf or 2   3" x 5 3/4" loaves

Per Serving	RCU	FU	Cal	% Ft	P	F	C	Na
	1	1	96	36	2	4	14	101

Applesauce-Banana Bread

This bread is a blue-ribbon winner.

1/3 cup shortening or oil
1/2 cup honey or 3/4 cup sugar
2 eggs
Applesauce
1 medium banana, mashed
1/4 cup sour milk or buttermilk

2 cups whole wheat flour
1/2 teaspoon soda
1/2 teaspoon salt
1 teaspoon baking powder
1/2 cup chopped nuts (optional)
1/2 cup raisins (optional)

Cream shortening, honey or sugar and eggs. Add enough applesauce to mashed banana to measure 1 cup. Combine with the creamed mixture. Add milk, dry ingredients, nuts, and raisins. Mix just until moistened. Pour into lightly greased loaf pans.
Bake: 350° 40 to 50 min
Yield: 1   4" x 8 1/2" loaf or 2   3" x 5 3/4" loaves

Per Serving	RCU	FU	Cal	% Ft	P	F	C	Na
	1	0	93	32	1	3	15	92

Applesauce Bread

Prepare Applesauce-Banana Bread as directed, using 3/4 cup brown sugar in place of the honey or white sugar. Use 1 cup applesauce in place of the mashed banana and applesauce.

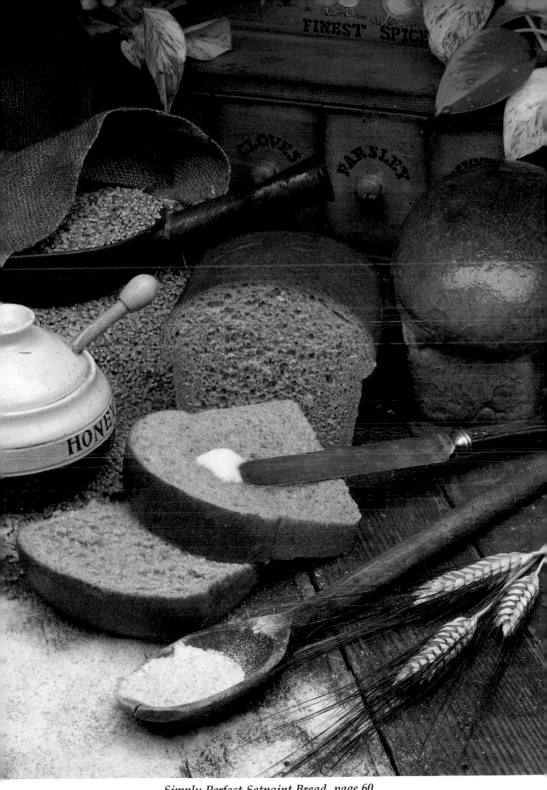

Simply Perfect Setpoint Bread, page 60.

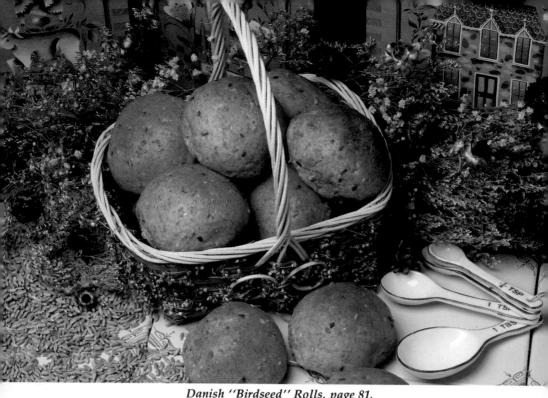

Danish ''Birdseed'' Rolls, page 81.

Assorted Muffins, pages 88 - 92.

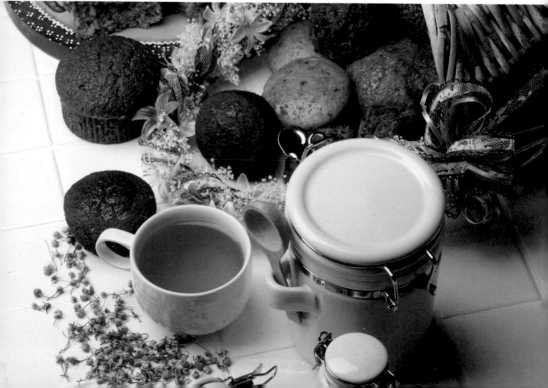

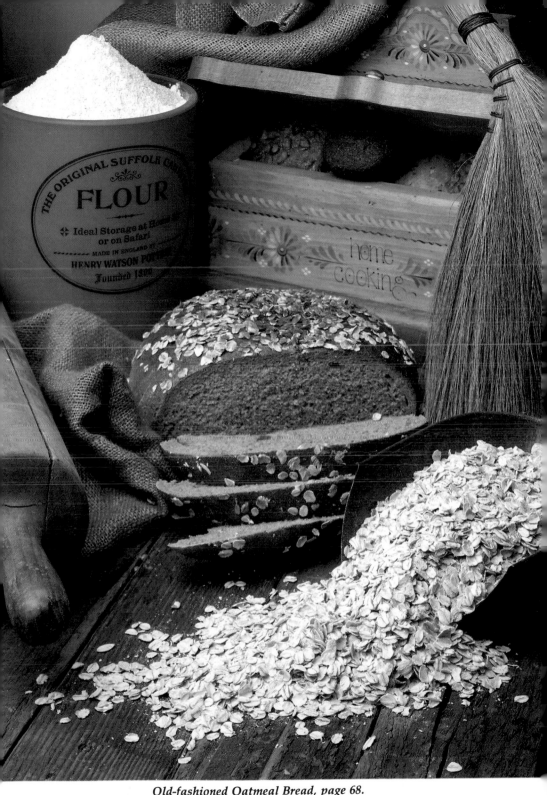

Old-fashioned Oatmeal Bread, page 68.

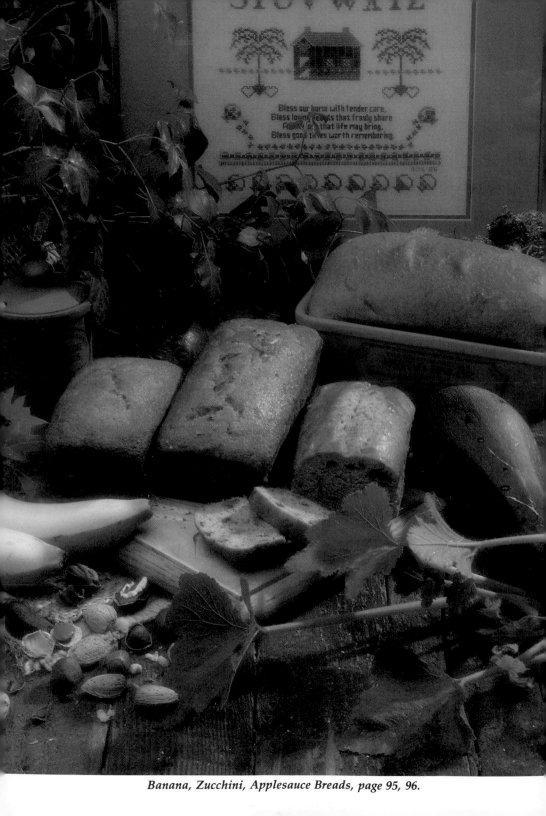

Banana, Zucchini, Applesauce Breads, page 95, 96.

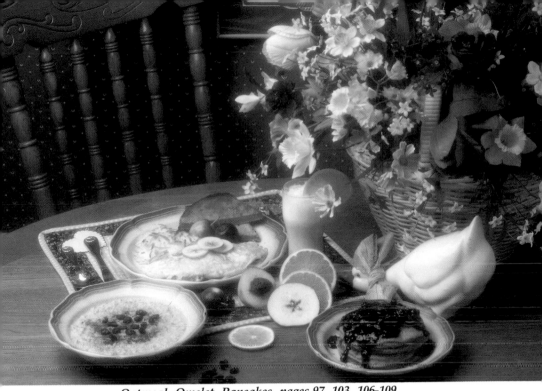

Oatmeal, Omelet, Pancakes, pages 97, 103, 106–109.

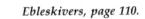

Ebleskivers, page 110.

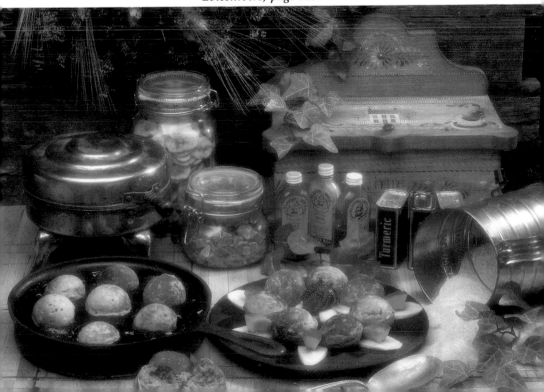

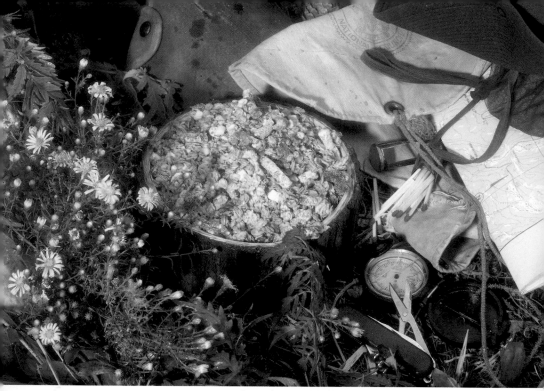

Granola, page 101.

Omelet, Muffins, pages 103, 88-92.

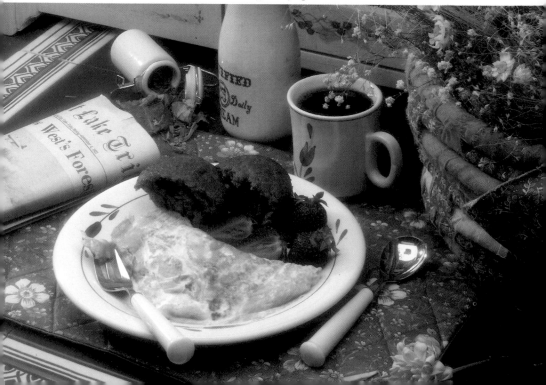

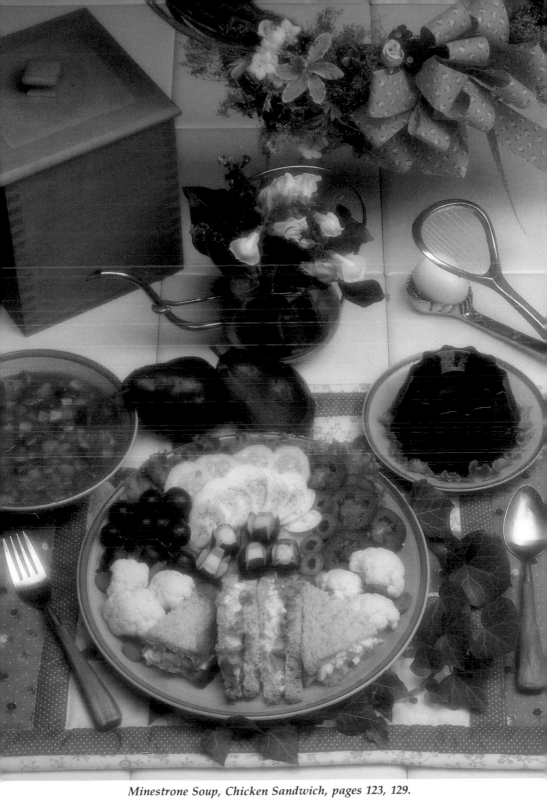

Minestrone Soup, Chicken Sandwich, pages 123, 129.

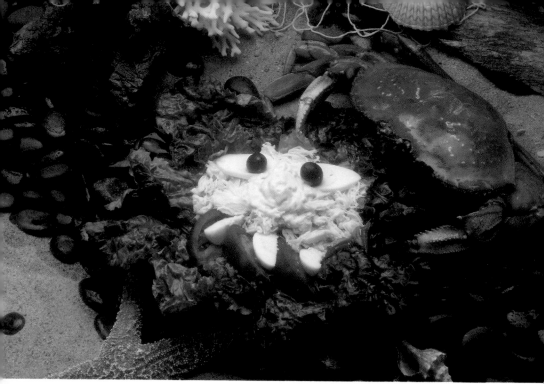

Crab Louis, page 142.

Tostada Party Dip, page 152.

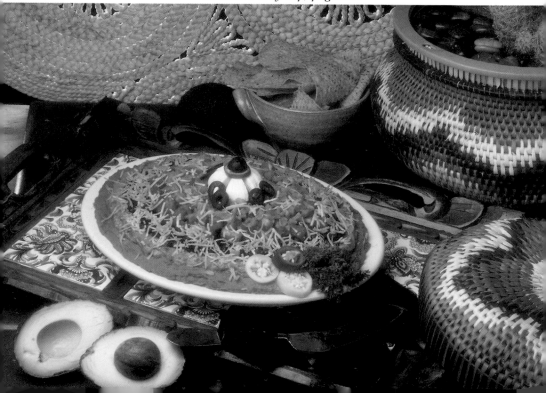

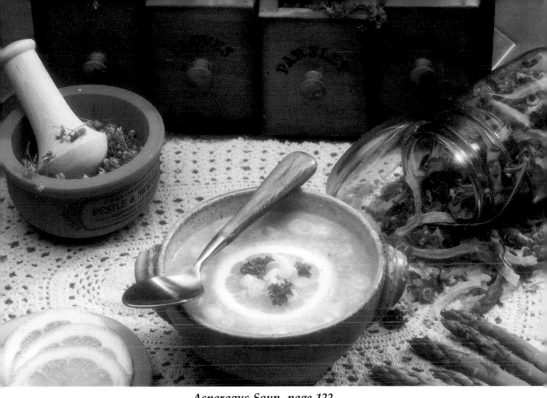

Asparagus Soup, page 122.

Summer Delight Salad, page 133.

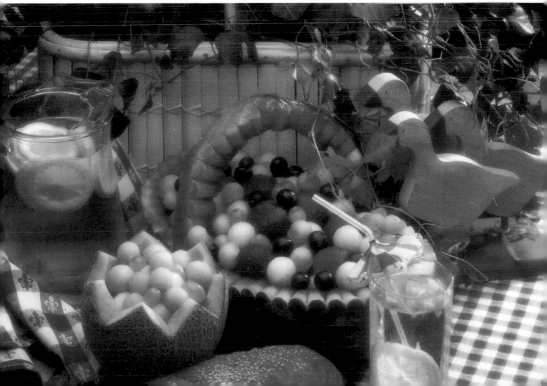

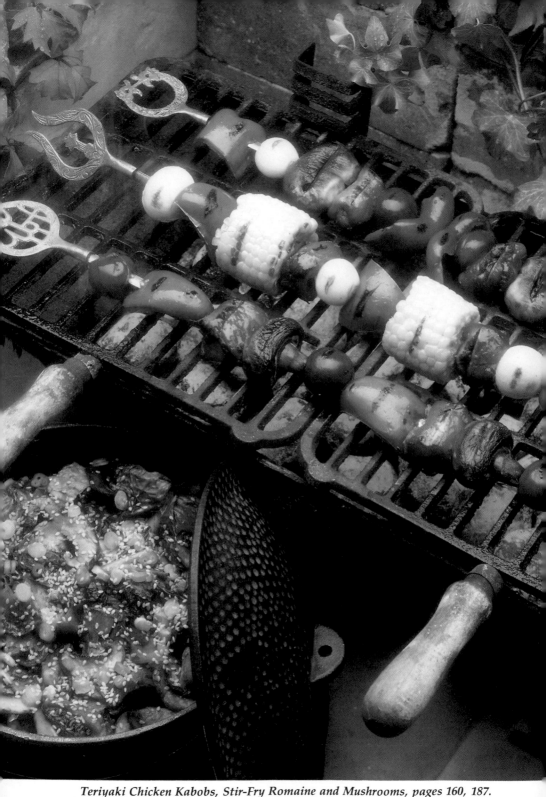

Teriyaki Chicken Kabobs, Stir-Fry Romaine and Mushrooms, pages 160, 187.

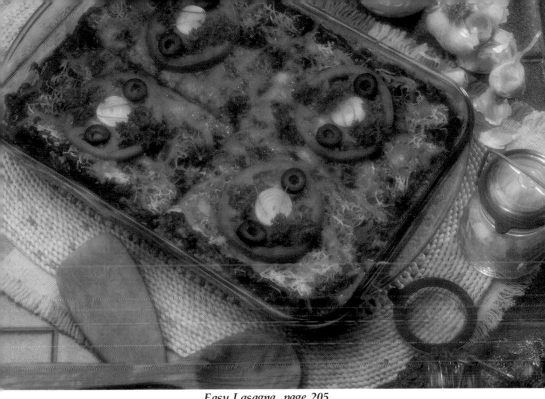

Easy Lasagna, page 205.

Quick Fix Chicken, Baked Potato, pages 157, 221-222.

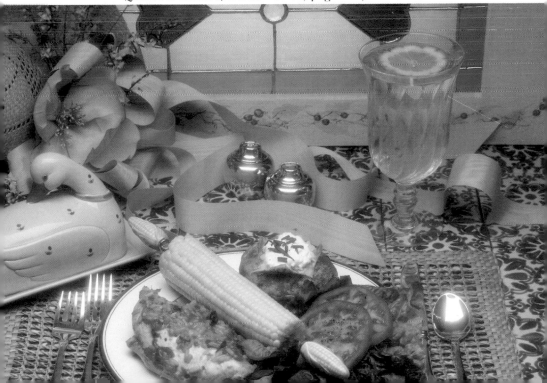

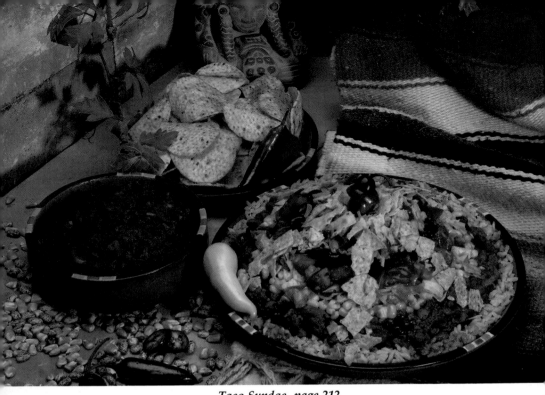

Taco Sundae, page 212.

Oriental Chicken and Shrimp, page 183.

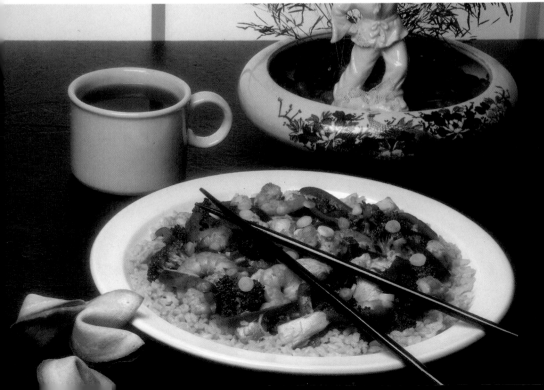

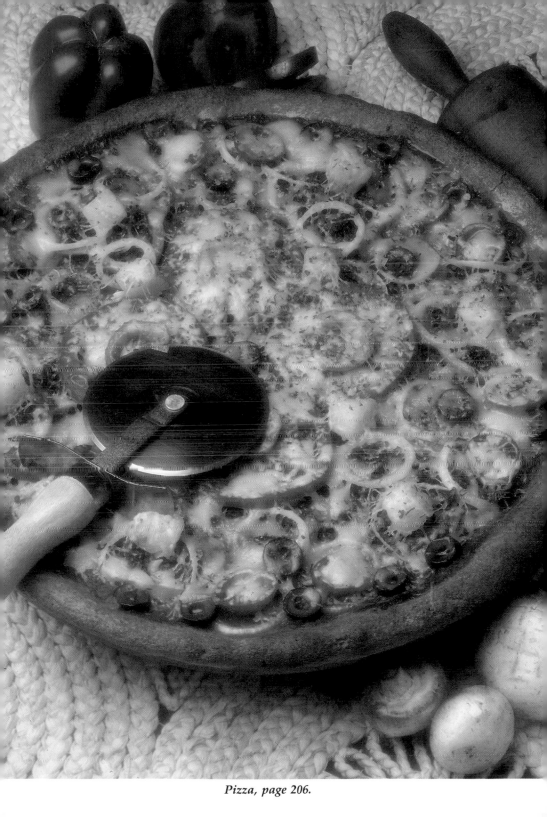

Pizza, page 206.

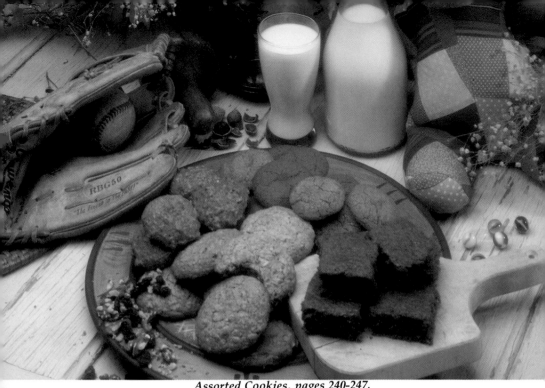

Assorted Cookies, pages 240-247.

Magic Fruit Cobbler, page 264.

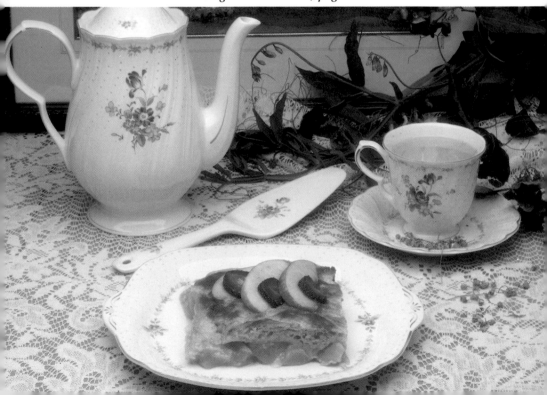

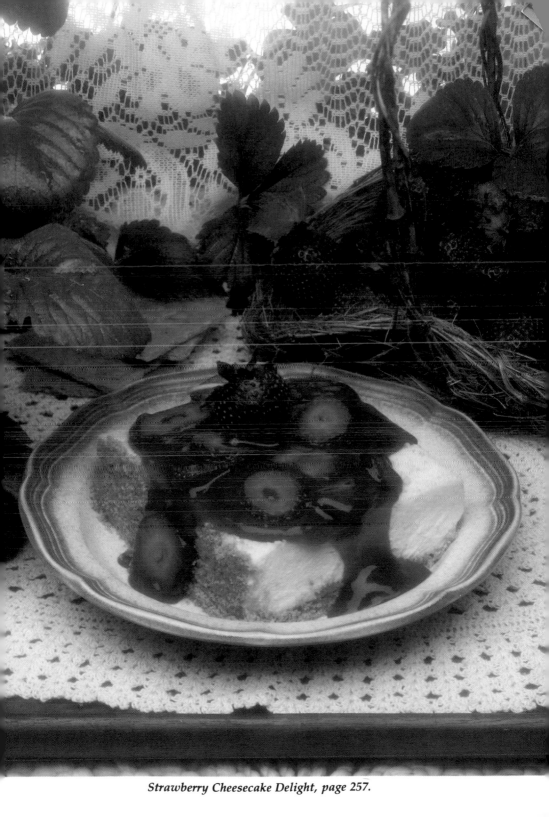

Strawberry Cheesecake Delight, page 257.

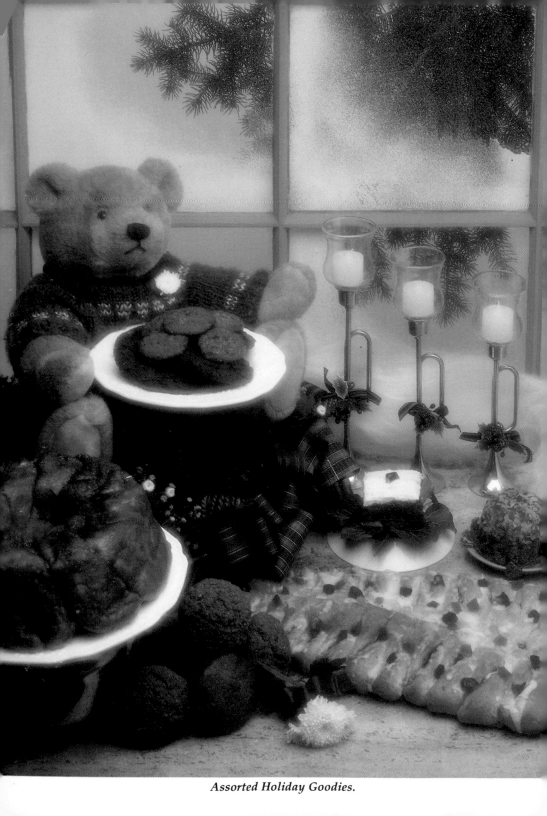

Assorted Holiday Goodies.

CHAPTER 7

What's For Breakfast?

Start The Day Right

Eating a whole-grain breakfast does marvelous things for your health and your weight. It also eliminates the mid-morning slump that gets many people into trouble. Something as simple as whole wheat toast or a dish of oatmeal will make a big difference in your energy level for the day. It will even affect your other food choices. Sweeten your oatmeal with half a banana or a few raisins and add a little cinnamon if desired. Top it with 1% or skim milk, and you'll feel satisfied and energetic all morning without needing a high-calorie snack.

True, whole grains may not be your favorite meal. They haven't always been mine but now I eat them often because they help me feel terrific for the rest of the day. In addition to oatmeal, try cracked wheat, millet, and brown rice. We've also listed some cold cereals which are convenient when you're in a hurry. However, they don't stay with you quite as long as the cooked cereals do.

Habits and food preferences are learned. Make a conscientious effort to eat a wholesome breakfast every day. Your tastes will change. Most importantly, so will your health and your weight!

HOT CEREALS

Oatmeal

A steamy bowl of oatmeal in the morning will keep you satisfied until lunch.

2 cups water
1/4 to 1/2 teaspoon salt

1 cup old-fashioned oats
1/4 teaspoon cinnamon (optional)

Stir oats and cinnamon into salted water. Simmer for 5 minutes. Remove from heat, cover, and let sit 5 minutes.

Cook: 5 min   Yield: 4   1/2-cup servings

Per Serving	RCU	FU	Cal	% Ft	P	F	C	Na
	0	0	38	2	1	1	6	118

Microwave Oatmeal

This can be cooking while you shower.

3/4 cup water
1/8 teaspoon salt
1/2 cup old-fashioned oats

Combine ingredients in 2-cup cereal bowl. Microwave at 50% power 5 to 6 minutes or until thickened or microwave on high for 2 1/2 to 3 minutes or until thickened. Stir before serving.
Cooking Time: 5 min   Yield: 1 serving
Microwave: 2 1/2 min

Millet Cereal

Millet is high in calcium and makes a healthy breakfast.

2 cups water
1/4 teaspoon salt
1/2 cup millet

Bring water and salt to a boil. Add millet. Reduce heat to low, cover, and steam 25 to 30 minutes. Do not raise lid during cooking. Serve with milk.
Cook: 25-30 min Yield: 4   1/2-cup servings

Note: For a fluffier cereal, soak millet overnight and cook in the morning. Cooking time will be reduced to 20 minutes.

Cracked Wheat Cereal

Here's a chewy cereal with a nut-like flavor.

1/2 cup whole wheat
2 cups water
1/4 teaspoon salt

Crack wheat in blender on high speed for 35 to 40 seconds. Bring water and salt to a boil. Using a wire whisk to avoid lumps, gradually stir in cracked wheat. Bring to a boil, stirring constantly. Reduce heat to low. Cover and simmer 15 to 20 minutes, stirring occasionally.

Microwave: Reduce water by 1/2 cup. Put in covered dish and cook on 50^6 power for 25 to 30 minutes. Requires no watching.

Cook: 15-20 min   Yield: 4   1/2-cup servings
Microwave: 25 to 30 min

Per Serving	RCU	FU	Cal	% Ft	P	F	C	Na
	0	0	53	8	2	0	11	119

Four-Grain Cereal

Combine 1 cup each of wheat, rye, brown rice, and millet. Crack 1/2 cup in blender, and prepare as directed for cracked wheat cereal. Store remaining cereal mix in an airtight container.

Whole Wheat Cereal

Plan on lots of chewing time for this good dish. Use leftovers in soups and casseroles.

2 cups boiling water
1/4 to 1/2 teaspoon salt
1 cup whole wheat

Thermos method: Place wheat in a 1- or 2-quart vacuum bottle. Add salt and boiling water. Screw on lid. Let sit overnight, 10 to 12 hours. The wheat will swell into plump, chewy kernels. Reheat just before serving; the microwave works well. Cover unused portion and store in refrigerator.

Conventional method: Bring water and salt to a boil in a small saucepan. Stir in whole wheat. Reduce heat to simmer. Cover and cook 45 to 60 minutes or until wheat kernels are tender and chewy.

Cook: 45-60 min   Yield: 6   1/2-cup servings

Per Serving	RCU	FU	Cal	% Ft	P	F	C	Na
	0	0	106	6	4	1	23	119

Brown Rice Cereal

Try making this cereal with milk; it tastes like rice pudding.

2 1/2 cups water or skim milk
1 cup brown rice
1/4 teaspoon salt
1 teaspoon cinnamon
1/2 teaspoon allspice
1/4 teaspoon nutmeg
1/4 cup raisins (optional)

Bring water or milk to a boil. Stir in brown rice. Reduce heat. Cover and simmer 45 minutes. Do not remove the lid during cooking or rice will be gummy. Stir in spices and raisins just before serving. Note: To shorten cooking time, soak rice in water at least 1 hour or overnight before cooking.

Cook: 45 min   Yield: 4   3/4-cup servings

Per Serving	RCU	FU	Cal	% Ft	P	F	C	Na
	0	0	206	4	4	1	40	126

Rice 'n Apple Breakfast

"Mmmmm, good!" is the best way to describe this cereal.

1/2 cup apple juice
2 cups cooked brown rice
1 tablespoon honey, optional
2 tablespoons raisins
1/2 teaspoon cinnamon
1 to 2 medium apples, peeled, quartered and thinly sliced

Combine all ingredients in a medium saucepan. Cover. Simmer 8 to 10 minutes over low heat.

Microwave: Use a microwave-safe bowl. Cover and cook on High for 4 to 5 minutes. Serve plain or with milk.

Cook: Stove: 8-10 min   Yield: 4   1/2-cup servings
Microwave: 4-6 min

Per Serving	RCU	FU	Cal	% Ft	P	F	C	Na
	0	0	160	3	2	1	34	5

COLD CEREALS

Favorite Granola

Take this high-energy mix on your next camping trip.

4 cups old-fashioned oats
2 cups rolled wheat
1 cup unprocessed oat or wheat bran
1 cup whole wheat flour
1/2 cup nonfat dry milk
1/2 teaspoon salt
1/2 to 1 cup raw sunflower seeds
1 to 2 cups slivered almonds
1 12-ounce can frozen apple juice concentrate, thawed
1 teaspoon vanilla
1 cup chopped dates
1 cup chopped dried apples or pineapple

[handwritten: ½ cup oil / 1 cup water / 3/4 cup brown sugar / vanilla ↓]

Mix the dry ingredients in a large bowl. Mix apple juice concentrate and vanilla. Pour over dry ingredients and stir until well mixed. Spread mixture on a large baking sheet. Bake in a 200° oven for 1 to 1 1/2 hours or until golden and almost dry. For chunky granola, do not stir during baking. Break into bite-size pieces and add dried fruit. Store in an airtight container. Serve as a cold cereal.
Bake: 200° 1 1/2 hours   **Yield: 12 cups   36   1/3 cup servings**

#2 Granola

High energy requirements? A low Setpoint? This cereal's for you.

Prepare Favorite Granola, making these changes: Omit apple juice concentrate and mix 1/2 cup oil, 1 cup water, 3/4 cup brown sugar and vanilla in blender. Mix on low and pour over dry ingredients. Mix well and bake as directed above.

Per Serving	RCU	FU	Cal	% Ft	P	F	C	Na
	0	0	134	22	4	3	22	38
#2	0	1	149	32	4	5	22	39

High Fiber Bran Mix

Try this quick, stick-to-your-ribs cereal. It's excellent for improving sluggish elimination. Blend it slightly and it makes a good breading for oven-fried chicken and other meats.

1 18-ounce box All-Bran, Bran Buds or 100% Bran cereal
1 16-ounce box 40% Bran Flakes
2 cups unprocessed wheat bran or oat bran

Mix all ingredients in a large bowl. Return to empty cereal boxes for storage. Serve cold with milk.
Yield: 60   1/3 cup servings

Per Serving	RCU	FU	Cal	% Ft	P	F	C	Na
	0	0	56	4	3	0	14	132

EGGS

With a little imagination, eggs can be served a dozen different ways. Make your own egg muffin or create a prize-winning omelet.

Poached-Fried Eggs

4 eggs
Dash of salt
Lemon pepper

Break eggs into a nonstick frying pan. Season with salt and lemon pepper. Cook over medium heat until whites are set. Add 2 tablespoons hot water. Place lid on pan, and cook 2 to 3 minutes until yolks are cooked to desired firmness. Watch closely.
Cook: 2-3 min   Yield: 4 servings

Per Serving	RCU	FU	Cal	% Ft	P	F	C	Na
	0	1	80	68	6	6	0	133

Perfect Stuffed Omelets

Reid and Beverly Merrill furnish these simple instructions for a perfect omelet. Let each person fill a small cup with their choice of fillings and you can feed a crowd in minutes.

2 eggs
2 tablespoons water
1 teaspoon butter or margarine
Omelet Fillings (see below)

Mix eggs and water with fork, wire whisk, or blender. Heat an omelet pan or 10-inch nonstick skillet over medium-high heat until a drop of water sizzles in the pan. Add butter. Pour in egg mixture (about 1/2 cup) and cook quickly, pushing cooked portion toward center with a pancake turner, and tilting pan to allow uncooked egg to flow to edges. While top is still moist and shiny, place 1/3 to 1/2 cup of desired fillings on left half of omelet. Using a pancake turner, fold the right half onto the filling and turn onto a platter with a quick flip of the wrist.

Cooking Time: 1-2 min   Yield: 1 omelet

Omelet Fillings

Precooked fillings:
Potatoes, diced or shredded
Asparagus or creamed asparagus
Broccoli
Peas and carrots
Mushrooms
Chicken, diced
Tuna or salmon, drained and flaked
Cottage cheese, low-fat
Refried beans

Raw vegetables:
Green onions, diced
Green peppers, chopped
Tomatoes, diced

Top with Salsa* if desired

Per Serving	RCU	FU	Cal	% Ft	P	F	C	Na
	0	2	327	44	17	16	31	198

Framed Eggs

Here's a fun change the kids will love.

2 eggs
2 slices whole wheat bread

Cut a circle in the center of each slice of bread. Wipe inside of nonstick skillet with stick of margarine. Place bread in skillet over low heat. Drop an egg into the center of each slice. Cook slowly until egg is set and underside of bread is brown. Turn and brown the other side. Season to taste. Toast bread cutouts and serve on the side.
Cook: 3 to 5 min   Yield: 2 servings

Per Serving	RCU	FU	Cal	% Ft	P	F	C	Na
	0	1	151	42	8	7	13	147

Egg Souffle Breakfast Casserole

Serve this for breakfast to overnight guests. It will be a hit!
Prepare the day before & microwave or bake just before serving!

1/4 cup diced green pepper
6 green onions, diced
4 slices whole wheat bread
1 2-1/2-ounce package thinly sliced lean ham, diced
2 potatoes, cooked, peeled, and diced
2 cups 1% or skim milk
6 eggs
1/2 teaspoon salt
1 teaspoon dry mustard
1 4-ounce can mushrooms, drained
1/4 cup Parmesan cheese

Microwave green pepper and onions in 1 teaspoon water until tender. While vegetables are cooking, cube bread and spread in the bottom of a 9 x 13-inch baking dish. Spread ham and potatoes evenly over bread. Combine milk, eggs, salt and dry mustard in blender. Blend on high speed until mixed and pour over bread, ham, and potatoes. Top with green pepper, onions, and mushrooms. Sprinkle with Parmesan cheese. Microwave or bake until eggs are just set.
Microwave: High   10 to 12 min.
Bake: 30 to 40 min   Yield: 12 servings

Per Serving	RCU	FU	Cal	% Ft	P	F	C	Na
	0	1	120	40	7	5	11	195

POTATOES

Fresh Potato Hash Browns

Hash browns prepared this Setpoint way are crunchy outside, tender inside.

4 potatoes, peeled if desired
1 teaspoon oil
Salt and pepper
2 tablespoons water

Grate raw potatoes with a grater or the large shredding blade on food processor. Heat oil in a frying pan until quite hot. Add potato shreds. Season to taste with salt and pepper. Turn heat to low and cover pan. *Do not stir.* Cook 5 to 8 minutes. Using a pancake turner, turn the whole pile of potatoes at once. Add water, season again, and replace lid. Continue cooking another 5 to 8 minutes. Potatoes should be crunchy and golden on the outside, tender on the inside.

Cook: 10-16 min   Yield: 4 servings

Per Serving	RCU	FU	Cal	% Ft	P	F	C	Na
	0	0	67	11	2	1	14	81

Cooked Potato Hash Browns

4 potatoes, baked or boiled
Salt and pepper

Remove skin from precooked potatoes, if desired. Shred potatoes with a grater or the large shredding blade on food processor. Wipe bottom of warmed nonstick fry pan lightly with a stick of butter or margarine. Add potatoes. Season to taste with salt and pepper or other seasonings. Add a tablespoon of water if potatoes are dry. Fry 3 minutes on each side, turning with a pancake turner.

Cook: 6 min   Yield: 4 servings

Per Serving	RCU	FU	Cal	% Ft	P	F	C	Na
	0	0	90	0	3	0	21	122

PANCAKES AND WAFFLES

Favorite Pancakes or Waffles

1 cup whole wheat flour
2 teaspoons baking powder
1/4 teaspoon salt
1 beaten egg
1 tablespoon honey or sugar
1 tablespoon oil
1 cup skim milk

Mix dry ingredients. Add egg, honey, oil, and milk, stirring just until flour is moistened. Batter will be slightly lumpy. For lighter pancakes or waffles, separate eggs, beat whites until stiff, and fold into batter the last minute. Bake immediately on a hot 375° griddle, turning once, or in a hot waffle iron.

Cook: 3-4 min   Yield: 12   2" pancakes

Buckwheat Pancakes

Prepare Favorite Pancakes as directed, substituting 1/2 cup buckwheat flour for 1/2 cup whole wheat flour.

Blueberry Pancakes

When underside of pancakes are browned, sprinkle with drained blueberries. Turn and cook the other side.

Per Serving	RCU	FU	Cal	% Ft	P	F	C	Na
	0	0	61	30	2	2	9	117

Oatmeal Pancakes

Good and good for you. Kids love 'em.

1 cup whole wheat flour
1 cup quick rolled oats
1 tablespoon brown sugar
1 teaspoon soda
1/2 teaspoon salt
2 eggs, slightly beaten
1 tablespoon oil
2 cups buttermilk

Combine dry ingredients. Add eggs, oil, and buttermilk; stir just until mixed. Spread 3 tablespoons batter on hot griddle.

Yield: 36   2" pancakes

Per Serving	RCU	FU	Cal	% Ft	P	F	C	Na
	0	0	28	28	1	1	4	70

Blender Pancakes

They're quick, easy, and have a great nutty taste.

1 1/4 cups water	2 tablespoons margarine or oil
1 cup whole wheat kernels	1 tablespoon honey or sugar
1/4 cup nonfat dry milk (optional)	1/4-1/2 teaspoon salt
1 egg	1 tablespoon fresh baking powder

In blender, mix water, wheat kernels, and dry milk on high for 3 minutes. Add egg, margarine, honey, and salt. Blend for 20 seconds. Add baking powder. Pulse three times, just enough to mix. Mixture should foam up and get very light. Cook immediately on a hot nonstick griddle.

Cook: 3-4 min   **Yield: 16   2" pancakes**

Tip: Skim milk may be used instead of the water and nonfat dry milk. Batter also makes delicious waffles.

Fruit-Filled Pancakes

Prepare Blender Pancakes as directed. Pour onto hot griddle and top with blueberries, sliced bananas, or other fruit.

Per Serving	RCU	FU	Cal	% Ft	P	F	C	Na
	0	0	64	33	2	2	9	87

Buttermilk Blender Pancakes

You just can't beat the sweet nutty flavor of freshly ground whole wheat, and your blender does it all!

1 1/2 cups buttermilk	1/4 teaspoon salt
1 cup whole wheat	1 tablespoon brown sugar
2 heaping tablespoons cornmeal	1 tablespoon baking powder
2 tablespoons margarine	1/4 teaspoon soda
1 egg	

In blender mix buttermilk and wheat kernels on high for 3 minutes. Add cornmeal, margarine, egg, salt, and brown sugar. Blend for 10 seconds. Add baking powder and soda. Pulse three times and let mix foam up and get light. Cook at once on a hot 375° nonstick griddle. Turn once. (If cornmeal is not readily available, omit it and use a rounded cup of wheat kernels.)

Cook: 3-4 min   **Yield: 18-20   2" pancakes**

Per Serving	RCU	FU	Cal	% Ft	P	F	C	Na
	0	0	53	30	1	2	8	89

Buttermilk Pancakes or Waffles

These family favorites melt in your mouth!

2 cups whole wheat flour
1 teaspoon baking powder
1 teaspoon soda
1/2 teaspoon salt
2 tablespoons sugar or honey
2 eggs
2 tablespoons oil
2 cups buttermilk

Mix dry ingredients. In blender combine sugar, eggs, oil, and buttermilk. Add liquid to dry ingredients, stirring just until mixed. Bake on a hot 375° griddle, turning once.
Cook: 3-4 min   Yield: 24   2'' pancakes

Apple Buttermilk Pancakes

Prepare Buttermilk Pancakes as directed. Fold in 1 cup finely grated apple.

Per Serving	RCU	FU	Cal	% Ft	P	F	C	Na
	0	0	57	29	2	2	8	86

Pancake Master Mix

Make up the mix and store it—or feed a crowd!

10 cups whole wheat flour
2 cups unbleached white flour (use all whole wheat flour if desired)
1/2 cup baking powder, rounded (10 tablespoons)
4 teaspoons salt
3/4 cup sugar
4 cups nonfat dry milk

Combine all ingredients and mix well. Store in a covered container in cool dry place. Use as directed in Master Mix Pancakes on page 109.
Yield: 275   3'' pancakes

Per Serving	RCU	FU	Cal	% Ft	P	F	C	Na
	0	0	26	4	1	0	4	73

Five-Grain Pancake Master Mix

Try LaVerne Larson's delicious pancake mix.

6 cups wheat
1 cup barley
1 cup rye
1 cup oat groats
1 cup brown rice

4 cups nonfat dry milk
1/4 cup sugar
4 teaspoons salt
1 cup baking powder

Mix dry grains together. Mill into flour. Add remaining ingredients and mix well. Place in covered storage container and freeze until needed. Use as directed below.
Yield: 350   3-inch pancakes

Per Serving	RCU	FU	Cal	% Ft	P	F	C	Na
	0	0	24	5	1	0	4	83

Master Mix Pancakes

Nutritious homemade pancakes are so easy to make this way.

1 cup Pancake Master Mix (either recipe)
1 tablespoon oil
1 egg, slightly beaten
1/2 to 3/4 cup water

Mix just until ingredients are combined, adding water to desired consistency. Bake on a 375° nonstick griddle, turning once.
Cook: 3-4 min   Yield: 15   3'' pancakes

Per Serving	RCU	FU	Cal	% Ft	P	F	C	Na
	0	0	39	32	2	1	5	77

Danish Ebleskivers

Serve ebleskivers for a fun weekend breakfast.

3 eggs, separated	1 teaspoon soda
2 cups buttermilk	1/2 teaspoon salt
2 cups whole wheat flour	2 tablespoons sugar or honey
1 teaspoon baking powder	

Mix egg yolks and buttermilk. Stir in dry ingredients. Whip egg whites until stiff but not dry. Fold egg whites into batter. Preheat ebleskiver pan over medium-low heat. Place 2 drops cooking oil in each cup. Fill cups 3/4 full of batter. Cook over medium-low heat until bubbly; turn carefully with a hat pin or toothpick and cook the other side. Serve with low-calorie syrup, fruit topping, or jam.

Cook: 3-4 min   **Yield: 40 Ebleskivers**

Per Serving	RCU	FU	Cal	% Ft	P	F	C	Na
	0	0	36	21	2	1	6	68

Apple Ebleskivers

Prepare Danish Ebleskivers as directed. Heat pan and fill cups 1/2 full. Add a teaspoon of applesauce or diced apples to each cup. Cover applesauce with batter to 3/4 full. Avoid spilling applesauce in cups, or Ebleskivers will stick. Cook as directed.

French Toast

1 egg
1/2 cup skim milk
Pinch of salt
6 slices whole wheat bread

Mix egg, milk, and salt with a wire whisk until frothy, or blend on low speed for 5 seconds. Transfer egg mixture to pie tin or other shallow pan. Quickly dip bread slices, one at a time, into the egg and milk mixture. Cook on a nonstick griddle until golden brown. Turn and cook the other side. Serve with a fruit topping if desired. French toast may be baked in a waffle iron.

Cook: 3-4 min   **Yield: 6 servings**

Per Serving	RCU	FU	Cal	% Ft	P	F	C	Na
	0	0	104	24	5	3	15	112

SYRUPS

Fruit Syrup

You determine the flavor by using different juice concentrates.

1/2 cup water
2 tablespoons cornstarch
1 12-ounce can frozen unsweetened fruit juice concentrate

Using a wire whisk, stir cornstarch into water in medium pan. Add juice concentrate. Bring to a boil and stir until thickened, 1 to 2 minutes.

Cook: 1-2 min   Yield: 2 cups   2 tablespoon servings

Per Serving	RCU	FU	Cal	% Ft	P	F	C	Na
	0	0	49	2	1	0	12	1

Spicy Apple Syrup

A tasty low-sugar syrup.

1 cup unsweetened apple juice
1 tablespoon cornstarch
1 teaspoon cinnamon
1/2 teaspoon allspice
1-2 tablespoons honey, optional

Using a wire whisk, stir cornstarch and spices into cold juice. Bring to a boil. Stir until thickened, 1 to 2 minutes.

Note: Any fruit juice may be substituted for the apple juice. Omit spices.

Cook: 1-2 min   Yield: 1 cup   2 tablespoon servings

Per Serving	RCU	FU	Cal	% Ft	P	F	C	Na
	0	0	26	4	0	0	7	0

Maple Syrup

It's easy and economical to make your own maple syrup.

1 cup sugar or honey
1 tablespoon cornstarch
1 1/2-2 cups water
1 teaspoon Mapleine flavoring (Crescent brand)

Mix sugar and cornstarch in a small pan and then stir in water. If using honey, mix cornstarch in a small amount of the water before adding honey and remaining water. Cook and stir over medium heat until mixture comes to a boil and is slightly thickened. Stir in maple flavoring. Serve hot.
Cook: 3-4 min   Yield: 2-3 cups   1 tablespoon servings

Plum, Grape or Berry Syrup

Use unsweetened fruit juice in place of water and omit flavoring.

Per Serving	RCU	FU	Cal	% Ft	P	F	C	Na
	1	0	24	1	0	0	6	0

TOPPINGS

Applicious Topper

You'll love this eat-all-you-want topping! Use fresh apples for a delicious fresh applesauce.

1 cup applesauce or 2 apples, peeled and quartered
1 ripe banana
1/2 teaspoon cinnamon
1/4 teaspoon allspice
apple juice or water

Place all ingredients in blender. Blend until smooth. Thin to desired consistency with apple juice. Warm before serving.
Yield: 3 cups   1/4 cup servings

Per Serving	RCU	FU	Cal	% Ft	P	F	C	Na
	0	0	26	2	0	0	6	1

Fruit Topping

1 cup pureed fresh or frozen fruit
 (apples, blueberries, raspberries,
 strawberries, strawberry-banana)

1/2 cup unsweetened apple juice
1 tablespoon cornstarch
1-2 tablespoons honey or sugar (optional)

Bring fruit, juice, and cornstarch to a boil in a small saucepan. Cook just until thick.
Cook: 3-4 min   **Yield: 1 1/2 cups**   **2 tablespoon servings**

Per Serving	RCU	FU	Cal	% Ft	P	F	C	Na
	0	0	17	9	0	0	4	0

Blueberry Sauce

1 1/2 cups fresh or frozen blueberries or any other fruit
3 tablespoons apple juice concentrate, sugar or honey
1/2 cup orange juice
1 tablespoon cornstarch
few grains salt

Combine berries, sugar, or honey and 1/4 cup orange juice in saucepan. Bring to a boil. Mix remaining juice with cornstarch. Stir into berries and cook until slightly thickened. Serve warm.
Cook: 3-4 min   **Yield: 2 cups**   **2 tablespoon servings**

Per Serving	RCU	FU	Cal	% Ft	P	F	C	Na
	0	0	16	3	0	0	4	0

Fresh Peach Topping

Mmmmm...juicy fresh peaches

6 large peaches, peeled
1/8 teaspoon almond extract

Puree peaches in blender. Blend in almond extract. Serve at room temperature or slightly heated.
Yield: 2 cups   **2 tablespoon servings**
Tip: One 16-ounce can of light peaches may be substituted for the fresh peaches. Drain off most of the syrup, puree, and add almond extract.

Per Serving	RCU	FU	Cal	% Ft	P	F	C	Na
	0	0	14	0	0	0	4	0

Tutti Frutti Topping

Apricots and pineapple are a pleasing combination.

1 cup canned apricots, drained and coarsely mashed or pureed
1/2 cup unsweetened crushed pineapple, undrained

Bring fruit to a boil in a small saucepan. Cook to desired thickness or just warm and serve.
Cook: 3-5 min   Yield: 1 1/2 cups   2 tablespoon servings

Fresh Fruit Tutti-Frutti
Puree 1 1/2 cups fresh, unpeeled apricots, strawberries or other fruit. Mix with the pineapple. Serve fresh or cook to desired thickness, and serve hot or cold.

Per Serving	RCU	FU	Cal	% Ft	P	F	C	Na
	0	0	16	0	0	0	4	0

Waffle & Pancake Topping

Use this delicious topping in place of traditional whipped cream and fruit.

1/2 cup nonfat vanilla yogurt
1/2 cup "lite" fruit jam or fresh fruit

Mix lightly and serve!

Yield: 1 cup   16 1 tablespoon servings

Honey Butter

Making good fluffy honey butter is almost a lost art.

1 cube butter or margarine, softened
1/2 cup honey
1 teaspoon vanilla (optional)

Whip butter until light and fluffy. *Slowly* add the honey and vanilla. Adding the honey too rapidly makes the butter lose its thick, fluffy consistency. Whip 2 to 3 minutes longer. Cover and refrigerate. Stores well.
Yield: 1 1/2 cups   1 teaspoon servings

Per Serving	RCU	FU	Cal	% Ft	P	F	C	Na
	0	0	18	60	0	1	2	15

CHAPTER 8

Lean Lunches

Whether your family takes brown baggers or eats lunch at home, we have something new for you. A crunchy Bible sandwich topped with sprouts is a tasty summer treat. On a frosty winter day, a steaming bowl of clam chowder is sure to warm chilled bones. For the teen on the run, pack a pita bread full of taco meat, lettuce, tomatoes, and salsa. This chapter gives dozens of suggestions for soups, salads, and sandwiches. Whichever you choose, it's sure to be a winner. The recipes marked with an asterisk* are included in this book.

SOUPS

Dry Soup Mix

Mix these together and add a cup to any soup or stew.

2 cups raw pearled barley
2 cups lentils
2 cups brown rice
2 cups vegetable macaroni (spinach, tomato, etc.)
1 to 2 cups split peas
2 cups instant minced onion

Mix all ingredients. Store in large, covered container in cool place. Add to any soup or stew. Simmer approximately 1 hour or until lentils are tender.
Yield: 11-12 cups

Per Serving	RCU	FU	Cal	% Ft	P	F	C	Na
	0	0	487	3	19	2	101	21

Slim Cream Soup Mix

Here's a lowfat, low-cost recipe for creamed condensed soup. It contains almost no fat and is lower in sodium. It's so convenient to use and adds a rich, creamy flavor to any cream soup or casserole. Keep the mix on hand for convenience.

2 cups instant nonfat dry milk
1 cup cornstarch
3 tablespoons low-sodium instant chicken boullion granules
2 tablespoons dried minced onion
1/2 teaspoon thyme leaves, crushed (optional)
1/4 teaspoon pepper

Mix together and store in an airtight container.
Yield: 3 1/2 cups

Slim Cream Soup

To reconstitute the mix to equal one can of condensed cream soup:

1/3 cup dry Slim Cream Soup Mix (see above)
1 1/4 cups water or skim milk

Combine soup mix and water or milk in small pan. Bring to a boil, and stir until thick. For a casserole or cream soup: Combine soup mix and water or milk. Add to casserole or soup, it will thicken as it cooks.
Yield: 1 1/4 cups   Equals 1 10 3/4-ounce can condensed soup

Per Serving	RCU	FU	Cal	% Ft	P	F	C	Na
1 1/4 cups	0	0	158	0	12	0	23	623

Variations:
Cream of Mushroom Soup Add 1 4-ounce can mushrooms, drained.
Cream of Vegetable Soup Add 1/2 cup diced cooked vegetables.
Cream of Chicken Soup Add 1/2 cup cooked and diced chicken.

Dry Onion Soup Mix

Here's the equivalent of one package of dry onion soup mix.

1 tablespoon instant beef bouillon granules
2 tablespoons instant minced onion
1/2 teaspoon onion powder

Mix all ingredients in a small bowl. Store in an airtight container.
Yield: 3 tablespoons

Per Recipe	RCU	FU	Cal	% Ft	P	F	C	Na
	0	0	95	0	4	0	20	1222

Cooked Chicken or Turkey and Broth

Buy poultry on sale. Cook...then freeze meat and broth for later use.

3 pounds chicken pieces or turkey hindquarters, skinned
8-10 cups water
3 carrots
2 stalks celery
1 onion, quartered

Place all ingredients in a large 5-quart pan. Simmer on low heat until meat is tender, about 1 hour. For best flavor, let meat cool slightly in broth. Remove meat from bones and refrigerate or place in 2-cup packages and freeze. Strain vegetables out of broth.

Pour the hot broth into a specially designed fat-skimmer cup. The fat rises to the top and you can pour off the fat-free broth immediately through the spout that attaches at the bottom. Or refrigerate broth until fat hardens on the top. Spoon off fat and discard. Freeze broth for later use in soups, gravy, etc.

Cook: 1 hour   **Yield: 8 cups**

Baked Onion Soup

Everyone raves about this simple-to-make soup.

3 medium onions, sliced in thin rings
2 teaspoons oil
2 to 4 tablespoons soy sauce

1 quart Chicken or Turkey Broth*
4 slices whole wheat bread
1 tablespoon Parmesan or cheddar cheese

In a large nonstick fry pan, cook onion rings in oil for 5-7 minutes or until onions are tender. Add soy sauce and broth. Cover and bake in a 250° oven for 1 hour. Or cover and simmer about 20 minutes. Ladle into bowls. Top with a slice of whole wheat bread and a sprinkle of cheese.

Oven: 250°   1 hour
Cook: 20-25 min   Yield: 4 servings

Per Serving	RCU	FU	Cal	% Ft	P	F	C	Na
	0	1	133	25	4	4	22	744

Hearty Turkey Frame Soup

Susan Ovitt shares her favorite way to finish up the turkey. This is a delicious soup.

1 leftover turkey carcass or 1 fryer chicken, cut and skinned
12-14 cups water
1 large chopped onion
1 to 2 teaspoons salt
1 teaspoon dried thyme leaves, crushed
1 teaspoon dried oregano leaves, crushed
3-4 cups canned tomatoes, slightly blended
6-8 cups fresh or frozen chopped vegetables (celery, carrots, potatoes, onion, mushrooms, or broccoli.)
2 cups broken whole wheat spaghetti, whole wheat noodles, or brown rice spirals
1-2 cups cooked white beans (optional)

Place turkey carcass or chicken in a large pan. Add water, onion, and salt. Bring to a boil, and simmer for 1 hour. Cool, and remove meat from bones. Strain broth, if desired. Use a specially designed fat-skimmer cup to separate fat from broth or chill broth until fat hardens on top. Skim off fat, discard, and add remaining ingredients. Add more water if needed. Cover and bring to a boil. Simmer 30 minutes. Add deboned meat, uncooked spaghetti or noodles, and beans. Simmer uncovered 15 minutes or until noodles are tender. This soup freezes well.

Cook: 1 hour 45 min   Yield: 12-15 servings

Per Serving	RCU	FU	Cal	% Ft	P	F	C	Na
	0	0	148	9	10	2	26	253

Ten Minute Chicken Noodle Soup

It's so soothing when you're under the weather!

1 quart Chicken or Turkey Broth*
1 teaspoon instant minced onion
1/2 teaspoon salt
1/2 teaspoon thyme
1 cup finely chopped chicken or 1 6 3/4-ounce can chicken, cubed
1/4 cup whole wheat spaghetti noodles, broken into 1-inch pieces

Bring chicken broth to a boil. Add remaining ingredients. Reduce heat and simmer 10 minutes.
Cook: 10 min   **Yield: 4 servings**

Per Serving	RCU	FU	Cal	% Ft	P	F	C	Na
	0	0	98	15	14	2	5	43

Golden Nugget Soup

Try Connie Watterson's unbelievably good summer soup!

3 medium yellow summer squash
2 medium carrots
2 medium onions
1 14 1/2-ounce can chicken broth or 2 cups Chicken or Turkey Broth*
1/2 teaspoon salt
1 12-ounce can evaporated skimmed milk
Snipped parsley

Slice squash, carrots, and onions by hand or in food processor. In medium pan combine all ingredients except milk. Cover and cook 15 to 20 minutes or until carrots are just tender. Blend soup slightly, if desired. Stir in evaporated skimmed milk. Heat through. Garnish with parsley.
Cook: 15-20 min   **Yield: 6 servings**

Per Serving	RCU	FU	Cal	% Ft	P	F	C	Na
	0	0	103	0	8	0	20	250

Potato Soup

This recipe makes a delicious basic soup that's easy to vary.

1 large onion, chopped
2 stalks celery
1 teaspoon salt
2 cups water
5-6 large potatoes, peeled and diced
3 to 4 cups skim milk

In blender puree onion, celery, and salt in water. Pour over diced potatoes in a 5- to 6-quart pan. Cook over low heat until potatoes are mushy tender. Stir in milk. Remove 2 cups of the potato mixture, and puree in blender if desired. Stir back into soup. Heat through and serve.

Cook: 20 min   Yield: 6-8 servings

Tip: For a thicker, creamier soup, add 1 can lowfat cream of celery soup. OR: Mix 1/2 cup Slim Cream Soup Mix (page 116) with the milk. Stir into soup, and cook until thickened.

Per Serving	RCU	FU	Cal	% Ft	P	F	C	Na
	0	0	135	7	7	1	26	319

Clam Chowder

Prepare Potato Soup as directed. After pureeing soup, add 2 6 1/2-ounce cans undrained chopped clams. Heat through before serving.

Seafood Chowder

Add to diced potatoes 1 pound white fish fillets (haddock, cod, etc.) cut into bitesize pieces. Prepare Potato Soup as directed but do not puree.

Tuna Chowder

Prepare Potato Soup as directed. Just before serving, add 2 6 1/2-ounce cans undrained water-packed tuna. Heat and serve.

Clam Chowder

Serve this creamy soup with hot bread sticks.

1 6 1/2-ounce can minced clams
1 small onion, chopped
2 stalks celery, chopped
2-3 large potatoes, peeled and cubed
1 teaspoon salt
1 rounded tablespoon shortening
1/2 cup unbleached flour
2-3 cups skim milk
1 tablespoon vinegar
Pepper to taste

Drain juice from clams, and pour over vegetables in a medium-size pan. Add salt and enough water to barely cover vegetables. Cover, and cook over medium heat until tender. Let cool slightly. Melt shortening in a large pan. Add flour and blend. Stir in milk and mix with a wire whip. Cook and stir over medium heat until smooth and thick. Stir in undrained vegetables, clams, vinegar, and salt and pepper to taste. Thin with more milk if needed. Heat through and serve.

Cook: 20-30 min   Yield: 6-8 servings

Per Serving	RCU	FU	Cal	% Ft	P	F	C	Na
	1	1	223	30	13	7	26	390

Fat-Free Chowders

#1 — Omit shortening and flour. Mix 1/2 cup Slim Cream Soup Mix with the milk before adding to soup. Cook until thick, stirring often. Add remaining ingredients and season to taste.

#2 — Omit shortening and flour. Mix 1/3 cup cornstarch with the milk before adding to soup. Cook until thick, stirring often. Add remaining ingredients and season to taste.

Per Serving	RCU	FU	Cal	% Ft	P	F	C	Na
	0	0	162	15	13	3	24	390

Cream of Asparagus Soup

Rose Kreiger's guests enjoy this elegant soup, which takes just minutes to make.

2 10-ounce packages frozen
  asparagus pieces
2 stalks celery, chopped
1/2 small onion, chopped
1 teaspoon salt
2 tablespoons flour

dash pepper
3 cups skim milk
1 10 3/4 ounce can or 1 1/4 cups chicken broth
1 lemon, sliced thin
2 green onions, finely sliced

Cook asparagus, celery, and onion in very small amount of water until tender. Place undrained vegetables, flour, and pepper in blender. Add 1 cup of the milk and pulse to blend. Asparagus can be left a little chunky if desired. Heat milk, broth, and asparagus mixture. Cook and stir over medium heat until hot and slightly thickened. Serve with a thin slice of lemon and a sprinkle of green onions if desired.

Cook: 15-20 min   Yield: 6-8 servings

Per Serving	RCU	FU	Cal	% Ft	P	F	C	Na
	0	0	82	11	7	1	12	317

Cream of Broccoli-Cauliflower Soup

Try this creamy, low-fat soup with a turkey sandwich.

1/2 medium bunch of broccoli
1/2 head cauliflower, chopped
1 stalk celery, finely chopped
1 large potato, diced
1 small onion
1 small carrot

1 teaspoon salt
1/4 cup cornstarch
2 cups skim milk
1/8 teaspoon white pepper
1 teaspoon instant chicken bouillon
1 teaspoon Worcestershire sauce

In a large saucepan, combine broccoli and/or cauliflower, celery, and potato. Peel, then cut onion and carrot in quarters. Place in blender with 1/2 cup water and pulse until finely chopped before adding to vegetables in pan. Add salt and enough water to barely cover vegetables. Cook until tender but not mushy. Mix cornstarch and milk. Stir into undrained vegetables and add pepper, bouillon, and Worchestershire sauce. Cook, stirring constantly, until thick. Thin with more milk if desired.

Cook: 15-20 min   Yield: 8 servings

Extra Creamy Soup: One-half cup Slim Cream Soup Mix* may be used to thicken soup in place of the cornstarch.

Per Serving	RCU	FU	Cal	% Ft	P	F	C	Na
	0	0	94	12	6	1	18	402

Minestrone Soup

Jan Huizinga taught me to make this outstanding minestrone soup. The flavor is even better the second day, if that's possible!

3 slices lean bacon, chopped
1 clove garlic, minced
1 medium onion, minced
1/4 cup minced parsley
2 stalks celery, diced
2 carrots, diced
1 large potato, diced
1/2 medium cabbage, finely sliced (use wide slice blade on food processor)
1 28-ounce can tomatoes, slightly blended
1 teaspoon basil
1 teaspoon salt (optional)
1 15-ounce can kidney beans or 2 cups cooked white or pinto beans
2 quarts soup stock or 2 quarts water plus 2 tablespoons beef or chicken bouillon
   granules
1/2 cup dry whole wheat spaghetti, broken into 1-inch pieces

In a large kettle, fry bacon thoroughly but not until crisp. Do not drain grease. Add garlic, onion, parsley, celery, carrots, potato, and cabbage. Saute' for 20 to 25 minutes, stirring often, until vegetables are tender but still crunchy. (This step is vital for full flavor.) Add tomatoes, basil, salt, beans and stock. Simmer about 45 minutes. Add spaghetti, and cook until tender, 10 to 12 minutes. Serve with fresh rye bread or bread sticks, hot from the oven.

Cook: 1 to 1 1/2 hours   **Yield: 1 gallon**

Per Serving	RCU	FU	Cal	% Ft	P	F	C	Na
	0	0	110	9	5	1	20	340

Lentil Soup

Children love this nourishing soup!

2 cups lentils
4 to 6 cups water
2 slices bacon or 1 ham bone (optional)
1 clove garlic, chopped
1 medium onion, chopped
1 carrot, chopped
1 stalk celery, chopped
1 16-ounce can tomatoes (optional)

1 chicken bouillon cube
2 tablespoons minced parsley
1 teaspoon salt
1/2 teaspoon pepper
1 bay leaf
1/4 teaspoon thyme
1 10-ounce package frozen chopped
    spinach (optional)

Combine lentils and water in a large pan. Bring to boil. Simmer uncovered for 15 minutes. Fry bacon until crisp; remove from pan. Saute garlic, onion, carrot, and celery in bacon grease until tender, about 5 minutes. Stir into lentils. Add tomatoes, bouillon, parsley, and seasonings. Heat to boiling. Reduce heat, cover, and simmer 1 hour. Add spinach during the last 20 minutes. Remove bay leaf before serving.

Cook: 1 1/2 hours   Yield: 6 servings

Per Serving	RCU	FU	Cal	% Ft	P	F	C	Na
	0	0	257	7	17	2	44	538

Love-Those-Lentils Soup

Serve homemade soup tonight made in just an hour!

2 cups lentils, sorted and washed
2 quarts chicken or beef broth or 2 quarts water
    and 1 to 2 tablespoons instant beef or
    chicken bouillon
1 quart water
1 large potato, peeled and diced

3 carrots, coarsely grated
1 large onion, chopped
3 tablespoons vinegar
1/8 teaspoon ground cloves
Salt to taste
Parmesan cheese (optional)

Place lentils, broth, water, potato, carrots, onion, vinegar, and cloves in a soup pot. Bring to a boil. Cook over low heat for 1 to 1 1/2 hours. (Soup will be done in 1 hour, but slow simmering improves the flavor.) Salt to taste. (Salt is not necessary if using bouillon.) Sprinkle with Parmesan cheese, if desired.

Cook: 1 to 1 1/2 hours   Yield: 1 gallon

Per Serving	RCU	FU	Cal	% Ft	P	F	C	Na
	0	0	129	2	9	0	23	219

Split Pea Soup

Here's a hearty soup that genuinely satisfies.

2 cups split peas
2 quarts water
1 large onion, diced
2 medium potatoes, cubed
2 carrots, diced or grated
3 celery stalks, thinly sliced

1 cup diced lean ham
1 teaspoon salt
1/2 teaspoon pepper
1/4 teaspoon dried marjoram
1/4 teaspoon dried thyme leaves

Place all ingredients in a large pan. Bring to a boil. Reduce heat to low, and simmer 1 to 2 hours.

Cook: 1-2 hours   Yield: 8-10 servings

Per Serving	RCU	FU	Cal	% Ft	P	F	C	Na
	0	1	233	21	15	5	32	300

Bean Soup

This flavorful soup is good year-round.

2 cups white beans, sorted and washed
10 cups water
1 onion, quartered, or 1 tablespoon dried minced onion
2 cloves garlic
1 lean, meaty smoked ham hock, ham bone or 1 cup diced lean ham
1 bay leaf
2 potatoes, peeled and cubed
2 stalks celery, thinly sliced
2 to 3 carrots, peeled and diced
1-2 teaspoons salt (optional if using ham hock)

Place beans and 9 cups of water in a large pan. In blender combine the remaining 1 cup water, onion, and garlic cloves. Pulse to finely chop. Pour into pan with beans, and add washed ham hock and bay leaf. Cover pan and cook until beans are almost done, about 2 hours. Remove ham hock. Cool slightly. Remove meat from bone, and discard bone and skin. Add ham, potatoes, celery, carrots, and salt. Cook 1 hour more or until beans and vegetables are tender. Remove bay leaf and serve.

Cook: 3 hours   Yield: 10-12 servings

Quick: Use 2 16-ounce cans beans, diced ham and instant onion. Add vegetables and follow recipe above. Soup is ready in less than 1 hour.

Per Serving	RCU	FU	Cal	% Ft	P	F	C	Na
	0	1	208	19	13	5	30	29

Taco Soup

Barbara Gerratt's spicy soup adds zip to your day! Serve with tortilla chips or cornbread.

1/2 pound (or less) extra lean ground beef (beef can be omitted)
1 small onion, chopped
1 28-ounce can tomatoes, slightly blended (3-4 cups)
1 15-ounce can kidney beans, undrained
1 17-ounce can whole-kernel corn, undrained
2 to 3 tablespoons taco seasoning mix (to taste)
2 cups water
Tortilla chips, optional   See page 215

   Brown ground beef and onion. Drain well. Add remaining ingredients. Simmer 15 minutes. Ladle soup into bowls and top each with a handful of crushed tortilla chips if desired.
Cook: 15 min   Yield: 8 1 cup servings

Per Serving	RCU	FU	Cal	% Ft	P	F	C	Na
	0	0	173	17	12	3	25	254

Hamburger Soup

This soup is satisfying all year round. Serve with hot crusty pan rolls.

1/2 pound lean ground beef
1 onion, chopped
3 stalks celery, diced
4 potatoes, cubed
3 carrots, diced
2 cups chopped cabbage
2 16-ounce cans tomatoes

1 cup whole kernel corn, optional
1/4 cup brown rice, noodles or macaroni
4 to 6 cups water
1 large bay leaf
2 to 3 teaspoons salt
1 tablespoon Worcestershire Sauce, optional
pepper to taste

   In a large pan brown ground beef and onion. Drain well. Add remaining ingredients. Soup should not be too thick so add more water if needed. Bring to a boil. Lower heat, and simmer about 1-1/2 hours. Remove bay leaf before serving.

Slow cooker: Browned ground beef and remaining ingredients may be combined in a slow cooker and simmered on low all day.
Cook: 1-1/2 hours   Yield: 12 servings

Per Serving	RCU	FU	Cal	% Ft	P	F	C	Na
	0	0	100	20	7	2	14	422

Vegetable Beef Stew

Serve hot biscuits with this nourishing meal.

1 pound lean stew meat, cut
  into 1 inch pieces
3-4 cups canned tomatoes
6 carrots, peeled and cubed
4 celery stalks, sliced in 1 inch pieces
6 large potatoes, peeled and cut

2 large onions, diced
1 teaspoon salt
1/4 teaspoon pepper
1/4 cup raw pearl barley
6 cups hot steamed brown rice
  (2 cups raw)

Trim all fat from stew meat and discard. Brown meat in a large heavy pan. Add vegetables, seasonings, and barley. Add water if needed. Simmer for 3 to 4 hours or cook in oven all day at 250°. Stew may also be prepared in a slow cooker. Cook on low 10 to 12 hours or on high for 4 to 5 hours. Serve over steamed brown rice.
Cook: Stove: 3-4 hours   Yield: 12 servings
Slow cooker: 10-12 hours

Per Serving	RCU	FU	Cal	% Ft	P	F	C	Na
	0	1	239	25	15	7	32	499

Chili Con Carne

Here's a very quick and tasty chili.

1/2 pound lean ground beef
1 onion, chopped
1 green pepper, chopped
1 16-ounce can tomatoes (2 cups) or 2 cups water
2 15-ounce cans pinto or red kidney beans, drained
  or 4 cups Ranchero Beans*

1 8-ounce can tomato sauce
1/2 teaspoon salt (optional)
1 tablespoon chili powder
1 bay leaf

In 6-quart pan, brown ground beef, onion, and green pepper until meat is lightly browned and vegetables are tender. Drain and discard fat. Stir in remaining ingredients. Cover and simmer for 30 minutes to 1 hour. Remove bay leaf before serving.
Cook: 1 1/2 hours   Yield: 6-8 servings
Tip: One 1 1/2-ounce package chili seasoning mix may be used instead of the salt and chili powder.

Per Serving	RCU	FU	Cal	% Ft	P	F	C	Na
	0	1	274	15	21	5	34	508

Meatless Chili
Omit ground beef and add 2 cups tofu before simmering.

Creative Nine Bean Soup

We ate this delicious soup at the home of Florence Bowman who lives and teaches the Setpoint lifestyle. A nine bean mix is available, but you can make your own and use it in most any bean soup recipe.

2 cups dry 9-bean mix	**Nine Bean Mix:**
2 quarts water	Pearled barley
1 lean ham hock or ham bone	Red Beans
1 large onion, chopped or	Pinto beans
1 tablespoon dried onion	Navy beans
1 clove garlic, minced	Great northern beans
1 4-ounce can diced green chile	Lentils
2 cups canned tomatoes	Split peas
Juice of 1 lemon	Black beans
1/2 to 1 teaspoon salt	Black-eyed peas

Chop onion and garlic in blender, using a small amount of the water. Put beans, water, ham hock, onion and garlic in slow cooker and cook three hours on high or all day on low, or until beans are just tender; soaking beans overnight reduces cooking time. Add remaining ingredients and cook one hour more. This soup is even better the next day.

Per Serving	RCU	FU	Cal	% Ft	P	F	C	Na
	0	0	146	16	9	3	21	199

Blender Gazpacho

This cool soup makes a refreshing summer meal.

3 cups tomato juice	1 medium onion, cut in pieces
2 tablespoons wine vinegar	4 sprigs parsley
1 clove garlic	1/2 teaspoon salt (optional)
2 medium tomatoes, peeled and quartered	1/8 teaspoon freshly ground pepper
1 small cucumber, cut in pieces	1 cup croutons
1 small green pepper, cut in pieces	Cucumber slices
3 stalks celery, sliced	

Combine 1 cup tomato juice, vinegar, and garlic in blender. Blend until garlic is finely chopped. Add half of the vegetables, and blend until vegetables are pureed. Transfer to another container. Puree remaining tomato juice and vegetables. Mix all together. Season with salt and pepper. Cover and chill thoroughly. Serve in chilled mugs or bowls topped with croutons and cucumber slices.

Chill: 1-2 hours   Yield: 6   3/4-cup servings

Per Serving	RCU	FU	Cal	% Ft	P	F	C	Na
	0	0	75	16	4	1	14	325

SANDWICHES AND SANDWICH FILLINGS—
PITA BREAD FILLINGS

Chicken Salad Sandwich Filling

Add this good standby to your Setpoint repertoire.

2 to 3 cups cooked diced chicken or turkey
1/2 cup cooked brown rice
1 stalk celery, thinly sliced
1/2 cup salad dressing or mayonnaise, fat free

   Mix all ingredients together. Chill thoroughly.
Yield: 2-3 cups filling   8   1/3 cup servings

Per Serving	RCU	FU	Cal	% Ft	P	F	C	Na
	0	0	88	12	15	1	3	109

Egg Salad Sandwich Filling

3 eggs, hard-boiled
1 stalk celery, thinly sliced
1 green onion, finely chopped
1/8 teaspoon dry mustard
1/4 cup salad dressing or mayonnaise, fat free

   Peel the hard-boiled eggs, and mash or finely chop. Add celery, onion, dry
mustard, and salad dressing. Mix well.
Yield: 1 1/2 cups filling   6   1/4 cup servings

Per Serving	RCU	FU	Cal	% Ft	P	F	C	Na
	0	0	45	60	3	3	1	89

Tuna Salad Spread

An old favorite takes on a new twist.

1 6 1/2-ounce can water-packed tuna, drained
1 cup cooked brown rice
1/4 head lettuce, shredded
2 stalks celery, thinly sliced
1 tomato, diced
2 tablespoons chopped dill pickle
1/2 cup salad dressing or mayonnaise, fat free

Mix ingredients in a medium-size mixing bowl.
Yield: 4-5 cups filling   8-10   1/2 cup servings

Per Serving	RCU	FU	Cal	% Ft	P	F	C	Na
	0	0	50	11	6	1	6	248

Chicken-Rice Spread

This filling is so good you'll want to eat it often. It's especially good in pita bread or stuffed tomatoes.

1 cup cooked brown rice
2 cups cooked diced chicken or turkey
2 to 3 small tomatoes, diced
1 avocado, peeled and chopped
1 cup fresh or frozen chopped broccoli, cooked and drained
1 hard-boiled egg, chopped
1/4 cup finely shredded cheese
3/4 cup mayonnaise, fat free
1 tablespoon Dijon-style mustard
1/4 teaspoon celery salt
1/2 teaspoon pepper
1/2 cup unsweetened crushed pineapple, drained

Combine all ingredients in a medium-size mixing bowl. Stir carefully and only enough to moisten ingredients. Cover and chill well.
Chill: 1 hour   Yield: 5-6 cups   1/3 cup servings

Per Serving	RCU	FU	Cal	% Ft	P	F	C	Na
	0	1	129	38	12	5	3	159

Crunchy Bible Sandwich

This is a popular pita bread filling.

1/2 head cabbage, finely sliced or coarsely shredded
1 avocado, chopped
1/2 cup sunflower seeds
2 tablespoons sesame seeds, optional
1 medium tomato, diced
1/2 cup mayonnaise, fat free
1/2 teaspoon Spike, Mrs. Dash, or seasoned salt
Dash cayenne
6 whole wheat pita breads, torn in half
Alfalfa sprouts

Slice or shred cabbage. Mix cabbage, avocado, sunflower seeds, sesame seeds, and tomato with mayonnaise and spices. Fill pita breads with mixture. Garnish with alfalfa sprouts.
Yield: 12   1/2 cup servings

Per Serving	RCU	FU	Cal	% Ft	P	F	C	Na
	0	1	136	30	4	5	21	150

Beefy Pita Pockets

You'll love the subtle blend of flavors in this filling.

1/2 pound extra-lean ground beef
1 medium onion, minced
1/4 cup coarsely cracked wheat (crack 30 seconds in blender)
2 cups tomatoes, canned or fresh
1 teaspoon sugar or honey
1/2 teaspoon oregano
1/2 teaspoon salt
1 tablespoon chopped parsley
4 whole wheat pita breads, torn in half
Alfalfa sprouts or shredded lettuce
1 tomato, chopped

Brown meat and onion. Drain and discard any fat. Stir in dry, uncooked wheat. Add tomatoes, sugar, oregano, salt, and parsley. Simmer 20 to 30 minutes, stirring often, until thick. Spoon into pita bread and top with alfalfa sprouts and chopped tomatoes or serve on whole wheat buns.
Cook: 20-30 min   Yield: 8 servings

Per Serving	RCU	FU	Cal	% Ft	P	F	C	Na
	0	1	166	22	12	4	22	259

gers

his burger.

...ce can water-packed tuna, drained
1/2 cup cooked brown rice
1 egg
1/2 cup whole wheat bread crumbs
2 tablespoons minced onion
2 tablespoons chopped pickle
1 teaspoon Dijon-style mustard
6 whole wheat hamburger buns
Lettuce leaves
Sliced tomatoes

Mix tuna, rice, egg, bread crumbs, onion, pickle, and mustard. Form into patties. Coat with whole wheat flour. Cook on a nonstick or lightly greased pan until lightly browned on each side, about 3 to 4 minutes. Serve on whole wheat buns with lettuce and tomatoes.

Cook: 3-4 min   Yield: 6 burgers

Per Serving	RCU	FU	Cal	% Ft	P	F	C	Na
	0	1	293	21	17	7	42	600

Creamed Tuna

Our favorite creamed tuna — quick and tasty.

2 tablespoons butter
1/4 cup flour
1/2 teaspoon salt

1 teaspoon instant minced onion
2 cups skim or 1% milk
2 6-ounce cans tuna, water-packed

Melt butter in pan over medium heat; blend in flour, salt and onion. Add milk slowly and cook over medium heat, stirring constantly until thick. Add undrained tuna. Heat through and serve over whole wheat toast or baked potatoes.

Yield: 6 servings

Per Serving	RCU	FU	Cal	% Ft	P	F	C	Na
	0	0	156	29	20	5	9	614

SALADS

Winter Fresh Fruit Salad

Who can resist this tempting blend of fresh fruits?

2 bananas, sliced
2 apples, cored and sliced
1 pineapple, cut into chunks, or 1 15 1/4-ounce can unsweetened pineapple chunks,
  drained (save juice)
2 oranges, peeled and cut into bite-size sections
2 seasonal fresh fruits (tangerines, pomegranates, etc.)
Pineapple juice or Fruit Salad Dressing*

Dip banana and apple slices in pineapple juice to prevent browning. Toss all fruits together. Pour juice or dressing over fruit; stir gently to coat. Chill or serve immediately.

Chill: 1-2 hours   **Yield: 10 servings**

Per Serving	RCU	FU	Cal	% Ft	P	F	C	Na
	0	0	102	0	1	0	27	2

Summer Delight Fresh Fruit Salad

This beautiful fruit combination makes a hit on any occasion.

1 watermelon
1 cantaloupe
1 honeydew melon
2 cups seedless grapes
2 bananas, sliced
Seasonal fresh fruit (peaches, nectarines, berries, etc.)
Lemon juice or pineapple juice

Slice watermelon in half lengthwise. Remove the fruit from the watermelon using a melon baller. Cut a saw-toothed or scalloped edge on the watermelon shell. Ball or chunk the cantaloupe and honeydew. Mix all the melons and grapes in a large bowl. Dip banana slices in lemon or pineapple juice to prevent darkening. Add to melons and grapes. Mix carefully. Spoon fruit into the watermelon shell. Cover with plastic wrap and chill.

Chill: 1-2 hours   **Yield: 12-15 servings**

Per Serving	RCU	FU	Cal	% Ft	P	F	C	Na
	0	0	169	7	3	1	37	26

Fruit Cup

This makes a nice dessert for a summer lunch.

2 apples, peeled and cubed
4 bananas, thickly sliced
1 cup cubed pears
1 cup cubed peaches
1 8-ounce can unsweetened pineapple tidbits, undrained
2 tablespoons fresh or frozen lemon juice
1/2 cup unsweetened coconut

Chill all fruits before preparing. Combine fruits and lemon juice. Fold in coconut. Serve immediately.
Yield: 6 servings

Per Serving	RCU	FU	Cal	% Ft	P	F	C	Na
	0	0	126	21	1	3	24	4

Pear Salad

This old favorite is a meal in one.

4 lettuce leaves
1 16-ounce carton low-fat cottage cheese
4 pear halves, canned
Mayonnaise, fat free
4 maraschino cherries

Place lettuce leaves on four individual plates. Put 1/2 cup cottage cheese in the center of each leaf. Top with a pear half, a dollop of mayonnaise, and a maraschino cherry.
Yield: 4 servings

Per Serving	RCU	FU	Cal	% Ft	P	F	C	Na
	0	0	159	11	15	2	18	444

Berry Patch Salad

Once you've tried it, you'll be hooked.

2 medium cantaloupe, chilled
1 16-ounce carton low-fat cottage cheese
1 8-ounce can unsweetened pineapple tidbits, drained
1/2 cup fresh strawberries
1/2 cup fresh red raspberries

Cut cantaloupe in half crosswise; remove seeds. Combine cottage cheese and pineapple. Spoon into melon halves. Top with strawberries and raspberries.
Yield: 4 servings

Per Serving	RCU	FU	Cal	% Ft	P	F	C	Na
	0	0	204	10	17	2	28	469

Chef Salad

This whole-meal salad tastes as good as it looks.

1 head red leaf, green leaf, or iceberg lettuce
2 green onions, sliced
2 carrots, sliced
2 celery stalks, sliced
1 cup cauliflower florets
1 cucumber, peeled and diced
1 green pepper, cut into rings
1 cup fresh mushrooms, sliced
2 hard-boiled eggs, quartered
1 cup kidney beans
1-2 cups cooked and cubed chicken, turkey, crab, shrimp or tuna

Toss the vegetables together in a large salad bowl. Attractively arrange eggs, beans, and meat or fish on top. Serve with desired low-calorie dressings.*
Yield: 6-8 servings

Per Serving	RCU	FU	Cal	% Ft	P	F	C	Na
	0	0	167	14	17	3	17	127

Marinated Vegetables

These are delicious. Serve with rolls for a luncheon or fix for everyday. Flavor improves as they marinate. Kids love 'em.

1/2 small cauliflower, cut into florets
3 stalks broccoli, cut into florets and chunks
4 large carrots, peeled and thinly sliced
4 medium stalks celery, thinly sliced on the diagonal
1 green pepper, cut into thin strips
1 small summer squash
1 cup raw mushrooms, sliced (optional)
1 cucumber, peeled, cut lengthwise and sliced
2 tomatoes, chopped, or 1/2 cup cherry tomatoes (optional)
8 radishes, thinly sliced
1 small sweet or red onion, sliced
1 16-ounce bottle nonfat Italian Dressing

Mix all vegetables except tomato, radishes, and red onion. (Red foods lose their color if marinated too long.) Pour dressing over vegetables, and toss to coat. Marinate in the refrigerator 12 to 24 hours. One hour or less before serving, add tomatoes, radishes, and red onion. Drain dressing and reuse if desired. Serve vegetables on a lettuce leaf.

Tip: For more zest, add a little dry Italian dressing mix to the dressing.

Chill: 12-24 hours   **Yield: 8-10 servings**

Per Serving	RCU	FU	Cal	% Ft	P	F	C	Na
	0	0	48	4	3	0	9	493

Pasta Salad

For a main dish salad, add 2 cups cooked whole wheat spaghetti noodles, broken into small pieces, or cooked brown rice spirals. Marinate with vegetables for at least 1 hour before serving.

Salad Bar For a Crowd

We've figured the amounts; all you do is assemble ingredients.

1/2 head red cabbage, coarsely shredded
3 large heads lettuce, torn into bite-size pieces
1 8-ounce package alfalfa sprouts
4 cucumbers, peeled and sliced
1 bunch green onions, sliced
6 carrots, grated
1 large cauliflower, cut into florets
1 bunch broccoli, cut into florets
4 large green peppers, diced
1 to 2 pounds mushrooms, sliced
1 20-ounce package frozen petite peas, thawed
1 dozen tomatoes, cut in eighths
6 to 8 hard-boiled eggs, sliced or chopped
1 15-ounce can garbanzo beans, drained
1 15-ounce can kidney beans, drained
1 16-ounce can shoestring beets, drained
2 pounds low-fat cottage cheese
1 20-ounce can unsweetened crushed pineapple, undrained
1 cup sliced olives
1-2 cups raw sunflower seeds (soak in water 20 minutes and drain)
1-2 quarts low-calorie salad dressings*

Toss shredded cabbage with lettuce in large salad bowl. Serve the remaining items in separate bowls.
Yield: 20-30 servings

Per Serving	RCU	FU	Cal	% Ft	P	F	C	Na
	0	1	165	22	11	4	21	224

Layered Green Salad

So delicious to eat — so quick to make.

1 small bunch red leaf lettuce, torn in bite-size pieces
1 cup watercress leaves, optional
1 small head iceberg lettuce, torn in bite-size pieces
1 1/2 cups celery, thinly sliced on the diagonal
8 green onions, finely sliced
1 large green pepper, diced
1 10-ounce package frozen petite peas, thawed and drained
1 to 1 1/2 cups mayonnaise, fat free
2 to 4 tablespoons milk
1 to 2 teaspoons cider vinegar (to taste)
1 to 2 tablespoons sugar
Finely grated cheddar or Parmesan cheese (optional)
2 tomatoes, cut into 6 wedges each
2 sliced hard-boiled eggs, optional

In a large clear glass serving bowl, layer salad greens, celery, onions, water chestnuts, green pepper, and peas. Mix mayonnaise, milk, vinegar, and sugar. Spread evenly over salad. Sprinkle lightly with cheese if desired. Cover and refrigerate at least eight hours or overnight. Before serving garnish with tomato wedges and sliced eggs. To serve, scoop to bottom of the salad bowl and lift out a portion of all layers.

Tip: For a main dish, add 3 cups cooked and cubed bite-size pieces of chicken or turkey between the layers of vegetables.

Yield: 15 servings

Per Serving	RCU	FU	Cal	% Ft	P	F	C	Na
	0	0	59	13	3	1	10	170

Creamy Coleslaw

The seasoning gives it that wonderful old-fashioned flavor.

1/2 head of cabbage, coarsely shredded
1/2 green pepper, diced (optional)
1 medium carrot, peeled and finely shredded
1/2 cup salad dressing or mayonnaise, fat free
1/2 teaspoon mustard
1 teaspoon honey or sugar
1 teaspoon apple cider vinegar
1/4 teaspoon salt
1/4 teaspoon celery seed, optional
2 tablespoons milk

Combine vegetables in a serving bowl. In small bowl mix mayonnaise, mustard, honey, vinegar, salt, celery seed, and milk. If too thick, thin with a little extra milk. Add dressing to salad, and stir until well mixed.
Yield: 8-10 servings

Per Serving	RCU	FU	Cal	% Ft	P	F	C	Na
	0	1	39	1	1	0	9	226

Waldorf Salad

Prepare Creamy Coleslaw as directed, deleting mustard and celery seed in dressing. Add 1 to 2 cups chopped raw apple and 1/4 cup chopped nuts.

Colorful Coleslaw

Prepare Creamy Coleslaw as directed. Add 1 medium cucumber, finly diced, and 1 chopped tomato.

Cucumbers in Sour Cream

2 large cucumbers, pared and diced   **1/2 cup sour cream, fat free**
1 green onion, sliced   **1 tablespoon vinegar (to taste)**
2 large tomatoes coarsely chopped (optional) **1 teaspoon dill weed**

Season sliced cucumbers, onion, and tomatoes with salt and pepper. Mix sour cream, vinegar, and dill weed; stir gently into vegetables. Serve immediately or chill no longer than 2 hours (cucumbers will weep).
Chill: 1-2 hours   Yield: 4 servings

Per Serving	RCU	FU	Cal	% Ft	P	F	C	Na
	0	0	28	0	1	0	6	6

Carrot Salad

4 carrots, peeled and finely shredded
1 8-ounce can unsweetened crushed pineapple, undrained
1/4 cup raisins
2 tablespoons frozen orange juice concentrate

Combine all ingredients, and mix gently. Chill.
Chill: 1 hour   Yield: 6-8 servings

Per Serving	RCU	FU	Cal	% Ft	P	F	C	Na
	0	0	47	0	1	0	9	19

Spinach Salad

1 bunch fresh spinach   **2 tablespoons sugar**
1 to 2 eggs, hard-cooked   **1/2 teaspoon salt**
1/4 cup Italian dressing, nonfat **Dash Tabasco sauce**
2 tablespoons wine vinegar   **2 tablespoons bacon bits, optional**

Wash, drain and dry spinach leaves. Tear leaves if desired. Peel and dice egg. Place spinach and egg in large serving dish. Mix dressing, vinegar, sugar, salt and Tabasco sauce. Pour over salad and mix until greens are coated. Garnish with bacon bits if desired.
Yield: 6 to 8 servings

Per Serving	RCU	FU	Cal	% Ft	P	F	C	Na
	1	0	31	3	2	0	6	365

Potato Salad

Here's a delicious potato salad for a summer picnic.
Menu: Oven fried chicken, baked beans, marinated vegetables.

6 large potatoes, boiled or baked in skins
4 large eggs, hard-boiled
1 small onion, chopped
2 dill pickles, finely chopped
1 cup salad dressing or mayonnaise, fat free
1 teaspoon mustard (to taste)
1 teaspoon honey or sugar
1 teaspoon apple cider vinegar
1 teaspoon salt
2 to 4 tablespoons milk

Peel potatoes and cut into bite-size chunks. Dice eggs and add to potatoes. Add onion and pickle. Toss gently. In another bowl mix dressing, mustard, honey, vinegar, and salt. Thin with milk to desired consistency. Pour over salad, and mix lightly. Chill well before serving.

Chill: 3-4 hours   Yield: 12 servings

Per Serving	RCU	FU	Cal	% Ft	P	F	C	Na
	0	0	106	17	4	2	19	440

Turkey Potato Salad

Follow above recipe and add:

2 cups cooked and cubed turkey or chicken
5 stalks celery, diced

Add to dressing:

1 teaspoon prepared horseradish (optional)
1/4 teaspoon dried rosemary leaves, crushed
Dash white pepper

Crab Louis

This is a wonderful treat from the sea. Add hot rolls to make it a complete lunch.

4 large lettuce leaves
8 cups shredded green or red leaf lettuce (1 large head)
2 cups crab meat or mock crab, chilled and drained
2 large tomatoes, cut in wedges
2 hard cooked eggs, sliced
Louis Dressing (see below)
8 large pitted olives

Louis Dressing

2/3 cup mayonnaise, fat free
2 tablespoons chili sauce
1/4 cup chopped green pepper
1 large green onion and top, finely sliced
1 teaspoon lemon juice
1/3 cup Dream Whip, Cool Whip, or nonfat vanilla yogurt

Combine all dressing ingredients. Chill thoroughly before serving.

Line four salad plates with lettuce leaves, forming a cup. Place shredded lettuce inside cup. Fill 1/2 full with crab. Garnish with tomatoes and eggs. Pour 1/4 cup Louis Dressing over each salad. Top with olives if desired.

Chill: 1-2 hours   Yield: 4 servings

Per Serving	RCU	FU	Cal	% Ft	P	F	C	Na
	0	1	207	23	21	5	17	309

Winter Green Salad

This colorful combination makes a delicious winter salad.

1/2 head of cabbage
1/4 small head red cabbage
2 medium carrots, peeled
1 green pepper, seeded and sliced
3 stalks celery, sliced
8-10 radishes, sliced
1/4 head cauliflower, sliced

Coarsely shred cabbage and carrots by hand or use food processor. Slice green pepper, celery, radishes and cauliflower by hand or use wide slice blade on food processor. Toss together. Serve with Creamy Coleslaw Dressing, page 139 or Reduced-calorie Ranch Dressing.

Yield: 8 to 10 servings

Shrimp 'n Rice Salad

Stuff tomatoes with Shrimp-Rice Salad for a perfect summer luncheon.

6 large tomatoes
2 cups cooked shrimp or 2 4 1/4-ounce cans shrimp, drained
1 cup cooked brown rice
2 stalks celery
2 to 3 tablespoons sliced ripe olives
1 tablespoon snipped parsley (optional)
1/2 cup mayonnaise, fat free
1 small clove garlic, diced
1/4 teaspoon dry mustard
1/4 teaspoon paprika
1/2 teaspoon salt

With stem ends down, cut tomatoes into 6 wedges, cutting to, but not through, bases. Spread wedges slightly apart. Carefully scoop out pulp. Dice and drain pulp. Chill tomato shells. Combine diced tomato, shrimp, rice, celery, olives, and parsley. Mix remaining ingredients for dressing; toss with shrimp mixture and chill. Just before serving, spoon rice mixture into shells.

Chill: 2-3 hours   **Yield: 6 servings**

Per Serving	RCU	FU	Cal	% Ft	P	F	C	Na
	0	0	131	16	13	2	17	525

Tuna Salad

Serve this on a bed of lettuce.

1 6 1/2-ounce can water-packed tuna, drained
4 stalks celery, diced
2 green onions, diced
2 hard-boiled eggs, peeled and diced
2 tablespoon chopped pickle
1/2 head lettuce, torn into bite-sized pieces
1/2 cup salad dressing, fat free
1 cup cooked brown rice
6 lettuce leaves

Carefully mix all ingredients except lettuce. Serve on lettuce leaves.

Yield: 6 servings

Per Serving	RCU	FU	Cal	% Ft	P	F	C	Na
	0	1	121	29	12	4	11	497

Gazpacho Salad

A zesty garden salad that complements any meal.

1 pint cherry tomatoes, cut in half
2 medium cucumbers, diced and seeded
1/2 red onion, finely chopped
2 green onions with tops, finely chopped
2 tablespoons shredded fresh basil leaves or 1 teaspoon dried basil leaves
1/2 cup Salsa* or picante' sauce
2 tablespoons Italian reduced-calorie dressing

Combine tomatoes, cucumbers, onions, and basil. Mix salsa and Italian dressing and pour over vegetables. Mix lightly and chill before serving.
Yield: 8 servings

Per Serving	RCU	FU	Cal	% Ft	P	F	C	Na
	0	0	54	0	3	0	12	68

Taco Salad

This main-dish salad is a good budget stretcher. Your guests will say, ''That's the best taco salad I've ever eaten.''

1/2 pound extra-lean ground beef
1 medium onion, chopped (optional if using taco seasoning mix)
1 1 1/4-ounce package taco seasoning mix or 1 tablespoon chili powder and 1/2 tea-
    spoon cumin
1 15-ounce can kidney or pinto beans, undrained
1 cup cooked brown rice
1 head lettuce, torn into bite-size pieces
4 medium tomatoes, diced
1 2 1/4-ounce can sliced olives (optional)
1 cup finely grated cheese (optional)
3 to 4 cups corn tortilla chips
Salsa or mild taco sauce
French or Ranch dressing, fat free

Brown the ground beef and onion. Drain off excess grease. Add taco mix and beans. Simmer 10 to 15 minutes. Stir in rice and let cool 5 to 10 minutes while you prepare remaining ingredients. Mix lettuce, tomatoes, olives, and cheese in large serving bowl. Add meat mixture and slightly crushed chips just before serving. Toss lightly. Serve immediately with Salsa and a low-calorie dressing.
Cook: 15-20 min   **Yield: 6-8 servings**

Per Serving	RCU	FU	Cal	% Ft	P	F	C	Na
	0	1	229	23	14	6	30	193

SET SALADS

Fruit Set Salad

This delicious recipe is so versatile. Be creative as you use your favorite juices and fruits. Try Fruit 'n Berry frozen fruit juice concentrate in place of the apple juice or use any of the frozen juice combinations that are available in your area.

2 envelopes unflavored gelatin
1 cup cold water
1 12-ounce can frozen unsweetened apple juice concentrate
2 bananas, cubed
1 8-ounce can unsweetened crushed pineapple, undrained
2 cups chopped fresh fruit (apples, peaches, apricots, oranges, berries, etc.) or drained lite canned fruit

Sprinkle gelatin over 1 cup of the cold water in a 2-cup measure. Let soften for 1 minute. Heat 1 1/2 minutes on high in microwave or in a pan on the stove. Stir to dissolve gelatin. Pour into a 2-quart dish. Stir in frozen fruit juice concentrate. Add fruit and mix well. Cover and chill until firm.

Chill: 3-4 hours   **Yield: 12-15 servings**

Per Serving	RCU	FU	Cal	% Ft	P	F	C	Na
	0	0	97	0	3	0	22	1

Orange-Pineapple Salad

A cool and beautiful salad.

1 1/2 cups unsweetened orange or pineapple juice
1 envelope unflavored gelatin
1 8-ounce can unsweetened crushed pineapple, undrained
1/4 cup frozen orange juice concentrate or 3 tablespoons sugar
2 oranges, peeled and sectioned or 1 cup mandarin oranges
1 banana, sliced
1 medium carrot, finely shredded

Sprinkle gelatin over juice and let soften 1 minute. Heat in microwave on high for 1 1/2 minutes. Stir to dissolve gelatin. Stir in orange juice concentrate. Add fruit and mix well. Pour into a 2-quart dish. Cover and chill until firm.

Chill: 3-4 hours   **Yield: 9 servings**

Per Serving	RCU	FU	Cal	% Ft	P	F	C	Na
	0	0	69	0	2	0	16	5

Apple Salad

This salad is deceptively delicious, even without the fruit.

1 envelope unflavored gelatin
2 cups apple juice
1/4 cup frozen apple juice concentrate or 2 tablespoons sugar
1 tablespoon fresh or frozen lemon juice
2 apples, coarsely shredded

Sprinkle gelatin over 1 cup apple juice. Let soften 1 minute. Heat 1 1/2 minutes on high in microwave. Stir to dissolve gelatin. Add remaining cup of juice, apple juice concentrate or sugar, and lemon juice. Stir in fruit. Pour into a 9 x 9-inch dish and chill.
Chill: 3-4 hours   Yield: 9 servings

Per Serving	RCU	FU	Cal	% Ft	P	F	C	Na
	0	0	59	3	1	0	14	1

Raspberry Set Salad

It's tart and delicious!

1 envelope unflavored gelatin
1 1/2 cups Cranberry-Raspberry or Cranberry Juice Cocktail
2 tablespoons apple juice concentrate, sugar, or honey
1 teaspoon fresh or frozen lemon juice
1 cup fresh or frozen raspberries
1 cup unsweetened crushed pineapple, undrained

Sprinkle gelatin over fruit juice. Let soften 1 minute. Heat 2 minutes on high in microwave. Stir to dissolve gelatin. Add juice concentrate and lemon juice. Stir in drained raspberries and crushed pineapple. Pour into a 2-quart dish. Cover and chill until set.
Chill: 3-4 hours   Yield: 10 servings

Per Serving	RCU	FU	Cal	% Ft	P	F	C	Na
	0	0	39	2	1	0	9	1

SALAD DRESSINGS

These dressings are quick and easy to prepare. They're so good no one will believe they are lowfat.

Basic Salad Dressing

This versatile lowfat dressing is good on potato and pasta salad as well as green salad. It's also a great potato topper and it stores well. The Ranch Dressing variation is a favorite.

1 cup lowfat cottage cheese
1/4 to 1/2 cup skim or 1% milk
1 to 2 tablespoons reduced-calorie mayonnaise, optional
1 teaspoon instant minced onion
1/4 to 1/2 teaspoon seasoned salt
1 teaspoon dill weed, optional

Tip: The amount of milk needed will be determined by the amount of liquid in the cottage cheese. Use buttermilk in place of skim milk for a tangy dressing. Add a pinch of sugar or honey when making potato or pasta salad dressing.

Mix all ingredients in blender until smooth. Thin with additional milk if necessary. Make dressing thicker for potato or pasta salad. Store in refrigerator.
YIELD: 1 1/2 cups   1 tablespoon servings

Per Serving	RCU	FU	Cal	% Ft	P	F	C	Na
	0	0	10	15	1	0	1	54

Ranch Dressing

Prepare Basic Dressing, omitting onion, salt, and dill weed. Add 1 to 2 teaspoons dry Ranch Dressing Mix. (Hidden Valley, Uncle Dan's, etc.)

Thousand Island Dressing

Prepare Basic Dressing as directed. Add 1/4 cup chili sauce,
2 tablespoons chopped sweet pickle, and 2 tablespoons chopped olives.

Blue Cheese Dressing

Prepare Basic Dressing as directed. Add 1 teaspoon sugar and 1-ounce crumbled blue cheese.

Slim Mayo

You may want to double the recipe for this good basic mayonnaise and store the extra in your refrigerator. It keeps well.

1 tablespoon sugar or honey
2 tablespoons unbleached flour
1 teaspoon dry mustard
1/2 teaspoon salt
1 egg, beaten
1 cup skim milk
1/4 cup vinegar
1 tablespoon margarine or butter

Mix dry ingredients in a medium saucepan. Add egg and milk. Mix well using a wire whisk. Slowly stir in vinegar. Cook over medium heat, stirring constantly, until mixture thickens. Remove from heat; stir in margarine. Cover and store in refrigerator. This is a concentrate. To use, dilute with milk and/or yogurt to desired consistency.

Cook: 5 min   Yield: 1 1/2 cups   1 tablespoon servings

Per Serving	RCU	FU	Cal	% Ft	P	F	C	Na
	0	0	20	39	1	1	2	64

Chili Mayonnaise

This is good on Taco Salad or Taco Sundaes.

1 cup Slim Mayonnaise
1/2 cup Salsa*

Mix together. Store in covered container in refrigerator.

Creamy French Dressing

It's especially good on Taco Salad and Taco Sundaes.

1 cup lowfat cottage cheese
1 10 3/4-ounce can tomato soup, undiluted
1/2 cup reduced-calorie Italian dressing
1 teaspoon Worchestershire sauce
1/4 teaspoon dry mustard
1/8 teaspoon paprika
1 tablespoon sugar or honey

Combine all ingredients and mix with a wire whisk or use a blender; mix until smooth. Thin with buttermilk if desired.
Yield: 3 cups   1 tablespoon servings

Per Serving	RCU	FU	Cal	% Ft	P	F	C	Na
	0	0	11	16	1	0	1	89

Mock Sour Cream

Use this as a potato topping or as the base for dips, salad dressings, etc. It is very versatile. It stores well refrigerated or frozen, but may need to be thinned with additional milk or buttermilk after storage.

1/4-1/2 cup buttermilk or nonfat yogurt
1 cup lowfat cottage cheese
1/2 teaspoon lemon juice, if desired

Puree all ingredients in blender until smooth. Add additional buttermilk or milk if needed to achieve desired consistency.
Yield: 1 1/2 cups   1 tablespoon servings

Per Serving	RCU	FU	Cal	% Ft	P	F	C	Na
	0	0	10	15	1	0	1	43

Fruit Salad Dressing

This versatile fruit dressing stores well.

1 cup pineapple or orange juice
1 to 2 tablespoons cornstarch
2 tablespoons sugar or honey
Pinch salt

Using a wire whisk, stir cornstarch into cold juice. Add sugar or honey. Bring to a boil over medium heat, stirring constantly. Cook 1 to 2 minutes until thick and clear. Chill. Thin with more juice if desired.

Cook: 1-2 min   **Chill: 1 hour**   **Yield: 1 1/4 cups**

Per Serving	RCU	FU	Cal	% Ft	P	F	C	Na
	0	0	14	4	0	0	4	4

Yogurt Dressing

Prepare Basic Fruit Salad Dressing as directed. Stir in 1/4 cup plain nonfat yogurt, 4 tablespoons frozen apple juice concentrate, and 1 additional tablespoon honey or sugar.

Snappy Fruit Salad Dressing

This favorite couldn't be easier!

1 cup nonfat vanilla or fruit-flavored yogurt

Drizzle over sliced fruit or fold into fruit salad.

DIPS AND SALSA

Vegetable Dip

Everyone loves it! Try it on your next baked potato, too.

1 cup lowfat cottage cheese
2 to 4 tablespoons skim or 1% milk
1 tablespoon reduced-calorie mayonnaise, optional
1 to 2 teaspoons dry Ranch Dressing Mix (Hidden Valley, etc.)
   Or use:
1 teaspoon dill weed
1 teaspoon instant minced onion
1 teaspoon parsley flakes
1/4 to 1/2 teaspoon seasoned salt

Tip: The amount of milk needed will be determined by the amount of liquid in the cottage cheese. Use buttermilk in place of skim milk if you like a tangy dip.
   Puree all ingredients in blender until smooth. Add additional milk if needed to achieve desired consistency. Chill at least 4 hours before serving.
Chill: 4 hours   **Yield: 1-1/4 cups 1 tablespoon servings**

Per Serving	RCU	FU	Cal	% Ft	P	F	C	Na
	0	0	12	14	1	0	1	62

Guacamole

Avocadoes are rich in natural fat and are a good food. Try this occasionally on whole wheat toast for a quick lunch, as a salad dressing, or as a dip for vegetables or corn chips.

2 large ripe avocados
2 teaspoons fresh lemon or lime juice
2 green onions, finely minced
1 small tomato, finely chopped
1/4 teaspoon seasoned salt
2 tablespoons Salsa* or taco sauce

   Pit and peel avocados, or scoop out pulp. Mash with a fork. Add lemon juice, onion, tomato, seasoned salt, and salsa, and mix well. Flavor is best at room temperature. If you are not going to serve guacamole immediately, return seed to bowl to help prevent discoloration. Cover tightly and refrigerate until ready to use.
Yield: Serves 8

Per Serving	RCU	FU	Cal	% Ft	P	F	C	Na
	0	1	101	80	1	9	5	62

Layered Tostada Party Dip

Guests will love this luscious blend of flavors. Serve with corn tortilla chips.

1 16-ounce can refried beans and 1 9-ounce can bean dip
  or 2 16-ounce cans spicy refried beans
1/2 - 1 teaspoon chili powder
2 large ripe avocados, peeled and mashed
2-3 tablespoons Salsa or taco sauce
2 green onions, finely diced
2 teaspoons fresh lemon or lime juice
1/4 teaspoon seasoned salt
1 to 2 tablespoons dry taco seasoning mix
1 cup sour cream, fat free
1 4-ounce can chopped green chiles, well drained
2 tablespoons finely shredded cheddar cheese
2 tablespoons sliced or chopped ripe olives
1-2 tomatoes, chopped
2 tablespoons finely shredded Monterey Jack cheese

Mix beans, bean dip, and chili powder. Set aside. Mash avocados with a fork (don't use a blender) and stir in salsa, onions, lemon juice, and seasoned salt. Set aside. Mix sour cream and taco seasoning mix; set aside. On a 10 to 12-inch glass or silver plate, layer bean mixture, avocado mixture, cream cheese mixture, green chiles, cheddar cheese, olives, and tomatoes. Leave a small border of each showing. Sprinkle lightly with cheese. Serve immediately.
Yield: 20 servings

Per Serving	RCU	FU	Cal	% Ft	P	F	C	Na
	0	0	102	37	5	4	14	82

Refried Bean Dip

Serve with tortilla chips for good low-fat snacking.

1 16-ounce can spicy or regular refried beans
2 tablespoons skim milk
2 green onions, finely chopped, or 1 teaspoon instant minced onion,
    softened in water and drained
2 tablespoons diced green chiles
1/2 to 1 teaspoon chili powder
2 tablespoons finely shredded Monterey Jack cheese
1/8 teaspoon cumin
Onion and garlic salt

Mix all ingredients. Season to taste with onion and garlic salt, if desired. Heat in microwave on 70 percent power for 2 to 3 minutes or until warm.

Cook: 2-3 min   Yield: 4-6 servings

Per Serving	RCU	FU	Cal	% Ft	P	F	C	Na
	0	0	90	6	6	1	19	23

Fresh Green Chile Salsa

Fresh salsa makes up in minutes and adds flavor to a multitude of dishes. It doesn't keep long unless it's frozen.

2 cups fresh tomatoes, chopped and drained
    or 2 cups canned tomatoes, drained
2 green onions, finely chopped
2 tablespoons chopped fresh cilantro (optional)
1 4-ounce can diced green chiles
1/4 teaspoon salt
1/2-1 teaspoon chili powder

Place tomatoes, onion, and cilantro in blender. Pulse to puree ingredients slightly if desired. Add to green chiles and seasonings. Keep salsa refrigerated or frozen.
Tip: If using canned tomatoes, add 1 fresh, diced tomato before serving.

Yield: 2 1/2 cups 1 tablespoon servings

Per Serving	RCU	FU	Cal	% Ft	P	F	C	Na
	0	0	6	0	0	0	2	7

Hot Salsa

Serve this delicious salsa with fresh corn tortilla chips.

2-4 jalapeno peppers (to taste)
1 teaspoon chicken bouillon granules
1/2 cup water
3-4 cups canned tomatoes, slightly drained
1/4 cup fresh cilantro or 1 teaspoon dried cilantro

Wash, remove stems, and cook jalapeno peppers until tender in bouillon and water. Place jalapenos and 1/4 cup cooking liquid in blender and puree. Add tomatoes and cilantro and blend to desired consistency. Keep refrigerated.
Yield: 4 cups salsa

Freezer Salsa

You can make up this thick, chunky salsa anytime.

8 cups fresh tomatoes, peeled and quartered
  or 2 28-ounce cans whole tomatoes
2 large onions
4 large green peppers
  or 8 large Anaheim chiles, unseeded
1 medium-size red beet, peeled and pureed (optional)
2 to 3 jalapeno peppers, unseeded
  or 1 to 2 teaspoons crushed dried hot red peppers
1 6-ounce can tomato paste
1 teaspoon garlic salt
2 to 3 teaspoons salt

Finely chop all vegetables in blender. Put in heavy pan. Add tomato paste and seasonings. Cook over medium heat about 30 minutes. Cool and freeze.
Cook: 30 min   Yield: 8-10 cups   1 tablespoon servings

Per Serving	RCU	FU	Cal	% Ft	P	F	C	Na
	0	0	4	0	0	0	1	47

For Fresh Salsa:

1 cup Freezer Salsa
1 diced tomato
3 tablespoons diced green pepper
2 diced green onions

CHAPTER 9

Delicious Dinners

At the close of the day, it is so pleasant to come home to the aroma of a home-cooked dinner. Whether it's a chicken roasting and rolls baking or stew bubbling in the slow cooker, your family will appreciate these delicious and easy-to-prepare dinners. Your friends will ask for seconds when they taste the Taco Sundaes or Chicken 'n Rice Bake. We've included a wide selection of main dishes and accompaniments to add variety and good nutrition to your main meal. If your meal is well-balanced, your plate will have a rainbow of colors. Menu suggestions are given with each of the main dishes and should be varied to fit the season. Eat from your garden whenever possible. Add bread and fresh fruit or dessert as desired. The recipes marked with an asterisk are included in this book.

MICROWAVE INSTRUCTIONS

Microwaves are popular and much preparation time may be saved by using one. In this section we have included instructions on preparing these dinner entrees and accompaniments in a microwave. Be aware, however, that *microwave ovens vary significantly*. For this reason, cooking times are given in ranges. Always begin with the minimum cooking time, check the food, and cook longer if necessary. Remember, food continues to cook after it is removed from the microwave. Consult your operator's manual for cooking and reheating times specific to your microwave.

SLOW COOKER TIPS

It's nice to have dinner ready when you walk in the door. Most main dishes can be cooked using a slow cooker. With a little practice, you'll become an expert. General instructions are included below.

All-day cooking: Use low-heat setting for 10-12 hours
Half-day: Use high-heat setting for 4-6 hours

If morning time is limited, prepare meat and vegetables the night before. Brown, drain, wrap, and chill meat if necessary. Clean and cut vegetables. Refrigerate until morning.

When cooking meat and vegetable combinations, place the vegetables in the bottom of the cooker. The liquid helps them cook and improves flavor. Sprinkle the vegetables with quick-cooking tapioca if desired. It's the best thickener for slow- cooking use; it needs no stirring and does not lump. Top with the meat.

CHICKEN AND TURKEY MAIN DISHES

Poultry is versatile, economical, low in fat, and a good source of protein. Chicken is always a good choice. Remember to skin it before cooking, as the fat clings to the skin. In all poultry, the light meat is lower in fat than the dark meat.

Turkey has always been recommended as being better for your health than beef, and it usually is. However, be careful what you buy and learn to read labels. Avoid butter-basted turkeys; they have added fats, salt, sugar, and preservatives. Raw, cooked, or cured turkey breasts are usually a good choice, but check for added salt and preservatives.

Just because a product is labeled "turkey" doesn't automatically mean it is low in fat. Read the labels. Ground turkey, turkey franks, turkey ham, and turkey salami are some of the new turkey products on the market. They are often 50 percent fat or higher. Use them sparingly, as you would beef.

Preparation tips: Cook chicken pieces or turkey hindquarters as directed under Cooked Chicken or Turkey in Chapter Eight. Freeze cooked meat in 2-cup portions in freezer containers. To thaw in microwave, place in baking dish covered with wax paper. Cook on high for 2-3 minutes or until thawed. Use this meat in many of the recipes in this chapter. Make gravy using Slim Cream Soup Mix*. Add this meat to the gravy and serve with Hawaiian Haystacks, as a potato topper, or in any other favorite poultry recipe.

Roast Chicken and Vegetables

Menu: Creamy Coleslaw, sliced tomatoes

1 3-pound whole or cut-up fryer, skinned
4 to 5 potatoes, scrubbed and halved
6 carrots, peeled and cut in large pieces
1 onion, sliced
1 medium yam, washed and cut into 2 inch pieces (optional)
1 fresh lime, juiced (optional)
1 teaspoon dried thyme leaves, crushed
Salt, pepper, and poultry seasoning

Place chicken in a small roaster or in a roasting bag. Arrange vegetables around chicken. Sprinkle chicken with lime juice and thyme. Season chicken and vegetables with remaining seasonings. Cover roaster. Bake in a 350° oven for 1 to 1 1/2 hours or as directed on roasting bag.

Bake: 350° 1 hour   **Yield: 6-7 servings**

Per Serving	RCU	FU	Cal	% Ft	P	F	C	Na
	0	1	340	11	40	4	32	155

Quick Fix Chicken

It's in the oven in 5 minutes!
Menu: Baked potatoes, steamed broccoli, raw vegetable plate

3 large chicken breasts, skinned and halved
1 10 3/4-ounce can chicken gumbo soup

Place chicken in a 7 x 12-inch baking dish. Pour undiluted soup over the chicken. Cover tightly. Bake until tender.
Microwave: Cover loosely. Rotate dish after 8 minutes. Let stand 5 minutes before serving.
Spoon sauce over baked potatoes or hot brown rice.

Bake: 300° 1 hour or until tender
Microwave: High 15-17 min   Yield: 6 servings

Per Serving	RCU	FU	Cal	% Ft	P	F	C	Na
	0	0	97	17	19	2	3	411

Crispy Oven-Fried Chicken

We fix this often because it is easy and delicious.
Menu: Potato salad, baked beans, green salad

1 cup High Fiber Bran Mix*, dry whole wheat bread crumbs or whole-grain cereal crumbs
1 teaspoon poultry seasoning or any favorite chicken seasoning
1/2 teaspoon pepper
1 teaspoon salt
2 tablespoons Parmesan cheese
1 tablespoon dry parsley flakes
1 chicken or 6 chicken pieces, cut and skinned
1 cup skim milk

Place Bran Mix, bread or cereal crumbs, and seasonings in blender and pulse until fine. Put breading mix in paper or plastic bag. Dip chicken in milk and let drain slightly. Place two or three pieces of chicken at a time in bag with breading, and shake to coat. Place on a foil-lined baking sheet. Bake in a 400° oven for 45 to 60 minutes.

Microwave: Arrange chicken pieces in a microwave dish with thick edges towards the outside. Cover with paper toweling. Cook on high 19-22 minutes. Rotate dish once or twice.

Bake: 400° 45-60 min
Microwave: High 19-22 min   **Yield: 6 servings**

Orange Chicken

Breading: Mix 1 cup fine whole wheat bread crumbs, 1 teaspoon paprika, 1 teaspoon grated orange peel and 1/2 teaspoon salt (use blender.) Mix 1 beaten egg and 1/3 cup orange juice. Dip chicken pieces into juice mixture and roll or shake in seasoned bread crumbs. Follow above directions to bake.

Per Serving	RCU	FU	Cal	% Ft	P	F	C	Na
	0	1	188	17	29	4	5	396

Jiffy Barbecue Chicken

This chicken is simple, yet special enough for any dinner party.
Menu: Baked potatoes, frozen petite peas, sliced tomatoes

2/3 cup water
1 onion, peeled and quartered or
   1 tablespoon dried onion
3/4 cup catsup
1/4 cup lemon juice
2 tablespoons sugar or honey

3 tablespoons Worcestershire sauce
2 tablespoons prepared mustard
1/2 teaspoon pepper
3 pounds chicken breasts, wings,
   or chicken pieces, skinned

Place water and onion in blender. Pulse to finely chop onion. Transfer to a saucepan and add other ingredients. Simmer uncovered for 15 minutes (this step can be omitted; if omitted, reduce water to 1/2 cup). Arrange chicken pieces in a 9 x 13-inch baking dish. Pour sauce over chicken. Cover, and bake 1-1 1/2 hours or until tender. If desired, uncover during the last 15 minutes of baking. Serve sauce over baked potatoes or steamed rice.

Microwave: Reduce water to 1/3 cup. Arrange chicken pieces in a 9 x 13-inch baking dish, placing thicker pieces on the outside. Pour sauce over chicken. Cover loosely with waxed paper. Cook on high for 20-25 minutes. Rotate dish twice.

Tip: This sauce is also good on hamburger patties.

Bake: **325° 1 1/2 hours**
Microwave: High 20-25 min   **Yield: 8 servings**

Per Serving	RCU	FU	Cal	% Ft	P	F	C	Na
	1	0	197	9	28	2	12	486

Microwave Barbecue Chicken

Lane Godfrey shares her 20-minute meal!
Menu: Creamed peas and potatoes, corn on the cob, gazpacho salad

1 3-pound cut-up chicken or
   chicken pieces, skinned
1/2 cup skim milk
1 cup whole wheat flour

1/4 cup cornmeal (optional)
3 tablespoons dry pizza sauce mix or
   taco seasoning mix

Dip chicken in milk. Combine dry ingredients in a plastic or paper bag. Add chicken, and shake to coat. Arrange chicken in a glass baking dish with thick edges towards the outside. Cover with waxed paper. Cook on high 10 minutes. Rotate dish and cook 7 additional minutes or until tender. Chicken can also be baked in a 400° oven for 45 to 60 minutes.

Microwave: High 17 min
Bake: **400° 45-60 min**   **Yield: 6-8 servings**

Per Serving	RCU	FU	Cal	% Ft	P	F	C	Na
	0	0	202	15	29	3	10	212

Teriyaki Chicken Kabobs—Barbecue Style

Serve this at your next patio party.
Menu: Stir-Fry Romaine and Mushrooms, Western Potato Strips, corn on the cob, sliced tomatoes, cucumbers

4 chicken breasts
1/4 cup soy sauce
1/4 cup water
2 tablespoons honey or sugar
1 teaspoon grated ginger root or 1/2 teaspoon ground ginger
2 cloves garlic, minced
2 tablespoons chopped chives or green onion
3 to 4 green peppers, cut in large pieces
12 to 18 cherry tomatoes
2 to 3 onions, cut in chunks
1/2 pound mushrooms
1 cup pineapple chunks

   Skin, remove bone, and cut chicken breasts into strips or bite-size chunks. Combine soy sauce, water, sugar, ginger, garlic, and chives. Place chicken in marinade. Cover, and refrigerate for 3 to 4 hours. Drain meat and thread on skewers, alternating with green pepper chunks, cherry tomatoes, onions, mushrooms, and pineapple. Broil on grill until tender, about 5 to 7 minutes.
   Kabobs may also be baked in a 400° oven for 6 to 8 minutes.
Broil: 5-7 min   Yield: 6-8 servings

Per Serving	RCU	FU	Cal	% Ft	P	F	C	Na
	0	0	138	7	16	1	15	342

Quick Lemon Chicken

Susan Robbins shares her top-of-the stove chicken recipe.
Menu: Potato Patties, creamed asparagus, tomato slices

2 chicken breasts	1 tablespoon soy sauce
2 tablespoons water	2 teaspoons Dijon mustard
2 tablespoons fresh or frozen lemon juice	1 teaspoon lime juice
1 tablespoon oil	Dash cayenne pepper

Skin and bone chicken breasts. Cut in half lengthwise and place in shallow dish. Mix water, lemon juice, oil, soy sauce, mustard, lime juice, and cayenne. Pour marinade over chicken. Cover and refrigerate several hours or overnight. Turn chicken in marinade at least once if possible. Drain marinade into skillet and bring to a boil. Add chicken and let simmer 15 to 20 minutes or until tender. Remove chicken from marinade and serve.

Cook: 20 min   Yield: 4 servings

Per Serving	RCU	FU	Cal	% Ft	P	F	C	Na
	0	0	131	20	21	3	1	306

Chicken 'n Rice Bake

You'll serve this dish often because it's inexpensive enough for everyday, elegant enough for guests, and very easy to prepare.
Menu: Petite peas, candied yams, creamy coleslaw

1 rounded cup raw brown rice
1 cup finely chopped celery (optional)
1 4-ounce can mushroom stems and pieces, drained (optional)
1 10 3/4-ounce can cream of mushroom soup, lowfat
2 cups chicken broth, homemade or made from bouillon cubes
1 - 1 1/4-ounce package dry onion soup mix (reserve 2 tablespoons)
1 cup-up chicken or 6-8 chicken pieces, skinned

Spread rice, celery, and mushrooms evenly in a 9 x 13-inch baking dish. Mix soup, chicken broth, and dry onion soup mix. Pour over rice and vegetables. Place chicken on top of mixture. Turn chicken pieces once to coat. Sprinkle remaining dry onion soup mix over chicken. Cover and bake in a 350° oven for 1 to 1 1/4 hours or until rice is done. Can bake at 275° for 3-4 hours.

Bake: 350° 1-1 1/4 hours or until rice is done
**   or 275° 3-4 hours   Yield: 8 servings**

Per Serving	RCU	FU	Cal	% Ft	P	F	C	Na
	0	0	294	13	30	4	28	647

Chicken Cacciatore

Fix it quickly in a large skillet.
Menu: Steamed brown rice, green beans, baked squash

4 chicken breasts, boned, skinned, and cut in half
  or 1 cut-up fryer, skinned
1 large onion, chopped or sliced
1 clove garlic, minced
2 to 3 cups canned tomatoes
1 teaspoon oregano
1/2 teaspoon salt
Pepper to taste
Cooked brown rice, noodles, or potatoes

Place chicken in a heavy pan or skillet. Combine remaining ingredients except rice, noodles or potatoes, and pour over chicken. Cover, and steam about 1 hour. If desired, uncover during the last 15 minutes of cooking to thicken sauce. Carrots and potatoes can be cooked with the chicken if desired.

Microwave: Use a 7 x 12 or 9 x 13-inch baking dish. Cover with waxed paper. Cook at 80% power 28-32 minutes or until meat near bone is no longer pink. Turn twice. Serve sauce over rice, noodles, or potatoes.

Cook: 1 hour
Microwave: 80% 28-32 minutes   Yield: 6 servings

Per Serving	RCU	FU	Cal	% Ft	P	F	C	Na
	0	0	209	7	23	2	26	315

Quick Chicken Cacciatore

In a nonstick skillet, brown chicken over medium heat for 15 minutes, turning often. Add 2 cups salsa. Cover and cook over low heat for 35 to 40 minutes or until chicken is tender. Chicken may also be covered loosely and microwaved on high heat for 18 minutes. Turn once.

Chicken Delight

You will love this chicken and dressing casserole.
Menu: Asparagas, carrots, gazpacho salad

1/4 cup cornstarch
3 cups seasoned Chicken or Turkey Broth*
1 tablespoon instant minced onion or 1 medium onion, chopped
4-5 cups whole wheat bread cubes
1/4 teaspoon salt
1-2 teaspoons poultry seasoning
Pinch of pepper
1 chicken, cooked and boned, or 2-4 cups chicken pieces
1 cup fine whole wheat bread crumbs (use blender)

Mix cornstarch with small amount of cold water and stir into hot broth. Add onion and cook until gravy is thick and clear. Set aside. To make dressing, mix bread cubes, salt, poultry seasoning, and pepper. Cover bottom of a 9 x 13-inch baking dish or 2 1 1/2-quart casserole dishes with a small amount of gravy. Place the dressing evenly over the gravy. Cover with a layer of bite-size chicken pieces. Pour sauce over all. Sprinkle fine bread crumbs over top. Cover, and bake in a 350° oven for 30 minutes. Uncover during the last 5 minutes of baking.

Microwave, cover with plastic wrap. Cook at 70% power for 14-16 minutes or until hot and bubbly. Rotate dish once.

Bake: **350° 30 min**
Microwave: 70% 14-16 min   **Yield: 12 servings**

Per Serving	RCU	FU	Cal	% Ft	P	F	C	Na
	0	0	104	15	11	2	11	112

Chicken Divan

Entertain guests with this elegant party dish.
Menu: Baked potatoes, frozen corn and green salad.

2 10-ounce packages frozen broccoli or asparagus spears
1/2 cup buttermilk
1 cup sour cream, fat free
2 teaspoons lemon juice
1/2 teaspoon curry powder (optional)
1 10 3/4-ounce can cream of chicken soup, low fat
2 cups cooked brown rice
2 cups cooked and cubed chicken or turkey breast
2 slices whole wheat bread
2 tablespoons Parmesan cheese

Slightly cook broccoli or asparagus. To microwave, place frozen packages of vegetables on paper towel in microwave and cook on high for 3-4 minutes. Drain well. Mix buttermilk, sour cream, lemon juice, and soup. In large baking dish, layer half the soup mixture, rice, chicken, and broccoli. Top with remaining soup mixture. Place bread and cheese in blender. Pulse to make fine bread crumbs. Sprinkle over casserole. Cover and bake in a 350° oven for 25 minutes. Uncover and bake 5 more minutes or until hot and bubbly.

Microwave: Cover with plastic wrap. Cook at 70% power for 12-15 minutes or until hot and bubbly.

Bake: 350° 30 min
Microwave: 70% 12-15 min   **Yield: 6 servings**

Per Serving	RCU	FU	Cal	% Ft	P	F	C	Na
	0	0	392	12	41	4	41	562

Hawaiian Haystacks

This creative delight comes from Janet Hales.
Menu: Birdseed rolls

4 cups seasoned chicken broth
1/4 cup cornstarch
2 to 3 cups cooked and cubed chicken or turkey
4 cups hot cooked brown rice
4 medium tomatoes, chopped
1 10-ounce package frozen petite peas, thawed
5 stalks celery, finely diced
1 to 2 green peppers, chopped
6 to 8 green onions, sliced
1 8-ounce can unsweetened crushed pineapple or pineapple tidbits
1/2 cup slivered almonds or sunflower seeds
1/2 cup shredded coconut, optional
1/2 cup sliced water chestnuts
1-2 cups Chinese noodles (optional)
1 cup finely grated cheddar cheese

Combine broth and cornstarch. Cook until thick and clear. Add chicken. Place remaining ingredients in individual bowls. Have guests build their own stack in the following order: rice, chicken in gravy, tomatoes, peas, celery, green pepper, onions, pineapple, almonds, coconut, water chestnuts, noodles, and cheese.
Yield: 6-8 servings

Per Serving	RCU	FU	Cal	% Ft	P	F	C	Na
	0	1	305	24	24	8	34	433

Sweet and Sour Chicken

Prepare this chicken in 10 minutes.
Menu: Steamed brown rice, baked squash, green beans

1 large green pepper, diced
3 green onions, thinly sliced
1 8-ounce can unsweetened pineapple tidbits, drained
1 cup chicken broth or 1 bouillon cube in 1 cup hot water
1-2 tablespoons soy sauce
3 tablespoons vinegar
3-4 tablespoons brown sugar or honey (to taste)
Pinch salt
2 tablespoons cornstarch
1/4 cup cold water
2 cups cooked and cubed chicken
3 cups cooked brown rice (1 cup raw)

Saute green pepper, onion, and pineapple tidbits in nonstick fry pan for 3-5 minutes. Add broth, pineapple juice, soy sauce, vinegar, and brown sugar or honey. Stir cornstarch into cold water. Add to mixture. Cook and stir gently until thickened. Add chicken, and heat through. Serve over hot brown rice.

Cook: 10 min   Yield: 6 servings

Per Serving	RCU	FU	Cal	% Ft	P	F	C	Na
	1	1	296	13	30	4	33	666

Quick Chicken and Noodles

Menu: Baked yams, steamed green beans, carrot sticks

2 chicken breasts, skinned
2 tablespoons low-sodium chicken bouillon
1 scant tablespoon instant minced onion
4 cups water
2 to 3 carrots, finely sliced
1 stalk celery, chopped
1 to 2 cups noodles

Combine all ingredients except noodles in a medium-size pan. Simmer 15 minutes. Remove chicken breasts, cool slightly, and remove meat from bones. Cut into bite-size pieces; return to broth. Add noodles. Simmer 10 to 12 minutes or until done. Add more water, if needed.

Cook: 25-30 min   Yield: 6-8 servings

Per Serving	RCU	FU	Cal	% Ft	P	F	C	Na
	0	0	156	7	14	1	23	199

Old-Fashioned Chicken and Noodles

This dish will be popular with the whole family.
Menu: Steamed broccoli and carrots, sliced cucumbers

1 large fryer chicken, cut and skinned
8 cups water
1 teaspoon salt
1 tablespoon instant minced onion
1 bay leaf

2 medium carrots, diced
1/2 teaspoon curry powder (optional)
Salt to taste
2 to 3 cups noodles
4-6 cups mashed potatoes

Wash chicken. Place in a large pan and add water, salt, onion, and bay leaf. Bring to a boil. Simmer chicken 1 hour or until tender. Let cool slightly in broth. Remove chicken from bones, leaving meat in large pieces. Discard bay leaf, bones, and skin. Cover and refrigerate meat. Put defatted broth in a large pan and bring to a boil. Add carrots and seasonings. Cook until carrots are tender, about 10 minutes. Add chicken pieces and noodles. Simmer until done, about 12 to 15 minutes. Serve over mashed potatoes if desired.

Cook: 1 hour   Yield: 8 servings

Per Serving	RCU	FU	Cal	% Ft	P	F	C	Na
	0	1	416	10	36	5	55	474

Chicken and Dumplings

Try these light and tender dumplings. They're easy to make.
Menu: Green beans, raw vegetable plate

1 fryer chicken or 6 chicken legs, cut and skinned
8 cups water
1 teaspoon salt
1 tablespoon minced dried onion
4 carrots, sliced
1/2 teaspoon poultry seasoning (optional)

Dumplings:
1 cup whole wheat flour
1 cup unbleached flour
1 tablespoon baking powder
1 scant teaspoon salt
2 to 3 tablespoons shortening
1 cup skim milk

Gravy:
2 tablespoons unbleached flour
1 cup skim milk

Wash chicken. Place in a large pan and add water, salt, onion, carrots and seasoning. Bring to a boil. Cover and simmer 45 to 60 minutes or until chicken is tender. Defat broth if needed.

Mix dumpling dry ingredients, and cut in shortening. Add milk and stir with a fork until mixed. Drop by spoonfuls onto chicken pieces in boiling broth. Cook 10 minutes, uncovered, and 10 minutes tightly covered. This is important for making light dumplings. Remove dumplings and meat to platter, and keep hot while making gravy. Mix flour and milk to make a smooth paste. Stir into hot broth. Cook and stir until smooth and thick. Serve immediately on a large platter. Garnish with parsley.

Cook: 1-2 hour   **Yield: 6-8 servings**

Per Serving	RCU	FU	Cal	% Ft	P	F	C	Na
	1	1	303	25	26	8	28	377

Chicken Pot Pie

A hearty chicken pie from Marge Merrill.
Menu: Steamed broccoli and cauliflower, green salad, hot biscuits

2 to 3 carrots, diced or thinly sliced	3 cups Chicken or Turkey Broth*
1 10-ounce package frozen petite peas	1 cup skim milk
1 tablespoon butter	1 teaspoon whole thyme leaves, crushed
1 small onion, finely minced	5 to 6 cups cooked and cubed chicken
3 stalks celery, thinly sliced	1 recipe Stir-n-Drop Biscuits*
1/2 cup flour	

Cook carrots for 3 to 5 minutes in a small amount of water. Add peas, and let stand for 3 minutes. Drain. Melt butter in a medium-sized frying pan. Add onion and celery, and saute. Add flour. Gradually stir in chicken broth and milk. Add thyme, and cook until thick, stirring constantly. Combine vegetables, gravy, and chicken. Place in a large 9 x 13-inch baking dish or two smaller ones. Top with biscuits. Bake in a 400° oven for 18 to 20 minutes until biscuits are brown.

Bake: 400° 18-20 min   **Yield: 12-14 servings**

Per Serving	RCU	FU	Cal	% Ft	P	F	C	Na
	1	1	252	29	19	8	24	280

Turkey Loaf

This light loaf is nice for a summer lunch or supper.
Menu: White beans, steamed summer squash and onion, tomatoes

2 to 3 cups cooked and cubed chicken or turkey	2 cups Chicken or Turkey broth*
1 cup whole wheat bread crumbs	2 eggs
1 cup cooked brown rice	1/4 teaspoon paprika
1/4 teaspoon salt	

Mix turkey, bread crumbs, rice, and salt. Place in an 8 x 8-inch baking dish or an 4 1/2 x 8 1/2-inch loaf pan. Mix broth and eggs in blender, and pour over mixture. Sprinkle with paprika. Bake in a 350° oven for 30 to 35 minutes or until set. Microwave: Reduce turkey broth to 1 1/2 cups. Place in a baking dish. Cover loosely with waxed paper, and microwave on 50 percent power for 13 to 14 minutes. Rotate dish twice.

Bake: 350° 30-35 min
Microwave: 50% 12-14 min   **Yield: 6-8 servings**

Per Serving	RCU	FU	Cal	% Ft	P	F	C	Na
	0	1	157	23	21	4	8	247

Tuna Loaf

Use 2 cans water-packed tuna, drained, in place of the turkey. Prepare and cook as directed for Turkey Loaf.

Quick Turkey Casserole

When you're in a hurry, remember this good recipe.
Menu: Baked squash, steamed green beans, raw cauliflower

2 cups large bite-sized pieces cooked turkey or chicken
3 cups cooked brown rice
1 tablespoon instant minced onion
1 4-ounce can mushrooms, drained
1 10 3/4-ounce can cream of mushroom soup, low fat
1/2 teaspoon poultry seasoning
2 slices whole wheat bread
1 teaspoon butter

Mix turkey, rice, onion, mushrooms, soup, and poultry seasoning. Pour into a 1 1/2-to 2-quart casserole. Combine whole wheat bread and butter in blender. Pulse to make crumbs. Sprinkle over casserole. Tip: For variety, add 1 cup cooked asparagus or broccoli. Cover and bake in a 375° oven for 25 to 30 minutes or until bubbly and hot.

Microwave: Cover and cook on high 8-10 minutes.

Bake: 375° 25-30 min
Microwave: High 8-10 min **Yield: 6-8 servings**

Per Serving	RCU	FU	Cal	% Ft	P	F	C	Na
	0	1	268	22	30	6	21	552

Stuffed Turkey

This favorite is good any time of the year.
Thanksgiving Menu: Mashed potatoes, gravy, frozen corn, fresh vegetable plate, candied yams, raspberry set salad, feather rolls

1 10- to 12-pound turkey, fresh or frozen
2 tablespoons butter or margarine
4 to 6 stalks celery, finely chopped
1 large onion, finely minced
1/3 cup chicken broth or water if needed
1 tablespoon poultry seasoning
1 to 1 1/2 teaspoons salt
1/4 teaspoon pepper
10 to 12 cups whole wheat bread cubes (approximately 1 large loaf of bread)

Thaw turkey and wash inside and out with cold water. Set aside. In a large frying pan, saute' celery and onion in butter for 5 minutes or until onions are transparent. Add seasonings and pour over bread crumbs. Toss lightly, and add broth if needed. Don't get dressing too moist. Stuff turkey. Insert into a large roaster or roasting bag. Bake in a 325° oven for 3 1/2 to 4 hours or as directed on roasting bag. Turkey may also be microwaved by following instructions in owner's manual.

Tip: *After removing cooked meat, put the bones in a large kettle and cook as directed for Hearty Turkey Frame Soup*. Use the stock for the soup or freeze for later use.*
Bake: 325° 3 1/2-4 hours or until tender
Microwave: Consult owner's manual   **Stuffing: 12 Servings**

Per Serving	RCU	FU	Cal	% Ft	P	F	C	Na
	0	0	112	25	33	3	18	303

Crusty Meat Braid

Everyone will want seconds, so make plenty.
Menu: Steamed carrots and cauliflower, fresh vegetable plate

Turkey or Beef Filling (see below)
2 to 3 cups whole wheat bread or roll dough
2 tablespoons finely grated cheese

Prepare filling as directed. Roll dough into a large rectangle, approximately 9 x 15 inches and 1/4 inch thick. Spread filling lengthwise down the center third of the dough. Using a pizza cutter or sharp knife, cut the dough into 1 inch strips on each side of the filling, cutting almost to the filling. Braid dough over meat, tucking in the last strip. Place on large, heavy baking sheet. Let raise 5 to 10 minutes. Bake in a 350° oven for 25 to 30 minutes. Pour remaining soup or sauce over top, and sprinkle with cheese. Serve immediately.

Bake: 350° 25-30 min   Yield: 6-8 servings

Turkey Filling
2 cups cooked and cubed turkey or chicken
1 teaspoon instant minced onion
1 cup frozen peas and carrots, slightly cooked and drained
1 4-ounce can mushrooms, drained
1 10 3/4-ounce can cream of mushroom soup, low fat
Salt and pepper

Mix turkey, onion, peas and carrots, and mushrooms. Add half the soup to the turkey mixture. Season with salt and pepper. Mix the remaining soup with a few tablespoons water or milk to achieve gravy consistency, and reserve for baked braid.

Per Serving	RCU	FU	Cal	% Ft	P	F	C	Na
	0	1	368	21	32	8	41	624

Beef Filling
1 pound extra-lean ground beef
1 onion, chopped, or 1 tablespoon minced dried onion
1 cup frozen mixed vegetables, cooked and drained (optional)
3 tablespoons taco or pizza sauce seasoning mix
1 8-ounce can tomato sauce
Salt and pepper

Cook ground beef and onion in a nonstick frying pan. Drain well. Stir in mixed vegetables, seasoning mix, and 1/2 cup tomato sauce. Season with salt and pepper. Reserve remaining 1/2 cup tomato sauce for top of baked braid.

Per Serving	RCU	FU	Cal	% Ft	P	F	C	Na
	0	1	340	24	23	9	44	468

Turkey Topper

What a nice way to use up left-over turkey. Use the Slim Cream Soup Mix* and you'll have a very creamy, lowfat meal.
Menu: Steamed broccoli, frozen corn, sliced tomatoes

2 cups cooked and diced turkey
1 teaspoon instant minced onion
1 10 3/4-ounce can cream of mushroom soup, low fat
1/2 cup skim milk
1 cup cooked mixed peas and carrots (optional)
4-6 baked potatoes, cooked brown rice, or whole wheat toast

Combine turkey, onion, soup, milk, and vegetables (if desired) in a medium-size saucepan. Cook until sauce is thick and hot. Thin with more milk if desired. Serve over baked potatoes.
Time: 10 min   Yield: 4-6 servings

Per Serving	RCU	FU	Cal	% Ft	P	F	C	Na
	0	0	211	17	28	4	13	342

FISH MAIN DISHES

Oven-Fried Fish

An easy way to fry fresh fish.
Menu: Creamed asparagus over baked potatoes, green salad

1 tablespoon butter or margarine   **2 teaspoons fresh minced onion**
2 tablespoons lemon juice   **8 to 10 fresh fish (8 to 11 inches long)**

Line a baking sheet with foil. Melt butter, and stir in lemon juice and minced onion. Spread on the foil-lined baking sheet. Place fish on baking sheet, turning once to coat. Bake in a 375° oven for 20 to 25 minutes or until fish flakes easily. Do not overbake. Serve at once.

Microwave: Use a 9 x 13-inch baking dish. Prepare as above. Put tails and thin pieces towards center. Cover loosely with waxed paper. Cook on high power for 6 to 8 minutes. Rotate dish once.

Bake: 375° 20-25 min
Microwave: High 6-8 min   Yield: 6-8 servings

Per Serving	RCU	FU	Cal	% Ft	P	F	C	Na
	0	0	141	21	30	3	1	127

Favorite Fish Dish

Preparation time is short for this beautiful lowfat dish.
Menu: Fried potatoes and onions, green salad, rolls

1 large onion, thinly sliced
1 cup fresh mushrooms, sliced or 1 4-ounce can mushrooms, drained
2 tablespoons water or chicken broth
1 1/2 pounds fish fillets (sole or any lowfat fish)
2 tablespoons fresh lemon juice
2 large tomatoes, thinly sliced or coarsely diced
1/2 medium green pepper, finely chopped
1/2 cup whole wheat bread crumbs (1 or 2 slices)
1/2 teaspoon dried basil

Place onion slices in the bottom of an 8 x 12-inch baking dish. Spread mushrooms evenly over onion and add water. Place fish in a layer over the mushrooms and season with lemon juice. Place tomato on the fish and sprinkle with green pepper. Put bread and basil in blender and pulse to make fine crumbs. Sprinkle crumbs over all. Bake uncovered for 25 minutes. Serve immediately.

Bake: 350° 25 min   **Yield: 6 servings**

Per Serving	RCU	FU	Cal	% Ft	P	F	C	Na
	0	0	140	2	22	0	10	120

Baked Fish Fillets

This gives a new taste to any fish fillets.
Menu: Oven potato fries, creamed carrots, green salad

2 pounds sole fillets, fresh or frozen
1/4 teaspoon salt
Dash pepper
1/4 teaspoon paprika
1/2 lemon, juiced

White sauce:
1 teaspoon butter
2 tablespoons flour
1/4 teaspoon salt
Dash pepper
1 teaspoon dry mustard
1 cup skim milk

2 slices whole wheat bread
1 teaspoon butter
1 tablespoon minced parsley

Line a baking sheet with foil, dull side up. Cut fish into serving pieces, and place on baking sheet. Sprinkle with salt, pepper, paprika, and lemon juice. Make white sauce by melting butter and adding flour, salt, pepper, dry mustard, and milk. Cook until thick. Pour white sauce over fish. Place bread and 1 teaspoon butter into blender. Pulse to make crumbs. Sprinkle over fish. Sprinkle with the parsley. Bake in a 350° oven for 25 to 30 minutes. Serve immediately.

Microwave: Use a 9 x 13-inch baking dish. Cover loosely with waxed paper. Cook on high for 10-12 minutes or until fish flakes easily with a fork. Do not overcook. Rotate dish once.

Bake: 350° 30-35 min
Microwave: High 10-12 min   **Yield: 8 servings**

Per Serving	RCU	FU	Cal	% Ft	P	F	C	Na
	0	0	128	9	21	1	5	309

Fish 'n Spinach Roll-ups

They're surprisingly easy and very gourmet!
Menu: Spanish rice, steamed broccoli, fresh vegetable plate

1 10-ounce package frozen chopped spinach
1 1/2 cups whole wheat bread crumbs (use blender)
3 eggs, slightly beaten
1 pound sole fillets
1 10 3/4-ounce can cream of mushroom soup, low fat
1/4 cup Parmesan cheese

Cook spinach according to package directions. Drain well. Combine spinach with bread crumbs and eggs. Evenly divide stuffing among fillets. Wrap fillet around stuffing, and place seam-side down in a flat baking dish. Heat soup and add cheese to make sauce. Cover fish with half the sauce. Bake uncovered in a 350° oven for 25 to 30 minutes. Pour remaining sauce over fish, and serve immediately.

Microwave: Cover with waxed paper. Microwave on high for 6-8 minutes. Don't overcook.

Bake: 350° 25-30 min
Microwave: High 6-8 min   **Yield: 4-6 servings**

Tip: Cut fish into serving-size pieces. Combine spinach, bread crumbs, and eggs. Spread 2 tablespoons sauce on bottom of 7 x 12-inch baking dish. Arrange half the fish on bottom of the dish. Cover evenly with the spinach mixture. Put remaining fish on top layer and cover with remaining sauce. Sprinkle with 1/2 cup bread crumbs.

Per Serving	RCU	FU	Cal	% Ft	P	F	C	Na
	0	1	191	27	20	6	13	461

Baked Whole Salmon

Menu: Rice pilaf, seasoned veggie combo tray, creamy coleslaw

1 whole fresh salmon

Place salmon on foil-lined baking sheet. Lightly coat fish with vegetable oil. Bake 10 minutes per pound in a 400° oven. Do not overcook. Serve immediately; fish becomes soggy if allowed to stand.

Bake: 400° 10 min per pound

Per Serving	RCU	FU	Cal	% Ft	P	F	C	Na
	0	2	220	61	21	15	0	51

Baked Fish Fillets

Place fillets on a foil-lined baking sheet.
Bake: 400° 20 min

Baked Fish Steaks

Place salmon steaks on a foil-lined baking sheet.
Bake: 400° 30 min or until fish flakes easily

Juicy Salmon Loaf

You can prepare this loaf in 5 minutes.
Menu: Creamed peas and potatoes, beets, fresh vegetables

1 15 1/2-ounce can salmon, undrained or 2 6 1/2 ounce cans tuna
1 egg, slightly beaten
1/3 cup skim milk
1 1/2 cups soft whole wheat bread crumbs (use blender)
1 cup cooked brown rice (optional)
2 teaspoons instant minced onion or 4 chopped green onions
1 tablespoon lemon juice
1/8 teaspoon salt
1/8 teaspoon pepper

Remove skin from salmon. Gently flake fish with a fork. Combine all ingredients. Press into a shallow 1-quart baking dish. Bake uncovered in a 350° oven for 30 minutes or just until set. Do not overbake. After baking, loosen sides of loaf with knife. Let stand in pan 5 minutes before serving.

Microwave: Use a glass baking dish. Cover with waxed paper. Cook on high power for 8-10 minutes. Rotate dish once.

Bake: 350° 30 min
Microwave: High 8-10 min   Yield: 6 servings

Per Serving	RCU	FU	Cal	% Ft	P	F	C	Na
	0	1	181	45	13	9	12	433

Salmon Patties

Prepare Juicy Salmon Loaf as directed. Shape into patties. Cook on a nonstick grill until golden brown on each side.

Tuna and Rice Quiche

This quiche can be varied using different meats and vegetables, such as cooked turkey or asparagus.
Menu: Baked yams, mushroom green beans, green salad

1 10-ounce package frozen chopped broccoli
1 1/2 cups cooked brown rice
1/2 cup finely shredded cheese
3 eggs

1/3 cup skim milk
1/4 teaspoon salt
1 6-ounce can water-packed tuna, drained

Place package of broccoli on paper towel in microwave; cook on high 5-6 minutes. Or cook broccoli following package directions until almost tender. Drain well. Combine rice, 1/4 cup cheese, and 1 egg. Press evenly over the bottom and 1/2-inch up the sides of a 9-inch glass pie plate or quiche dish. Layer broccoli and tuna evenly over rice mix. Beat remaining 2 eggs with milk and salt. Pour egg mixture over tuna. Sprinkle with remaining cheese. Bake uncovered in a 350° oven for 25 to 30 minutes.

Microwave: Cover with paper towel. Cook at 70% power for 14-16 minutes or until center is just about set. Rotate dish once. Let stand 5 minutes before serving.

Microwave: 70% 14-16 min
Bake: 350° 25-30 min   Yield: 6 servings

Per Serving	RCU	FU	Cal	% Ft	P	F	C	Na
	0	1	174	38	16	7	12	587

Tuna Macaroni Bake

Here's just the dish for a quick supper.
Menu: Ranchero beans, petite peas, carrot salad

2 eggs
1/2 cup water
3/4 cup evaporated low-fat milk
1 scant teaspoon dry mustard
1 teaspoon instant minced onion
1/2 teaspoon salt

3 cups cooked vegetable macaroni (spinach or tomato)
1 6 1/2-ounce can water-packed tuna, drained
2 tablespoons finely shredded cheese
1 cup chili sauce or green chile salsa

Beat eggs, and add remaining ingredients except cheese and chili sauce. Gently fold together. Place in a medium-size baking dish. Sprinkle with cheese. Cover, and bake in a 375° oven for 25 to 30 minutes. Top with chili sauce and serve immediately. Microwave: Cook on 80 percent power for 12 to 14 minutes. Rotate dish twice. Let stand 5 minutes before serving.

Bake: 375° 25-30 min
Microwave: 80% 12-14 min   Yield: 6 servings

Per Serving	RCU	FU	Cal	% Ft	P	F	C	Na
	0	1	319	12	20	4	52	820

Broccoli with Tuna or Chicken Sauce

Tuna and broccoli make a tasty combination.
Menu: Frozen corn, green salad

2 tablespoons butter or margarine
1/4 cup flour
1/2 teaspoon salt
Pinch of pepper
1 teaspoon instant minced onion
1/2 teaspoon chicken bouillon granules
2 cups skim milk
2 6 1/2-ounce cans water-packed tuna, drained
 or 2 cups cooked chicken pieces
1/2 cup slivered almonds
1 20-ounce package frozen broccoli spears, cooked
 or 1 bunch (4 cups) fresh broccoli spears, cooked
2 tablespoons Parmesan cheese (optional)

Melt butter, and blend in flour, salt, pepper, onion and bouillon. Add milk and cook over medium heat, stirring constantly until thick. Add tuna or chicken and half the almonds. Arrange broccoli in a 2-quart casserole dish and pour meat sauce over broccoli. Top with cheese and remaining almonds. Serve immediately, or bake in a 375° oven for 15 minutes.

Microwave: Cover with waxed paper. Microwave on high for 5 to 7 minutes or until hot and bubbly. Sprinkle with cheese.

Bake: **375° 15 min**
Microwave: High 5-7 min **Yield: 6 servings**

Per Serving	RCU	FU	Cal	% Ft	P	F	C	Na
	0	1	145	35	17	6	9	438

One-Dish Macaroni and Cheese

This is an unusually good macaroni and cheese recipe.
Menu: Marinated vegetables

1 tablespoon butter or margarine
1 onion, chopped
2 cups uncooked vegetable macaroni
1/2 teaspoon salt
Dash pepper
1/8 teaspoon oregano
1/2 teaspoon dry mustard
2 cups water
2 tablespoons flour
1 12-ounce can evaporated lowfat milk
1/2 cup finely shredded sharp cheese

In electric fry pan, melt butter. Add onion, uncooked macaroni, salt, pepper, oregano and dry mustard. Cook on low, stirring occasionally for 5-7 minutes or until onion looks clear. Add water and bring to a boil. Cover and simmer on low for 8 to 10 minutes or until macaroni is tender. Sprinkle flour over macaroni. Stir to mix well. Stir in milk and cheese, adding additional milk if needed to thin to desired consistency. Heat through and serve.

Cook: 25 minutes   **Yield: 6-8 servings**

Per Serving	RCU	FU	Cal	% Ft	P	F	C	Na
	0	1	177	21	9	4	27	243

WOK COOKERY

Once you have tried this simple method of cooking, you will use it often to prepare quick, nourishing, lowfat meals. These recipes are truly "eat yourself thin" dishes. Try them all for the variety they provide. Your choices should vary according to the season and the foods available to you.

A heavy, nonelectric wok is preferred because you can control the high temperature much easier, and the sides get hot. This aids in quality stir-fry cooking. However, any heavy frying pan or wok will do.

Use high heat. Put a little chicken broth or water in the pan before adding ingredients. Cut meat into thin strips. Diagonal slicing is great for vegetables. Stir-fry the slowest-cooking meats and vegetables first, adding the remaining ingredients as you go.

Continually stir the food as it cooks.

The key to stir-frying success is to have everything ready *before* you start. Cooking time is minimal; there's not time to stop and prepare ingredients as you go. However, if you have forgotten something, don't panic! Take the wok or fry pan off the heat. Remove the ingredients, and toss them to cool slightly and slow the cooking process. Prepare and stir-fry the forgotten item. Add your partially cooked foods, and continue. No one will know that you had a momentary pause.

Quick Chicken Broccoli Stir Fry

This pleasing combination of flavors cooks in a hurry. Keep some cooked brown rice on hand for a quick meal.
Menu: Ranchero beans or white beans, hot rolls or muffins

2 whole chicken breasts, boned and skinned
2 to 3 tablespoons soy sauce
1 tablespoon cornstarch
1/4 cup chicken broth or water
1 bunch green onions, sliced, or 1 large onion, sliced
1 20-ounce package frozen broccoli, slightly thawed
    or 4 cups fresh broccoli florets
3 cups cooked brown rice (1 cup uncooked)

Cut chicken crosswise into 1/2-inch strips. Put soy sauce in a 2-cup measuring cup, and add enough water to make 1 cup. Stir in cornstarch, and set aside. Prepare all ingredients as directed. Heat wok, and add chicken broth or water. Stir-fry chicken until meat is white, 1 to 2 minutes. Add vegetables, and stir-fry over high heat until vegetables are tender-crisp. Cover, and steam 1 to 2 minutes. Add cornstarch mixture, and stir until sauce is thick and clear. Serve immediately over hot brown rice.

Tip: Use 1 cup canned chicken chunks in place of chicken breasts if desired. Add chicken after vegetables are tender.
Cook: 5 min   **Yield: 3-4 servings**

Per Serving	RCU	FU	Cal	% Ft	P	F	C	Na
	0	0	154	15	22	3	16	708

Stir-Fry Veggies

Use your fresh garden vegetables—any or all. This is a basic recipe, so add your own variations.
The meat is optional.
Menu: Add bread, and you have a complete meal.

1 cup water
2 to 4 tablespoons soy sauce
1 rounded tablespoon cornstarch
1/4 cup chicken broth or water
1-2 chicken breasts, skinned and thinly sliced
  or 1/2 pound lean beef, thinly sliced
  or 1/2 pound extra-lean ground beef (meat is optional)
1 medium onion, sliced
3 stalks celery, diagonally sliced

Add any of the following vegetables as desired:
1 green pepper, sliced
2 carrots, coarsely shredded or sliced into matchstick pieces
1 small zucchini, sliced or cut into julienne strips
1/2 small yellow summer squash, sliced
1 cup shredded cabbage
1 cup broccoli florets
1 cup cauliflower florets
1 cup snow peas

3 cups cooked brown rice (1 cup uncooked)

Mix water, soy sauce, and cornstarch. Set aside. Heat wok, and add chicken broth or water. Stir-fry meat until tender, 1 to 2 minutes. Remove meat, and add vegetables. Stir-fry over high heat 2-5 minutes or until vegetables are tender-crisp. The time will depend on how many vegetables you use. Return meat to wok. Cover, and let steam 1 to 2 minutes. Add water-cornstarch mixture. Cook and stir until sauce is thick and clear. Serve immediately over hot brown rice.

Tip: Two 3-ounce packages whole wheat or brown rice ramen noodles may be added for variety. Soak noodles in very hot water for 5 minutes. Drain well. Add noodles when meat is returned to wok. Stir the flavor packets into the cornstarch-water mixture for added flavor.

Cook: 8-10 min   **Yield: 6-8 servings**

Per Serving	RCU	FU	Cal	% Ft	P	F	C	Na
	0	0	165	7	11	1	28	380

Oriental Chicken and Shrimp

Shrimp makes this delightfully different.
Menu: Baked yams or ranchero beans, hot bread or rolls

1 cup chicken broth
1 tablespoon cider vinegar
1 teaspoon brown sugar
1 teaspoon grated fresh ginger root
1 clove garlic, minced
1 tablespoon cornstarch
1/4 cup chicken broth or water
1 to 2 chicken breasts, boned, skinned and cut into 1 inch pieces
12 medium shrimp, shelled and deveined
2 cups fresh broccoli florets
1 small red bell pepper, cut into thin strips
4 green onions, sliced
3 cups cooked brown rice (1 cup uncooked)

Mix broth, vinegar, brown sugar, ginger root, garlic and cornstarch in a 2-cup measure. Set aside. Heat wok to very hot. Add chicken broth or water. Stir-fry chicken and shrimp for 1 to 2 minutes. Remove from wok and set aside. Add broccoli and red bell pepper. Stir-fry 1 to 2 minutes or until peppers are tender-crisp. Return chicken and shrimp to wok. Cover and let steam 1 to 2 minutes. Pour over vegetables. Cook and stir until sauce thickens and coats mixture. Sprinkle with green onions. Serve over hot brown rice.

Cook: 6-10 min   **Yield: 4 servings**

Per Serving	RCU	FU	Cal	% Ft	P	F	C	Na
	0	0	263	7	17	2	46	37

Chicken Pineapple Stir-Fry

Sweet 'n sour chicken never tasted better.
Menu: Baked squash or white beans, hot muffins

1 15-ounce can unsweetened pineapple tidbits
1 cup chicken broth or water
1 to 2 tablespoons soy sauce
1 tablespoon cornstarch
2 to 3 tablespoons brown sugar or honey (to taste)
1/4 cup chicken broth or water
2 medium carrots, thinly sliced
2 stalks celery, sliced diagonally
1 small onion, quartered or sliced
1 cup fresh broccoli florets
1 cup snow peas (optional)
1/4 teaspoon ground ginger
2 6 3/4-ounce cans chicken
3 cups cooked brown rice (1 cup uncooked)

good

Drain juice from pineapple. Reserve pineapple. In a 2-cup measure, combine pineapple juice, 2/3 cup chicken broth, soy sauce, cornstarch, and brown sugar. Set aside. Heat wok to hot, and add 1/3 cup chicken broth or water. Add carrots, celery, onion, broccoli, and ginger. Stir-fry until vegetables are tender-crisp, 3 to 4 minutes. Add peas, pineapple, and chicken. Cover, and steam 1 to 2 minutes. Stir in cornstarch mixture. Cook and stir until sauce is thick and clear. Serve over brown rice.

Cook: 6 to 7 min   Yield: 6 servings

Per Serving	RCU	FU	Cal	% Ft	P	F	C	Na
	0	0	165	12	20	2	15	316

Chicken Cantonese

Try this Cantonese cuisine for a nice change of flavor.
Menu: Baked yams, refried beans, hot biscuits

1 cup chicken broth
2 tablespoons cornstarch
2 to 3 tablespoons soy sauce
2 chicken breasts
1/2 teaspoon garlic salt
1 teaspoon paprika
1/4 cup chicken broth or water
1 large onion, cut in half lengthwise and sliced
2 medium green peppers, cut in thin strips
2-3 stalks celery, diagonally sliced
2-3 large fresh tomatoes, cut in eighths
3 cups hot cooked brown rice (1 cup uncooked)

Mix 1/2 cup broth with cornstarch and soy sauce. Skin and bone chicken breasts. Cut meat in thin strips. Sprinkle with seasonings. Prepare vegetables as directed. Heat wok to hot, and saute chicken in chicken broth or water about 2 minutes. Add onion, green peppers, celery, and 1/2 cup broth. Stir-fry for 2-3 minutes. Cover and steam 2 minutes. Stir cornstarch mix into chicken and vegetables. Add tomatoes; cook and stir about 2 more minutes or until sauce is hot and slightly thickened. Serve immediately over hot rice.

Cook: 6 to 7 min   **Yield: 5-6 servings**

Per Serving	RCU	FU	Cal	% Ft	P	F	C	Na
	0	0	207	7	14	2	35	648

Chow Mein 'n Noodles

This is a flavorful meal.
Menu: Fried rice, hot rolls or muffins

1/2 to 1 pound boneless raw chicken
1 tablespoon soy sauce
1 tablespoon water
1/4 teaspoon garlic powder
1 teaspoon oil
1 teaspoon cornstarch
2 3-ounce packages whole wheat or brown rice ramen noodles
1/4 cup chicken broth or water
2 green onions, sliced
2 cups shredded cabbage
2 carrots, cut into julienne strips or coarsely grated
3 stalks celery, diagonally sliced
1 cup snow peas (optional)

Cut chicken into very thin strips. Mix soy sauce, water, garlic powder, oil, and cornstarch. Marinate meat in the sauce. Cover ramen noodles with very hot water. Let sit a few minutes. Drain and set aside. Heat wok or frying pan to very hot. Add chicken broth or water. Add meat, and stir-fry until meat loses its color, about 2 minutes. Remove meat from wok. Add green onions and stir-fry for a few seconds. Add cabbage, carrots, celery, and peas. Stir-fry 1 to 3 minutes. Return meat to wok; add the noodles. Cover and let steam for 1 minute. Sprinkle flavor packets from ramen noodles over all. Toss. Serve immediately.

Cook: 5-6 min   Yield: 6-8 servings

Per Serving	RCU	FU	Cal	% Ft	P	F	C	Na
	0	0	221	10	20	2	31	296

Stir-Fry Romaine and Mushrooms

Vall Gene Mill's stir-fry is great for patio entertaining.
Menu: Teriyaki chicken kabobs, potato salad, rolls, summer delight fresh fruit salad

2 tablespoons soy sauce
1 tablespoon sesame oil
2 teaspoons white wine vinegar
1 teaspoon sugar
1 scant tablespoon peanut oil

2 heads romaine lettuce, sliced in 1-inch strips
1/3 pound mushrooms, sliced
3 scallions or green onions, minced
2 tablespoons sesame seeds, toasted

Mix soy sauce, sesame oil, vinegar, and sugar in a small bowl. Set aside. Heat wok to hot and add peanut oil. Reduce heat to medium-high, and add lettuce and mushrooms. Toss lightly, and stir-fry 2 minutes. Pour sauce mixture over lettuce and mushrooms. Remove from heat, cover, and let stand 2 minutes. Sprinkle with scallions and sesame seeds. Serve immediately.

Cook: 4-5 min   Yield: 6-8 servings

Per Serving	RCU	FU	Cal	% Ft	P	F	C	Na
	0	1	77	53	3	5	6	337

Summer Medley

This dish complements any meal.
Menu: Steamed brown rice, lemon chicken

1/4 cup chicken broth or water
2 large onions, chopped
1 large green pepper, chopped
2 cups fresh mushrooms, sliced
2 medium zucchini, chopped
1 cup snow peas (optional)

1/4 to 1/2 teaspoon garlic salt
1 teaspoon leaf oregano or 1/2 teaspoon
  powdered oregano
3 large tomatoes, chopped
2 tablespoons Parmesan cheese

Heat wok or large fry pan until hot. Add broth and saute' onions, green peppers, mushrooms, and zucchini for 3 to 4 minutes. Season with garlic salt and oregano. When vegetables appear almost transparent, add tomatoes. Cook an additional 2-3 minutes. Sprinkle with cheese. Cover and simmer for 3-4 minutes. Serve immediately over hot brown rice if desired.

Cook: 10 min   Yield: 6-8 servings

Per Serving	RCU	FU	Cal	% Ft	P	F	C	Na
	0	0	48	7	3	0	10	81

Fried Rice

You will soon learn to vary this to suit your own taste.
Serve with stir-fry or as a side dish at any meal.

2 tablespoons chicken broth or 1 tablespoon oil
1 small onion, finely chopped
1 small green pepper, finely chopped
1/2 cup sliced mushrooms
4 cups cold cooked brown rice
2 tablespoons Tamari or soy sauce
1 cup finely cooked and diced meat (optional)
1 egg, slightly beaten
1 green onion, minced

Heat wok to hot; add broth or oil. Add onion, green pepper, and mushrooms. Stir-fry 1 minute. Add rice, Tamari or soy sauce, and meat, if desired. Stir-fry 2 minutes or until hot. Pour egg over rice, and stir-fry 1 to 2 minutes or until eggs are set. Sprinkle with minced green onions.

Cook: 5 min   **Yield: 4-6 servings**

Per Serving	RCU	FU	Cal	% Ft	P	F	C	Na
	0	0	160	16	5	3	33	549

BEEF MAIN DISHES

We've included a large number of beef recipes because beef is popular and easily available. These recipes combine beef with vegetables, whole grains, and other complex carbohydrates, often using the beef more as a condiment than as a main ingredient.

Buy extra-lean ground beef. For convenience, brown the meat, drain it well, and discard the fat. Place in a colander and rinse with hot water to remove additional fat if desired. Package cooked meat in recipe size portions for the freezer. One cup cooked and drained ground beef is approximately 1/2 pound.

Roast Beef and Veggies Dinner

A heart-warming one-dish meal for a cold day.
Menu: Frozen corn, creamy coleslaw, hot rolls

1 3- to 4-pound lean pot roast
Garlic salt and pepper
Whole wheat flour
8 medium carrots, peeled and cut into strips
6-8 potatoes, peeled and cut in half
2 large onions, peeled and sliced
2 to 3 tablespoons cornstarch

Trim and discard all fat from meat. Season roast with garlic salt and pepper. Sprinkle with whole wheat flour. Brown on both sides in a heavy pan. Add carrots, potatoes, and onion. Sprinkle vegetables with salt and pepper. Cover and bake 3 to 4 hours, adding a little water if needed. (For longer, slower cooking, bake in a 250° oven or electric fry pan for 5 to 6 hours or in a slow cooker.) Remove meat and vegetables. Defat drippings.* Add additional water if needed for gravy. To make gravy, mix cornstarch with a small amount of water. Add to hot liquid, stirring until thick. Season to taste. Use leftover meat to make pepper steak.
Bake: 325° 3-4 hours or 275° 5-6 hours   Yield: 8-10 servings

Per Serving	RCU	FU	Cal	% Ft	P	F	C	Na
	0	2	358	33	30	13	32	84

Mushroom Swiss Steak

This fork-tender meat is smothered with vegetables and gravy.
Use the Slim Cream Soup Mix* to lower the fat content.
Menu: Vegetable relish tray, petite peas, hot rolls

2 pounds venison or beef round steak
1/2 teaspoon garlic salt
1 cup whole wheat flour

Mushroom Sauce:
1 10 3/4-ounce can cream of mushroom soup, low fat
1 soup can water
1 4-ounce can mushrooms, undrained
1 medium onion, finely chopped
6 potatoes, peeled and halved
6 carrots, peeled and cut in chunks

Cut steak in small serving pieces. Season with garlic salt, and coat with whole wheat flour. Brown in a nonstick frying pan without adding any oil. In a large roasting pan, combine and heat sauce ingredients. Drop browned steak into sauce; add potatoes and carrots. Cover. Meat may be simmered on stove for about 1 1/2 hours, baked in a 250° oven for 4 to 5 hours, or baked in a 325° oven for 2 hours.

Microwave: Put ingredients into a large baking dish. Cover and cook on high for 10 minutes. Rotate dish and cook at 50 percent power for 35 to 40 minutes or until tender.

Simmer: 1 1/2 hours
Bake: 325° 2 hours
Microwave: High 10 min   50% power 35-40 min   Yield: 10-12 servings

Per Serving	RCU	FU	Cal	% Ft	P	F	C	Na
Venison	0	1	227	23	21	6	28	334
Beef	0	2	352	36	30	14	26	298

Spanish Swiss Steak

Follow directions for Mushroom Swiss Steak, omitting the mushroom sauce using the following:

1 28-ounce can tomatoes, slightly blended
1 large onion, thinly sliced
1 green pepper, diced
   or use 2 cups mild salsa and 1 cup tomatoes

Per Serving	RCU	FU	Cal	% Ft	P	F	C	Na
Venison	0	1	247	23	21	6	40	244
Beef	0	2	369	35	30	14	30	251

Pepper Steak with Rice

The subtle blending of flavors makes this a mouth-watering treat.
Menu: Baked squash, petite peas, carrot sticks

1 pound beef or venison round steak, cut into thin strips
1 tablespoon paprika
2 cloves garlic, minced
1 1/2 cups beef broth or 1   14 1/2-ounce can beef broth
1 cup sliced green onion, including tops
2 green peppers, cut in strips
2 tablespoons cornstarch
1/2 cup water
1/4 cup soy sauce
2 large fresh tomatoes, cut in eighths
3 cups hot cooked brown rice (1 cup uncooked)

Put rice on to cook. Sprinkle meat with paprika; let stand while preparing other ingredients. Brown meat in a nonstick frying pan. Add garlic and broth. Cover and simmer 30 minutes. Stir in onion and green pepper. Cover and cook 5 minutes. Mix cornstarch, water, and soy sauce. Stir into meat mixture. Cook and stir until thick and clear, about 2 minutes. Add tomatoes, and stir gently. Serve over brown rice.

Cook: 35 min   Yield: 6 servings

Per Serving	RCU	FU	Cal	% Ft	P	F	C	Na
	0	2	351	31	25	12	34	908

Moist Meatloaf

Those good old-fashioned flavors really come through.
Menu: Scalloped potatoes, steamed green beans, raw vegetables

3 slices whole wheat bread or 1 cup oatmeal
1 cup tomato sauce or skim milk
1 pound extra-lean ground beef
1 egg
1 onion, chopped or 1 tablespoon instant minced onion
1/2 teaspoon salt
1/2 teaspoon pepper
1 8-ounce can tomato sauce

Break bread into small pieces and soak in tomato sauce or milk for 5 minutes. Add remaining ingredients. Mix lightly but well. Place in a loaf pan. Cover with tomato sauce. Bake in a 350° oven for 1 hour.

Microwave: Place in 8 x 8-inch baking dish. Cover with waxed paper. Cook on 70 percent power for 16 to 18 minutes. Rotate dish twice.

Bake: 350° 1 hour
Microwave: 70% 16-18 min   Yield: 6-8 servings

Per Serving	RCU	FU	Cal	% Ft	P	F	C	Na
	0	1	184	37	17	8	11	506

Porcupine Meatballs

These meatballs make hearty eating. This recipe works well in a slow cooker.
Menu: Steamed broccoli, sliced tomatoes and cucumbers.

1 pound extra-lean ground beef   **4 cups tomato juice**
1 cup cooked brown rice   **2-4 tablespoons Worcestershire or soy sauce**
2 tablespoons finely diced onion   **1 teaspoon sugar**
1/2 teaspoon salt   **Salt and pepper**
1 egg, slightly beaten   **6 baked potatoes**

Mix the first five ingredients, adding 1/4 cup of the tomato juice if mix seems dry. Shape into small balls. Mix tomato juice, Worcestershire Sauce and sugar in a medium saucepan; season to taste with salt and pepper. Bring mixture to a boil and add meatballs. Simmer about 20 minutes or until meat is tender. Serve over baked potatoes.

Cook: 20 min   Yield: 6 servings

Per Serving	RCU	FU	Cal	% Ft	P	F	C	Na
	0	2	338	27	27	10	37	541

Poor Man's Steak

This is more tender and has better flavor than any cubed steak!
Menu: Baked potatoes, frozen petite peas, green salad

Steaks:
1 pound extra lean ground beef
1 1/2 cups whole wheat bread crumbs (3-4 slices bread)
1/2 cup skim milk
1/2 1 1/4-ounce package dry onion soup mix
1 egg
Salt and pepper (optional)

Sauce:
1 10 3/4-ounce can cream of mushroom soup, low fat
1 soup can skim milk
1/2 - 1 1/4-ounce package dry onion soup mix
1 4-ounce can mushrooms, drained

6 large potatoes, baked

Put bread in blender to make fine crumbs. Combine the steak ingredients and mix well. Press into a 7 x 12-inch pan. Chill 30 minutes to 1 hour. Cut meat into 6 pieces. Coat each piece with whole wheat flour. Brown in a nonstick pan, and place in a 9 x 13-inch baking dish. To make sauce, mix soup and milk. Add the remaining 1/2 package onion soup mix and mushrooms. Pour over meat and cover. Simmer on stove or bake in a 325° oven for 1 hour.

Microwave: Cover with plastic wrap, cook on high for 10 minutes, then at 50 percent power for 35 to 40 minutes, turning dish twice.

Simmer: 1 hour
Bake: **325° 1 hour**
Microwave: High 10 min or 50% 35-40 min   **Yield: 6 servings**

Per Serving	RCU	FU	Cal	% Ft	P	F	C	Na
	0	1	336	25	23	9	39	772

Sweet 'n Sour Meatballs

Use this for entertaining or for everyday eating.
Menu: Seasoned veggie combo, baked beans

2 cups long grain brown rice
5 cups water

1 pound extra-lean ground beef
1/2 cup uncooked wheat, finely cracked (use blender)
1/2 cup water chestnuts, drained and chopped
1/2 cup crushed pineapple (use 16-ounce can; reserve remaining fruit and juice)
1/2 teaspoon ginger
1/4 teaspoon sage
1 egg
1/4 cup milk
1 teaspoon salt

Steam brown rice for 45-50 minutes while preparing meatballs.
Place ground beef in mixer bowl. Put dry wheat into blender and turn to high speed for 30-40 seconds. Add wheat to beef. Drain water chestnuts and put in blender. Pulse to chop coarsely. Drain pineapple. Reserve liquid and remaining fruit for sauce. Add remaining ingredients to beef and mix well. Chill 30 minutes. Form into balls size of walnuts. Place on large foil-lined baking sheet and bake at 375° for 20 minutes.

Sauce:
2-3 tablespoons soy sauce
1/4 cup vinegar
1/2 cup brown sugar
1 1/2 cups pineapple and juice (use remainder of 16-ounce can)
2 teaspoons beef bouillon granules
3 cups water
2 tablespoons cornstarch

Put soy sauce, vinegar, brown sugar, pineapple and juice, beef bouillon and 2 cups water in pan. Mix cornstarch with 1 cup water. Stir into other ingredients. Cook over medium heat, stirring constantly until thick. With tongs, lift meatballs out of drippings and put into sauce. Discard drippings. Cook gently in sauce 10-12 minutes. Serve over brown rice.

Bake: 375° 20 min
Cook: 10-12 min   Yield: 50 meatballs   Serves 10

Per Serving	RCU	FU	Cal	% Ft	P	F	C	Na
	1	1	310	20	17	7	45	567

Swedish Meatballs

Fine for company.
Menu: Brussel sprouts, green salad, fruit 'n berry compote

Meatballs:
1 egg
1 onion, chopped, or 1 tablespoon instant minced onion
1 cup mashed potatoes
1/4 cup whole wheat bread crumbs
1 pound lean ground beef
1/2 teaspoon salt

Gravy:
1 10 3/4-ounce can cream of mushroom soup, low fat
1 4-ounce can mushrooms, drained
1/2 cup plain nonfat yogurt or buttermilk

3 cups cooked brown rice (1 cup raw) or 6 baked potatoes
Fresh parsley

Mix meatball ingredients and shape into walnut-size balls. Place on a large, foil-lined baking sheet. Bake in a 400° oven for 15 minutes or until done. To microwave, place in a baking dish and cover with waxed paper. Cook at 70 percent power for 8 to 10 minutes or until meatballs are no longer pink. Turn dish twice. While meat is cooking, heat soup. Add yogurt or buttermilk, and blend until smooth. Using kitchen tongs, add meatballs to gravy. Serve over rice or potatoes. Garnish with fresh parsley.

Bake: 400° 15 min
Microwave: 70% 1-10 min   Yield: 6-8 servings

Per Serving	RCU	FU	Cal	% Ft	P	F	C	Na
	0	2	304	28	22	10	33	698

Beef Stroganoff

This favorite also makes a good baked potato topper.
Menu: Frozen petite peas, white beans, carrot salad.

1 pound extra-lean ground beef
   or round steak cut into thin, narrow strips
1 onion, minced
1 clove garlic, minced
1/4 cup flour
1/2 teaspoon salt
1/4 teaspoon pepper
1 8-ounce can mushrooms, sliced
1 1 1/2-ounce package Stroganoff Sauce Mix (optional)
1 10 3/4-ounce can cream of mushroom soup, low fat
1 cup nonfat sour cream or buttermilk
3 cups cooked brown rice, noodles or 6-8 baked potatoes
2 tablespoons minced parsley

    Brown ground beef with onion and garlic. Drain well. Add flour, salt, pepper and mushrooms. Cook 5 minutes. Stir in sauce mix and soup. Simmer uncovered for 10 minutes. Just before serving, stir in sour cream or buttermilk and heat through. Thin with a little milk if desired. Serve over hot rice, noodles, or potatoes. Garnish with parsley.

Cook: 20 min   **Yield: 6 servings**

Per Serving	RCU	FU	Cal	% Ft	P	F	C	Na
	0	1	343	26	25	10	35	607

Swedish Hot Dish

This hearty one-dish meal has a delicious combination of flavors.
Menu: Saucy beets, creamy coleslaw

4 medium potatoes, peeled and sliced
1/4 cup raw brown rice or 1 cup cooked rice
1 onion, diced or sliced
1 pound extra-lean ground beef
1/2 teaspoon salt
5 medium carrots, peeled and grated
2 cups cooked tomatoes, slightly blended or tomato juice
Pepper to taste

Place potatoes on the bottom of a 9 x 13-inch baking dish. Sprinkle raw rice, onion, and half the salt over potatoes. Break raw ground beef into small chunks and layer it over the onion. Season with remaining salt. Layer grated carrots over meat. Pour tomatoes evenly over carrots, and season lightly with pepper. Cover and bake in a 325° oven for 1 1/2-2 hours. Microwave: Prepare as above but use cooked rice. Cover with plastic wrap. Cook on 70 percent power for 34 to 38 minutes, turning dish twice. Let stand 5 minutes before serving.

Bake: 325° 1 1/2-2 hrs
Microwave: 70% 34-38 min   Yield: 8 servings

Per Serving	RCU	FU	Cal	% Ft	P	F	C	Na
	0	1	226	27	19	7	23	248

Savory Goulash

The name may not sound spectacular, but the eatin' is.
Menu: Baked squash, steamed broccoli, green salad

2 cups uncooked noodles
1/2 pound extra-lean ground beef
1 large onion, minced
2 cups diced celery

2 cups cooked tomatoes
2 carrots, peeled and thinly sliced
1/2 teaspoon salt
Dash of pepper

Cook noodles in boiling salted water. Drain. Brown ground beef, onion, and celery. Drain well. Add noodles, tomatoes, and carrots. Season with salt and pepper if desired. Cover and simmer for 20 to 30 minutes.

Microwave: Cover with waxed paper, and cook at 80 percent power for 14 to 16 minutes.

Stove: 20-30 min
Microwave: 80% 14-16 min   Yield: 6-8 servings

Per Serving	RCU	FU	Cal	% Ft	P	F	C	Na
	1	1	167	23	12	4	21	258

Oh Boy Casserole

This good year-round dish comes from Mary Merrill.
Menu: Swiss chard 'n lemon juice, summer squash, tomatoes

1 pound extra-lean ground beef
1 large onion, chopped
4 stalks celery, thinly sliced or chopped
1 10 3/4-ounce can cream of chicken soup, low fat
1 10 3/4-ounce can cream of mushroom soup, low fat
2 to 4 tablespoons soy sauce
2 cups cooked brown rice
1 14-ounce can bean sprouts, drained
1 4-ounce can water chestnuts, drained and sliced (optional)
1 4-ounce can mushrooms, drained
2 cups Chinese noodles (optional)

Brown the ground beef, onion, and celery. Drain well. Add soup and soy sauce. Stir to mix. Fold in rice, bean sprouts, water chestnuts, and mushrooms. Pour into a 9 x 13-inch casserole dish. Cover. Bake in a 350° oven for 25 minutes or until hot and bubbly. Sprinkle with chinese noodles if desired. Bake 5 more minutes uncovered before serving.

Microwave: Cover loosely with waxed paper and cook on 80 percent power for 14 to 16 minutes.

Bake: 350° **20-30 min**
Microwave: 80% **14-16 min**   **Yield: 6-8 servings**

Per Serving	RCU	FU	Cal	% Ft	P	F	C	Na
	0	1	209	30	16	7	22	910

Taglarinni

Barbara Payne's large family enjoys this quick flavorful dish.
Menu: Marinated vegetables

1/2-1 pound extra-lean ground beef
1 onion, chopped
1 4-ounce can mushrooms, drained
1 17-ounce can corn, drained
1 2 1/4-ounce can sliced olives (optional)

1 10 3/4-ounce can cream of tomato soup
1 1 1/2-ounce package spaghetti sauce mix
1/2 cup water
3 cups noodles, cooked and drained

Brown ground beef and onion. Drain well. Add mushrooms, corn, olives, and soup. Dissolve spaghetti sauce mix with water. Add to meat mixture. Mix well. Alternately layer noodles and meat sauce in a large casserole dish, ending with the sauce. Cover, and bake in a 350° oven for 25 to 30 minutes.

Microwave: Cover casserole with a lid or plastic wrap. Bake on high power for 12 to 14 minutes or until hot and bubbly.

Bake: 350° 25-30 min
Microwave: High 12-14 min   **Yield: 6-8 servings**

Per Serving	RCU	FU	Cal	% Ft	P	F	C	Na
	0	1	188	22	12	5	26	380

Garden Fresh Casserole

Vary this casserole using in-season fresh vegetables.
Menu: Hot rolls, fresh fruit salad

1/2 pound extra-lean ground beef
1 small onion, chopped
1 green pepper, coarsely chopped
1 beef bouillon cube

1 cup hot water
1 1/2 cups cooked brown rice
2 tomatoes, cut in eighths
2 thin slices cheese (optional)

Brown ground beef and onion. Drain well. Add green pepper. Dissolve bouillon in water and pour over beef mixture. Simmer 15 minutes. Add rice and tomatoes. Steam 10 minutes. Pour into casserole. Cut cheese diagonally and lay in shape of a pinwheel and serve.

Variation: Add sliced zucchini, cabbage, peas, or grated carrots.

Cook: 30 min   **Yield: 4 servings**

Per Serving	RCU	FU	Cal	% Ft	P	F	C	Na
	0	1	305	21	21	7	40	155

Shepherd's Pie

It's just as good as it is thrifty!
Menu: Cooked carrots, green salad

1/2 pound extra-lean ground beef
1 large onion, chopped, or 1 tablespoon instant minced onion
1/2 teaspoon salt
1/4 teaspoon pepper
1/8 teaspoon oregano
2 cups cooked green beans, drained
1 10 3/4-ounce can cream of tomato soup
1/2 cup water
3 cups mashed potatoes
Paprika

Brown the ground beef and onion until meat is brown. Drain well. Stir in seasonings, green beans, soup, and water. Heat through. Pour into an 8 x 12-inch baking dish. Spread mashed potatoes on top, and sprinkle with paprika. Bake in a 350° oven for 25 minutes or until bubbly and hot.

Microwave: Cover with waxed paper and cook on high power for 14 to 16 minutes, turning dish once.

Bake: 350° 25 min
Microwave: High 14-16 min   **Yield: 4-6 servings**

Per Serving	RCU	FU	Cal	% Ft	P	F	C	Na
	0	1	298	30	25	10	27	387

Stuffed Green Peppers

Stuff these yummies in the fall. Wrap each one in foil and freeze for winter eating pleasure.
Menu: Baked potatoes, steamed carrots, creamy coleslaw

1/2 pound extra-lean ground beef
1 small onion, chopped or 1 tablespoon instant minced onion
2 fresh tomatoes, chopped or 1 8-ounce can tomato sauce
1 cup cooked brown rice
1 cup whole-kernel corn
1 teaspoon mild chili powder
1/2 teaspoon salt
4 large green peppers

Brown beef and onion. Drain well. Add tomatoes, rice, corn, chili powder, and salt. Stir to mix well. Remove tops, seeds and pulp from peppers. Fill peppers with meat mixture. Place peppers in muffin tins, and bake in a 350° oven for 30 minutes.

Microwave: Arrange peppers in custard cups. Cover with waxed paper. Microwave on high for 8 to 10 minutes or until peppers are tender.

Bake: 350° 30 min   **Yield: 6-8 servings**

Per Serving	RCU	FU	Cal	% Ft	P	F	C	Na
	0	1	250	26	19	7	29	343

Beef 'n Things

This is a popular potato topper.
Menu: Baby lima beans, sliced tomatoes and cucumbers

1 pound extra-lean ground beef
  or round steak cut into narrow strips
1 large onion, sliced
1 green pepper, sliced thin
1 tablespoon flour

1/2 to 3/4 cup water
1/4 teaspoon salt
Dash pepper
4 baked potatoes
1 cup lowfat cottage cheese

Brown beef, onion, and green pepper in nonstick fry pan. Cook until all are tender. Drain well. Sprinkle flour over meat. Mix well, and add water. Cook and stir until sauce is thick and clear. Season with salt and pepper. Serve over baked potatoes, and top with cottage cheese.

Cook: **10 min**
Microwave: High 8-10 min   **Yield: 3-4 servings**

Per Serving	RCU	FU	Cal	% Ft	P	F	C	Na
	0	1	318	27	31	10	26	343

Sloppy Joes or Barbecue

Everyone loves this old favorite. It also makes a good potato topper or pita bread filling.
Menu: Potato salad, baked beans, raw vegetable plate

1 pound extra-lean ground beef
1 onion, chopped
1 cup cooked brown rice
1 10 1/2-ounce can chicken gumbo soup
1 tablespoon chili powder
1/2 teaspoon salt (optional)
2 tablespoons catsup
2 tablespoons hickory-flavored barbecue sauce (optional)
8 whole wheat hamburger buns

Brown ground beef and onion. Drain fat. Add rice, soup, seasonings, catsup, and barbecue sauce. Simmer slowly, uncovered, for about 15 minutes. Serve between whole wheat buns.

Cook: 20 min   Yield: 8 servings

Per Serving	RCU	FU	Cal	% Ft	P	F	C	Na
	0	1	332	31	31	11	37	473

Spaghetti

If you haven't tried whole wheat spaghetti, you're missing out. It is delicious and very satisfying. Dona Jo Osterhout shares her fool-proof way to cook spaghetti.

3 quarts boiling water
1 teaspoon salt
1 teaspoon cooking oil
1 large handful whole wheat spaghetti (approximately 8 ounces)

Bring salted water to a boil. Add cooking oil and spaghetti. Stir well. Return water to boiling. Cover and remove from heat. Let stand 15 minutes. You'll have perfect spaghetti every time with no boil-overs!

Vegetarian Spaghetti

Prepare spaghetti and sauce as directed, omitting meat and using 1 chopped medium-size zucchini or 1 cup cooked lentils.

Spaghetti Sauce

The sauce and the spaghetti can be fixed in 30 minutes.
Menu: Steamed broccoli, green salad, french bread

1/2 pound extra-lean ground beef
1 tablespoon instant minced onion or 1 small onion, chopped
2 cloves garlic, minced
1 1 1/2-ounce package dry spaghetti sauce mix
   or 1 tablespoon brown sugar and 1 teaspoon oregano
2 tablespoons dried parsley flakes
1 28-ounce can tomatoes, slightly blended
1 16-ounce can tomato sauce
1 4-ounce can mushrooms
6 to 8 ounces whole wheat spaghetti

Brown ground beef with onion. Drain. Add seasonings, tomatoes, tomato sauce, and mushrooms. Stir to mix. Simmer 25-30 minutes. Cook spaghetti according to directions below.

Cook: 30 min   Yield: 4-6 servings

Per Serving	RCU	FU	Cal	% Ft	P	F	C	Na
	0	1	266	25	21	8	31	557

Spaghetti Pie

An old favorite takes on a new look.
Menu: Steamed carrots and cabbage, mixed vegetables, green salad

1/3 cup grated Parmesan cheese
2 eggs, well-beaten
6 ounces whole wheat spaghetti, cooked and drained
1/2 pound extra-lean ground beef
1 small onion, chopped, or 1 tablespoon instant minced onion
1/4 cup chopped green pepper
2 cups canned tomatoes, slightly blended
1 6-ounce can tomato paste
1 teaspoon sugar
1 teaspoon oregano, crushed
1/2 teaspoon garlic salt
1/2 teaspoon salt
1 cup low-fat cottage cheese
1/4 cup mozzarella cheese (optional)

Mix Parmesan cheese and eggs into hot, cooked spaghetti. Form into a crust in a large 10-inch buttered pie dish. Cook meat, onion and green pepper until meat is brown. Drain well. Stir in tomatoes, tomato paste, sugar, and seasonings. Simmer 5 to 10 minutes. Spread cottage cheese over bottom of spaghetti crust. Fill pie with meat-tomato mixture. Sprinkle with mozzarella cheese, if desired. Bake in a 350° oven for 20 minutes.

Microwave: Cover with waxed paper. Cook at 50 percent power for 12 to 14 minutes or until hot and bubbly. Let stand 5 minutes before serving.

Bake: 350° 20 min
Microwave: 50% 12-14 min   Yield: 6-8 servings

Per Serving	RCU	FU	Cal	% Ft	P	F	C	Na
	0	1	313	30	27	11	28	481

Easy Lasagna

The noodles don't require precooking!
Menu: Seasoned Veggie Combo, green salad, pickles

1 pound extra lean ground beef
1 medium onion, chopped (optional)
1 1 1/2-ounce package spaghetti sauce mix or 1 teaspoon basil leaves, 1 teaspoon
    oregano leaves, 1 teaspoon salt, 1/8 teaspoon garlic powder and 1/2 teaspoon sugar
2 cups canned tomatoes, slightly blended
1 6-ounce can tomato paste
1 cup water
8 spinach or whole wheat lasagna noodles, uncooked
1 egg, slightly beaten
1 tablespoon dried parsley flakes
2 tablespoons Parmesan cheese
2 cups lowfat cottage cheese
1/4 cup finely shredded mozzarella cheese

Brown beef and onion. Drain well. Stir in seasonings, tomatoes, tomato paste, and water. Mixture may be used immediately, but for richer flavor, simmer uncovered for 15 to 20 minutes. Stir occasionally. Mix egg, parsley flakes, Parmesan cheese and cottage cheese.

In a 9 x 13-inch baking dish layer 1 cup of sauce, 4 dry noodles (break to fit), and half of the cottage cheese-egg mixture, spreading it evenly over the noodles. Repeat the sauce, noodles and cottage cheese mixture. Top with remaining sauce. Cover and bake in a 350° oven for 50 to 60 minutes or until noodles are tender. Let stand 10 minutes. Sprinkle with cheese and serve.

Microwave: Cover with plastic wrap and cook on high for 12 minutes. Cook at 50 percent power for 18 to 22 more minutes or until noodles are tender. Turn dish twice. Let stand 10 minutes before serving. Sprinkle with cheese and serve.

Tip: As a transition, use spinach noodles for the first layer and regular lasagna noodles for the second layer.

Bake: 350° 1 hour
Microwave: High 12 min and 50% 18-22 min   Yield: 12 servings

Per Serving	RCU	FU	Cal	% Ft	P	F	C	Na
	0	1	211	28	19	7	19	410

Favorite Pizza

Debbie Hunt makes the best pizza in town. She says the secret of crisp homemade pizza is to use a very hot oven and to prebake the crust.

Quick Sauce:
1 to 2 tablespoons dry pizza sauce mix
1 6-ounce can tomato paste
6 ounces water

Dough:
2 1/2 cups whole wheat flour
   or 2 cups whole wheat flour and 1/2 cup white flour
1 tablespoon sugar
1 tablespoon dry yeast
1/2 teaspoon salt
1 cup comfortably hot water (120° to 130°)
2 tablespoons oil

Suggested Toppings:
1 cup cooked baby shrimp
1/2 pound extra-lean ground beef, cooked and drained
1 chopped onion (cook with ground beef above)
1 4-ounce can mushrooms, drained
1 2 1/4-ounce can sliced olives, drained
1 green pepper, diced
2 tomatoes, diced
1 8-ounce can unsweetened pineapple tidbits
1 cup shredded skim mozzarella cheese
1 cup sliced broccoli or cauliflower, microwaved 3 minutes

Mix pizza sauce mix, tomato paste, and water. Let stand while preparing dough. Mix 2 cups flour, sugar, yeast, and salt. Add water and oil; mix well. Add remaining flour as needed to make a soft dough. Knead 5 minutes; let dough rest 5 minutes. Use a pizza roller to roll dough about 1/4-inch thick on a lightly greased heavy pizza pan or baking sheet. To prevent soggy crust, prebake at 500° for 3 to 4 minutes, just until puffed but not brown. After baking, spread dough with sauce and add desired toppings. Bake in a 500° oven for 10 to 12 minutes for a large pizza or 5 to 7 minutes for a medium or small pizza.

Tip: For later use, prebake crust as above. Cool, cover and freeze if desired. Top with sauce and toppings just before baking. If pizza pan is light weight, lower baking temperature to 450°.

Bake: 500° 10 min 1 large pizza
      500° 5-7 min 2 medium or small pizza

Per Serving	RCU	FU	Cal	% Ft	P	F	C	Na
	0	0	118	25	6	3	17	113

Pizza Sauce Supreme

Lynn and Clarence Johnson are pizza lovers who share this exceptionally good pizza sauce recipe.

Greens:
1/2 cup celery (1 large stalk)
1/2 cup chopped green onion (3 green onions and tops)
1/3 cup chopped green pepper (1/2 medium green pepper)
2 cloves garlic or 1/2 teaspoon garlic powder
1/4 cup water

Sauce:
2 cups canned tomatoes, slightly blended
1 12-ounce can tomato paste
1/4 cup greens (above)
1 tablespoon dry Italian seasoning
1/2 teaspoon salt
1/2 teaspoon black pepper

Place greens in blender and liquify. Measure 1/4 cup. Freeze unused portion in 1/4 cup portions in plastic sandwich bags. Mix all sauce ingredients and refrigerate until needed.
Yield: 4 cups pizza sauce

Per Serving	RCU	FU	Cal	% Ft	P	F	C	Na
	0	0	52	4	2	0	11	22

Pizza By the Yard

This pizza is as beautiful as it is delicious.
Menu: Mushroom green beans, green salad

1 pound extra-lean ground beef
1 6-ounce can tomato paste
1/3 cup grated Parmesan cheese
1/4 cup chopped green onion
1/4 cup chopped black olives
1/2 teaspoon dry crushed oregano
1/2 teaspoon salt
2 cups roll or bread dough*
2 tomatoes, sliced
1 green pepper, cut in rings
1/4 cup finely shredded cheese

Brown beef and drain well. Add the next six ingredients. Simmer 8 to 10 minutes. Prepare roll dough as directed, or use bread dough. (For convenience, keep 2-cup portions of dough in the freezer. Thaw until warm and pliable.)

Lightly oil a large baking sheet and roll dough into a 14 x 16-inch rectangle. Place the meat filling lengthwise down the center, covering only the center third of the dough. With a knife or kitchen shears, cut into the dough every 2 inches on each side. Cross the strips diagonally over the filling, creating a braided look; tuck in the ends. Let raise 5 to 10 minutes. Bake in a 350° oven for 25 minutes. Top with tomato and green pepper slices, and sprinkle with grated cheese. Bake 5 additional minutes.

Bake: 350° 30 min   **Yield: 10-12 servings**

Per Serving	RCU	FU	Cal	% Ft	P	F	C	Na
	0	1	199	31	15	7	20	263

Easy Crazy Crust Pizza

You'll enjoy this quick pizza version
Menu: Mushroom green beans, green salad

1 8-ounce can tomato sauce
2 teaspoons dry pizza sauce mix
  or 1 teaspoon oregano and 1 teaspoon basil
1/2 pound extra-lean ground beef
1 tablespoon minced dry onion
2/3 cup skim milk
2 eggs
1/2 teaspoon salt
1/4 teaspoon pepper
1 cup whole wheat flour
1 4-ounce can mushrooms
1/2 cup finely shredded mozzarella cheese

Mix tomato sauce and dry pizza sauce mix or oregano and basil. Set aside. Brown ground beef and onion. Drain well and set aside. In blender combine milk, eggs, salt, pepper, and flour. Pulse, then blend until smooth. Pour this batter onto a lightly greased 12-inch pizza pan, spreading to cover bottom. Top evenly with meat and onion mix, mushrooms, or any other lowfat toppings of your choice such as pineapple tidbits, diced tomato, or green pepper. When topping is complete, drizzle sauce over the toppings. Sprinkle with cheese if desired. Bake at 375° for 15 to 20 minutes or until crust is golden brown.

Bake: 375° 15-20 min   **Yield: 1   12-inch pizza**

Per Serving	RCU	FU	Cal	% Ft	P	F	C	Na
	0	1	156	32	13	6	14	407

MEXICAN DISHES

Ranchero Beans

You'll be missing a treat if you don't try these beans! They're simple to prepare; delicious as a main dish, a side dish, or in combination dishes. Double the recipe and freeze some for later. Use for chili, refried beans, tacos, or other dishes. Thanks to Florence Johnson for this versatile recipe that can be used to prepare any dried beans.

5 cups water
1 onion, peeled and quartered, or 1 tablespoon instant minced onion
1 clove garlic, peeled
1 carrot, peeled and cut into chunks
2 cups dry pinto beans, sorted and washed
Sprinkle of cayenne pepper
1/2 teaspoon ginger
1/2 teaspoon salt
1 teaspoon honey
1 cup salsa* or mild taco sauce

In blender place 1 cup of the water, onion, garlic, and carrot. Pulse until vegetables are finely chopped. Place chopped vegetables, the remaining 4 cups water, beans, cayenne, and ginger in a 5- to 6-quart pan. Cover and cook 8 hours or overnight in a 200° oven. Add salt, honey, and salsa. Return to oven for at least 1 hour and up to 4 hours. To cook in a slow cooker, cook on high for 8 hours. Add seasonings and cook on low about 8 hours or as desired.

Bake: 200° 12 hours
Slow cooker: High 8 hours or Low 8 hours   **Yield: 6 cups**

Per Serving	RCU	FU	Cal	% Ft	P	F	C	Na
	0	0	214	2	13	1	40	184

Mexican Beef and Beans

Prepare Ranchero beans as directed. Add 1/2 to 1 pound extra-lean ground beef, fried and well-drained, and 1 1 1/4-ounce package taco seasoning mix plus water as directed. Simmer 15 to 20 minutes. Can freeze for later use in taco sundaes, salads, or tacos.

Per Serving	RCU	FU	Cal	% Ft	P	F	C	Na
	0	1	226	19	19	5	27	141

Quick Mexican Beef and Beans

These beefy beans add zing to all your Mexican cooking. They're good in tacos, burritos, and as a side dish.

1/2 pound extra-lean ground beef
1 1 1/4-ounce package taco seasoning mix
2 16-ounce cans refried beans or pinto beans

Brown beef and drain well. Stir in seasoning mix and beans. Cook on low for 10 to 15 minutes.
Yield: 5 cups

Per Serving	RCU	FU	Cal	% Ft	P	F	C	Na
	0	1	175	19	15	4	25	21

Refried Beans

Prepare Ranchero Beans as directed. Mash and use for bean dip, burritos, etc. Add chili powder if desired.

Chili Beans

Prepare Ranchero Beans as directed. Add 1 1½-ounce package chili seasoning mix, 1 16-ounce can tomatoes, and 1/2 pound extra-lean ground beef, fried and well-drained. Mix and simmer 20 to 30 minutes.

Taco Seasoning Mix

1/3 cup dry minced onion
2 teaspoons salt
2 tablespoons chili powder
2 tablespoons paprika
1 teaspoon garlic powder
1 teaspoon cumin
1/2 teaspoon oregano
2 tablespoons flour

Mix ingredients. Cover and store in cool dry place.
2 to 3 tablespoons equal 1 package taco seasoning mix.
Stir seasoning mix into meat or beans. Add 1/2 cup water and simmer 10 minutes.
Yield: 3/4 cup

Taco Sundaes

Kathy Thompson introduced us to this "eat yourself thin" meal.
Menu: This is a complete meal.

1 pound extra-lean ground beef
1 1 1/4-ounce package taco seasoning mix
1/2 cup water
4 cups cooked kidney, pinto, or red beans
1 cup raw brown rice, steamed
1 17-ounce can whole-kernel corn, heated and drained
1 head lettuce, shredded (use French-fry blade on food processor)
4 to 6 tomatoes, chopped
1 2 1/4-ounce can sliced olives, drained
1 cup finely grated cheese
1 cup salsa or mild taco sauce
Catalina or Ranch Dressing, fat free
2 to 4 cups slightly crushed corn tortilla chips

Brown beef and drain. Add taco seasoning, water, and beans. Cook for 15 minutes. Let guests build their own sundae in the following order: steamed rice, meat-bean mixture, corn, lettuce, tomatoes, olives, cheese, salsa, and salad dressing. Add tortilla chips as the topping for the sundae.
Cook: 20 min   Yield: 10 servings

Per Serving	RCU	FU	Cal	% Ft	P	F	C	Na
	0	2	421	26	26	12	57	343

Tacos

They're always a crowd-pleaser!
Menu: Spanish rice, sliced cucumbers and tomatoes

1 pound extra-lean ground beef
1 onion, chopped
2 cups pinto or kidney beans, drained
1/2 cup water
1 1 1/4-ounce package taco seasoning mix
1/2 cup cooked brown rice
1 cup whole-kernel corn (optional)
24 corn tortillas or taco shells
4 tomatoes, diced
1/2 head lettuce, shredded
Salsa

In a nonstick fry pan, brown ground beef and onion. Drain well. Add beans, water, seasoning mix, brown rice, and corn. Simmer 15 minutes. For soft-shell tacos, fold 6 corn tortillas in half. Microwave on high for approximately 1 1/2 minutes. Repeat with the remaining tortillas. Or wrap tortillas in foil and warm in 350° oven for 5 to 10 minutes. Spoon meat mix into tortillas. Top with tomatoes, lettuce, and salsa.

Cook: 10-15 min   **Yield: 24 tacos**   **3 tablespoons filling per taco**

Per Serving	RCU	FU	Cal	% Ft	P	F	C	Na
	0	0	118	22	16	3	16	161

Chicken Fajitas

Prepare these sizzling fajitas in minutes.

2 cups chicken breast, raw or cooked
1/2 cup nonfat Italian salad dressing
1 onion
1 green bell pepper

1 red bell pepper
1/4 head cabbage (about 3 cups)
6 corn or lowfat flour tortillas
Green salsa or mild taco sauce

Cut chicken into strips and marinate in the Italian dressing while preparing vegetables. Cut onion lengthwise and then slice. Cut peppers into thin strips. Coarsely chop cabbage or cut in thin slices.

Pour chicken and marinade into large hot skillet or wok. Stir-fry until meat is almost tender. Add vegetables and stir-fry over hot heat until vegetables are tender crisp. Don't overcook. Serve with warm tortillas and green salsa.

Cook: 6-8 min   **Yield: 6 servings**

Per Serving	RCU	FU	Cal	% Ft	P	F	C	Na
	0	0	151	14	14	2	17	390

Lazy Day Mexican Casserole

Mae Nelson's layered casserole makes a hit at any potluck dinner.
Menu: Frozen mixed vegetables, carrot and celery sticks

1/2-1 pound extra lean ground beef
1 small onion, minced, or 1 tablespoon instant minced onion
1 package (1 1/4-ounce) taco seasoning mix
1/2 cup water
2 cups lightly crushed tortilla chips
2 cups cooked pinto beans or refried beans
1 cup mild enchilada sauce or spicy tomato sauce
1/2 head lettuce, shredded
2 tomatoes, diced
2 tablespoons sliced olives

Brown ground beef with onion. Drain well. Add taco seasoning mix and cook 5-7 minutes. In a large casserole dish, make a layer of tortilla chips. Top with a layer of beans. Next a layer of browned ground beef. Pour enchilada or tomato sauce over all. Sprinkle with finely crushed tortilla chips. Bake in a 375° oven for 18 to 20 minutes or until casserole is bubbly.

Microwave: Cover casserole with waxed paper. Cook on high for 8 to 10 minutes or until hot and bubbly. Turn dish twice.

Garnish with shredded lettuce, tomatoes, and sliced olives. Serve immediately.

Bake: 375° 18-22 min
Microwave: High 8-10 min Yield: 5-6 servings

Per Serving	RCU	FU	Cal	% Ft	P	F	C	Na
	0	1	293	26	21	9	38	358

Chicken Enchilada Casserole

Grandma Payne often served this quick dish to unexpected company.
Menu: Petite peas, fresh vegetable plate, rolls.

1 10 3/4-ounce can cream of chicken soup, lowfat
1 soup can 1% or skim milk
1 medium onion, chopped
1 4-ounce can diced green chiles, drained
1 to 2 cups chicken chunks (optional)
10 to 12 corn tortillas, torn into large pieces
1/2 cup finely shredded cheese

   Combine soup and milk. Stir in onion, green chiles, chicken, and tortillas. Pour into casserole dish. Cover and bake in a 350° oven for 30 minutes. Sprinkle with cheese and serve.
Tip: Chop onion in blender using 1/2 cup of the milk.
Bake: 350°   30 min
Microwave: High 10-14 min   Yield: 5-6 servings

Per Serving	RCU	FU	Cal	% Ft	P	F	C	Na
	0	0	187	22	6	5	30	618

Tortilla Chips

1 dozen corn tortillas
Seasoned salt (optional)

   Using a pizza cutter, cut corn tortillas into 6 or 8 pie-shaped pieces. Place on a large baking sheet. With a spray bottle, lightly mist tortillas with water. Sprinkle with seasoned salt, if desired. Bake in a 350° oven for 7 to 8 minutes or until crisp.

Fiesta Bake

This tasty casserole provides long-lasting energy. It's a large recipe, so you'll have extra to share or freeze.
Menu: Seasoned veggie combo, finely shredded lettuce

1 pound extra-lean ground beef
1 clove garlic, minced
1 onion, diced
1/2 teaspoon salt
1/4 teaspoon pepper
1 10-ounce can enchilada sauce, mild or hot
1 8-ounce can tomato sauce
2 15-ounce cans chili beans or 4 cups Ranchero Beans*
1 17-ounce can whole-kernel corn, undrained
1 4 1/4-ounce can chopped olives (optional)
8 to 10 corn tortillas, torn into large pieces
1/2 cup finely shredded cheese

Brown ground beef, garlic and onion. Drain off fat. Season with salt and pepper. Add sauces, beans, corn, and olives. Place 1 cup meat mixture in the bottom of a large casserole or two smaller ones. Add a layer of corn tortillas. Repeat layers until meat mixture and tortillas are used, ending with meat mixture. Cover and bake in a 350° oven for 30 minutes. Sprinkle with cheese and let stand 10 minutes before serving.

Microwave: Layer as directed. Cover loosely. Cook on 80% power for 15-18 minutes. Turn dish twice. Let stand 5 minutes before serving. Top each serving with lettuce.

Bake: **350° 30 min**
Microwave: 80% 15-18 min   **Yield: 8-10 servings**

Per Serving	RCU	FU	Cal	% Ft	P	F	C	Na
	0	1	305	24	21	8	41	663

Enchilada Pie

This contest winner from Edna Christensen provides hearty eating.
Menu: Green beans, green salad

1 pound extra-lean ground beef or 2-3 large chicken breasts, skinned, boned, and cut
  into cubes
1 large onion, diced
1 clove garlic, diced
1 10-ounce can enchilada sauce, mild or hot
1 28-ounce can tomatoes, slightly blended
1 8-ounce can tomato sauce
1/2 teaspoon salt
1 teaspoon chili powder
1 4 -ounce can chopped olives
16-18 corn tortillas
1/2 cup shredded Monterey Jack cheese

Brown ground beef or chicken, onion, and garlic. Drain well. Add enchilada sauce,
tomatoes, tomato sauce, salt, and chili powder. Simmer uncovered for 20 minutes.
Add olives. Put 1/2 to 1 cup sauce in the bottom of a large 9 x 13-inch baking dish or
two smaller ones. Line pan with half the tortillas, torn in 3 or 4 strips each. Cover with
half the sauce mixture. Repeat with tortillas and sauce. Top with cheese. Cover. Bake
in a 350° oven for 25 to 30 minutes until hot and bubbly.
Microwave: Cook on high for 12-15 minutes. Turn dish twice.

Bake: 350° 25-30 min
Microwave: High 12-15 min   **Yield: 12-14 servings**

Per Serving	RCU	FU	Cal	% Ft	P	F	C	Na
	0	1	183	33	12	7	18	616

Mexican Beef Burger

It's mighty good and mighty filling.
Menu: Petite peas, green salad

Filling:
1 pound extra lean ground beef
1 small onion, chopped
2 cups kidney, pinto, or red beans, undrained
1 8-ounce can tomato sauce
1 teaspoon chili powder
1/2 teaspoon salt

Crust:
3/4 cup comfortably hot water (120 to 130°)
1 egg
2 tablespoons oil
1 1/2 cups whole wheat flour
1/2 tablespoon dry yeast (1/2 packet)
1 tablespoon sugar or honey
1/2 teaspoon salt
1/2 teaspoon chili powder

Brown ground beef and onion in a deep 12-inch skillet. Drain well. Stir in kidney beans, tomato sauce, chili powder, and salt. Cover and simmer 10 minutes.

Place all crust ingredients in blender. Pulse, then blend until well mixed. Pour or spoon batter evenly over filling in skillet. Let rise 8 to 10 minutes. Bake in preheated oven until golden brown. Let stand 5 minutes and serve.

Bake: 350° 25-30 min   Yield: 6 servings

Variation: Use 2 cups cooked chicken in place of the ground beef.

Per Serving	RCU	FU	Cal	% Ft	P	F	C	Na
	0	2	421	32	31	15	39	608

Chicken Enchiladas

These make up in minutes.
Menu: Ranchero Beans, black beans or Spanish rice, green salad

1 1.5-ounce package enchilada sauce mix, prepared as directed on package
2 cups diced cooked chicken
1 4-ounce can diced green chiles
3 green onions, finely chopped
8 corn tortillas
1/4 cup finely grated cheese

Prepare sauce as directed. Heat to a simmer. Mix 1/2 cup of the sauce with the chicken, green chiles, and onion. Dip each of the corn tortillas into remaining sauce and drain. Place about 1/4 cup chicken filling on each. Roll tortilla around filling and place seam side down in 8 x 12-inch baking dish. Spread remaining sauce evenly over enchiladas and top with cheese. Cover and bake in 350° oven 15 to 18 minutes, until hot. Microwave: Reduce water in sauce by 1/4 cup. Prepare as above. Cook on high for 7 to 9 minutes or until hot and bubbly.
Bake: **350° 15-18 min**
Microwave: High 7-9 min   **Yield: 8 enchiladas**

#2 Beef Enchiladas:

Use 1/2 lb. extra lean ground beef, browned and drained and 1 cup cooked pinto or kidney beans in place of the chicken and green chiles; prepare as above.

Per Serving	RCU	FU	Cal	% Ft	P	F	C	Na
#1	0	0	167	20	15	4	15	540
#2	0	1	179	28	12	6	21	512

Turkey Chili

These hot and spicy flavors make delicious eating.
Menu: Lowfat cottage cheese, raw vegetable plate

1 tablespoon salad oil
1 small onion, diced
1 medium-sized green pepper, diced
1-2 teaspoons chili powder
1 16-ounce can tomatoes
1 16-ounce can red kidney beans, undrained
1 cup water
2 cups diced cooked turkey
1/4 teaspoon salt
1 teaspoon sugar
1/2 teaspoon crushed red pepper

Saute' onion and green pepper in salad oil until tender. Stir in chili powder and cook 1 minute. Add tomatoes, kidney beans, water, turkey, salt, sugar, and crushed red pepper. Heat to boiling, then simmer 10 minutes to blend flavors, stirring occasionally.

Cook: 15 minutes   Yield: 8 servings

Per Serving	RCU	FU	Cal	% Ft	P	F	C	Na
	0	1	203	23	22	5	14	204

Mexi-Corn Zucchini

Zucchini becomes a real meal in this tasty summer dish.
Menu: Refried beans, cucumber slices

1/2 pound extra-lean ground beef
1 medium onion, chopped, or 1 tablespoon instant minced onion
1/2 green pepper, chopped
3 cups sliced zucchini, 1/2 inch thick
1 8-ounce can tomato sauce
2 to 3 fresh tomatoes, chopped
1 to 2 cups whole-kernel corn
1/2 teaspoon salt
1 teaspoon mild chili powder

Brown ground beef, onion, and green pepper. Drain well. Add remaining ingredients. Cover and simmer 15 minutes or until zucchini is tender.
Cook: 20 minutes   Yield: 4-6 servings

Per Serving	RCU	FU	Cal	% Ft	P	F	C	Na
	0	1	163	25	13	5	19	486

POTATO, RICE, BEANS, AND PASTA ACCOMPANIMENTS

Baked Potatoes and Potato Toppers

Potatoes make a satisfying meal any time.

4 medium potatoes
Potato Topper*

Scrub potatoes well. Prick each potato with a fork.
Microwave: Turn once during cooking. Potatoes will feel firm when baked. Wrap in plastic wrap and let stand 5 minutes.
Bake: 425° 50 min
Microwave: High 9-12 min   Yield: 4 servings

Per Serving	RCU	FU	Cal	% Ft	P	F	C	Na
	0	0	90	1	3	0	21	4

Potato Toppers

Vegetables:
Any frozen mixed vegetable or stewed tomatoes topped with Mock Sour Cream* or lowfat cottage cheese
See Vegetable Accompaniments for the following:
Creamed asparagus
Creamed beans
Creamed carrots
Creamed peas

Beans:
Ranchero Beans
Refried beans (add tomatoes, lettuce, and salsa)

Main Dish Meat Combinations:
Turkey Topper
Beef 'n Things
Chili Con Carne
Beef Stroganoff
Mexican Beef and Beans
Old-Fashioned Chicken and Noodles
Porcupine Meatballs
Sloppy Joes

Soups and Stews (for a main dish):
Canned chunky soup
Homemade stew

Other:
Mock Sour Cream*
Lowfat cottage cheese
Basic Dressing*
Buttermilk
Green Chile Salsa*
Plain nonfat yogurt

Scalloped Potatoes

This recipe always brings compliments.

6 to 8 medium potatoes, peeled and cubed
2 tablespoons butter or margarine
1 large onion, minced
1 teaspoon salt
1/2 teaspoon paprika
1/2 teaspoon dry mustard
1/4 cup flour
2 cups 1% or skim milk
1 2-ounce bottle diced pimento, drained
1/2 cup finely grated cheese (optional)

Tip: Use the french-fry blade on food processor to cube potatoes.

To prepare sauce: Melt butter, add onion and cook one minute. Stir in salt, paprika, dry mustard, and flour. Add milk and pimento; cook until thick, stirring constantly. Pour sauce over potatoes, and mix gently. Put in large covered casserole and bake in 325° oven for 1 1/2 hours or until potatoes are tender. Sprinkle with cheese and serve.

Tip: To cut baking time, microwave on high for 10 minutes before baking in oven for 30 to 40 minutes, or until potatoes are tender.

To microwave: Cook on high for 10 minutes; stir mixture and continue microwaving on 80 percent power for 14 to 16 minutes or until potatoes are tender. Let stand 5 minutes. Sprinkle with cheese and serve.

Bake: 325°   1 1/2 hours
Microwave: High 10 min   80% power 14-16 min
Yield: 8-10 servings

Per Serving	RCU	FU	Cal	% Ft	P	F	C	Na
	0	0	198	11	3	2	21	116

Western Potato Strips

One of the simplest, yet best, go-with-barbecue dishes. Bake in heavy foil in the oven and then keep it hot on the edge of the grill. Place in a basket and fold back foil for serving.

4 large potatoes
1/2 teaspoon salt
1 tablespoon dry parsley flakes
1/2 cup evaporated milk
2 tablespoons finely grated cheese (optional)

Peel potatoes and cut into strips as for French fries (use French fry blade on food processor). Place in center of a large piece of heavy foil Shape foil to form baking dish. Sprinkle with salt and parsley. Pour evaporated milk over potatoes. Seal foil but do not flatten. Or prepare in baking dish and cover tightly before baking. Bake at 400° for 40 to 45 minutes or until potatoes are tender. Sprinkle with cheese if desired.

Microwave: Use baking dish and cover tightly. Cook on high 8-10 minutes. Let stand 5 minutes before serving.

Bake: 400° 40-45 min
Microwave: High 8-10 min   Yield: 6-8 servings

Per Serving	RCU	FU	Cal	% Ft	P	F	C	Na
	0	0	59	8	3	1	12	132

Potato Patties

Patties are a good way to enjoy the last of the mashed potatoes.

2 to 3 cups cold mashed potatoes
1 egg, slightly beaten
2 green onions, minced
2 tablespoons diced green chiles or green pepper (optional)
Pinch salt and pepper

Combine all ingredients and mix well. Lightly rub the bottom of a nonstick frying pan with a stick of margarine. Drop potatoes by spoonfuls into pan, and fry until golden brown on each side.

Cook: 5 min   Yield: 6 patties

Per Serving	RCU	FU	Cal	% Ft	P	F	C	Na
	0	0	84	21	4	2	13	323

Potato Boats

Often called twice-baked potatoes, they're a Christmas Eve tradition at our house. Leftovers rewarm well.
Menu: Ham or turkey ham, baked beans, frozen petite peas, frozen corn, green salad, fresh fruit salad

4 large baked potatoes
1/3-1/2 cup hot skim milk
4 green onions, finely minced
1/2 teaspoon salt
Dash pepper
Paprika and parsley flakes
1/2 cup finely grated cheese (optional)

Slightly cool baked potatoes. Cut each in half lengthwise, and carefully scoop out potatoes. Be careful not to break the skins. Place the skins in the oven on a baking sheet for a few minutes to slightly crisp the shells. Place potato, milk, onion, salt, and pepper in a bowl. Whip until potatoes are light and fluffy, about 2 to 3 minutes. Add milk, onion, salt, and pepper. Fill shells with mashed potato mixture. Sprinkle top of each potato with paprika and parsley flakes. Bake 5-7 minutes or until hot and golden. Sprinkle lightly with cheese if desired.

Variation: Add one cup low-fat cottage cheese while whipping potatoes.

Bake: 400° 5-7 min   **Yield: 5 servings**

Per Serving	RCU	FU	Cal	% Ft	P	F	C	Na
	0	0	84	2	3	0	18	205

Potatoes and Onions

You can fix this old standby in a hurry.

1 teaspoon oil
2 large potatoes, sliced
1 medium onion, peeled and sliced

Heat oil in nonstick fry pan. Add potatoes and onion. Sprinkle with a little salt and pepper. Cook over medium heat until potatoes are slightly brown, stirring occasionally. Add 2 tablespoons water, cover and steam 5 minutes or until potatoes are tender.

Cook: 10-15 minutes   **Yield: 4 servings**

Per Serving	RCU	FU	Cal	% Ft	P	F	C	Na
	0	0	88	12	3	1	18	6

Oven French Fries

These fries are lower in fat than traditional fries, but eat sparingly.

3 to 4 medium potatoes
1 scant tablespoon oil
Seasoned salt

Cut potatoes into long fries. Roll in oil, and sprinkle with seasoned salt. Bake on a nonstick baking sheet in a 400° oven for 15 to 20 minutes.

Bake: 400° 15-20 min   **Yield: 4 servings**

Per Serving	RCU	FU	Cal	% Ft	P	F	C	Na
	0	1	121	26	3	4	21	122

Steamed Brown Rice

An automatic rice cooker is a good investment. If you don't have one, follow this recipe for fluffy brown rice. Keep plenty in the refrigerator or freezer for quick meals.

2 1/2 cups water
1 cup long-grain brown rice
1/2 teaspoon salt (optional)

Combine ingredients in a 2-quart saucepan. Bring to a boil. Reduce heat, cover tightly, and simmer for 40 minutes. Remove from heat without lifting lid. Allow to sit for 10 minutes before using. To shorten cooking time, soak brown rice in water at least 1 hour or overnight before cooking.

Cook: 45 min   **Yield: 3 cups**

Tip: Cooked rice keeps refrigerated for about a week and also freezes well. Defrost in microwave. Stir once or twice.

Per Serving	RCU	FU	Cal	% Ft	P	F	C	Na
	0	0	111	5	2	1	24	3

Rice Pilaf

What a marvelous way to serve rice. It's so good with chicken, pheasant, salmon loaf, or almost any meal.

1 tablespoon butter
1 small onion, minced
1 clove garlic, minced
1 cup raw brown rice
1 4-ounce can mushrooms, undrained
1/8 teaspoon oregano
1/2 teaspoon salt, scant
1 1/2 cups water
1 8-ounce can tomato sauce

Melt butter in a 10-inch skillet. Saute' onion, garlic, and rice until transparent. Add mushrooms, oregano, salt, water, and tomato sauce and mix well. Pour into a 3-quart casserole dish. Cover, and bake in a 325° oven for 1 1/2 hours or until rice has completely absorbed the liquid and is tender.

Bake: 325° 1 1/2 hr   **Yield: 6-8 servings**

Per Serving	RCU	FU	Cal	% Ft	P	F	C	Na
	0	0	113	14	2	2	22	354

Rice Pilaf

On busy days you'll welcome this quick version.

2 cups cooked brown rice
1 8-ounce can tomato sauce
1 4-ounce can mushrooms, drained
1 teaspoon instant minced onion
1/8 teaspoon oregano
1/4 teaspoon garlic salt
1/2 teaspoon sugar

Mix together in pan and simmer over low heat about 10 minutes.

Cook: 10 minutes   **Yield: 5 servings**

Per Serving	RCU	FU	Cal	% Ft	P	F	C	Na
	0	0	81	9	2	1	18	358

Spanish Rice

Serve Spanish Rice as a side dish or add meat to make it a meal.

1 onion, chopped
1/2 green pepper, chopped
2 cups stewed tomatoes
1 cup uncooked brown rice
1 cup tomato juice or water
1/2 teaspoon salt, optional
1 teaspoon chili powder
1/4 teaspoon curry powder (optional)

In large nonstick frying pan, saute onion and green pepper for 3 minutes. Add remaining ingredients. Reduce heat. Cover and simmer for 40 to 45 minutes or until rice is tender. Add additional juice if needed.
Cook: 40-45 min   Yield: 6 servings

#2 Main Dish Spanish Rice

Cook 1/2 pound extra-lean ground beef with the onion and green pepper. Drain well. Follow recipe as directed above.

Quick Spanish Rice

Saute onion and green pepper as directed for Spanish Rice. Add 2-3 cups cooked brown rice, 8 ounces tomato sauce, and 1/2 teaspoon chili powder. Cover, and simmer 10 to 15 minutes. Add water if needed.

Per Serving	RCU	FU	Cal	% Ft	P	F	C	Na
	0	0	140	6	3	1	30	288
#2	0	1	223	21	14	5	30	307

Baked Beans

These savory beans are always popular at any dinner or picnic.

1 31-ounce can pork and beans
2 tablespoons brown sugar or molasses
1/4 teaspoon dry mustard
1/4 cup catsup
1 tablespoon instant minced onion or 1 onion finely chopped
1/8 teaspoon salt
2 tablespoons smoked barbecue sauce (optional)

Combine all ingredients in a bean pot or casserole dish. Bake uncovered in a 350° oven for 45 to 60 minutes.

Microwave: Use a 1 1/2-quart casserole. Cover loosely with waxed paper. Cook on 80 percent power for 10 to 12 minutes.

Bake: 350° 45-60 min
Microwave: 80% 10-12 min   **Yield: 8-10 servings**

#2 Calico Beans

Replace the 31-ounce can pork and beans with a 16-ounce can pork and beans. Add 1 16-ounce can of each: red kidney beans, butter beans, and lima or garbanzo beans, all drained. Double the remaining ingredients. Add 1 pound browned and drained extra-lean ground beef if desired. Bake as directed.

Per Serving	RCU	FU	Cal	% Ft	P	F	C	Na
	0	0	103	7	5	1	20	485
# 2	0	0	154	18	11	3	20	297

White Beans

These beans are simple to prepare and are a satisfying side dish.

5 cups water
2 cups white beans, washed
2 cloves garlic, peeled and cut in half
1 small onion, peeled and quartered
1 small stalk celery, cut
1 large whole bay leaf
1-1 1/2 teaspoons salt
1/4 teaspoon pepper

Soak beans overnight in cooking water, or bring beans and water to a boil in medium saucepan; turn off heat, cover, and let stand 1 hour. Place garlic, onion, and celery in blender with 1/2 cup of the water. Blend on high until vegetables are finely chopped. Pour into beans. Add bay leaf and 1/2 teaspoon cooking oil to prevent foaming. Bring to a boil, lower heat, and simmer gently until almost done, about 2 hours. Add salt and pepper and cook 15-20 minutes more or until tender. Remove bay leaf and serve.

Slow cooker: Soak beans overnight in water. Add remaining ingredients and cook on high for 5-6 hours or at low heat for 10-12 hours. Remove bay leaf, season, and serve.

Cook 2 1/2 hrs   **Yield: 8 servings**

Per Serving	RCU	FU	Cal	% Ft	P	F	C	Na
	0	0	200	2	13	1	37	243

Santa Fe Black Beans

These beans are a tasty side dish.

4 large cloves garlic, cut in half
1 small onion, cut in quarters
1 small green pepper, cut in quarters
6 cups cold water
2 cups black beans (do not soak)
2-3 teaspoons cumin
1 large whole bay leaf
1-1 1/2 teaspoons salt
1/4 teaspoon pepper

Place garlic, onion, and green pepper into blender with 1/2 cup of the water. Blend on high until vegetables are finely chopped and pour into medium saucepan. Add remaining water, washed beans, cumin, and bay leaf. Bring to a boil; lower heat, cover, and simmer gently until almost done, about 1 hour. Add salt and pepper. Cook 25-30 minutes more or until tender. Remove bay leaf, drain well, and serve.

Cook: 1 1/2 hours   Yield: 8 servings

Per Serving	RCU	FU	Cal	% Ft	P	F	C	Na
	0	0	202	2	13	1	38	244

Homemade Noodles

If you want to make your own, here's how to do it.

1 egg
1/2 scant teaspoon salt, optional
2 tablespoons water or skim milk
1 to 1 1/4 cups whole wheat flour

Beat egg, salt, and water or milk until frothy. Add flour, and mix to make a medium-stiff dough. Form noodles in a pasta maker or roll dough out to a very thin rectangle on a lightly floured surface. Dust with flour. Cut into strips 1/4 inch wide. Let dry, if desired.

Yield: 3 cups noodles

Per Serving	RCU	FU	Cal	% Ft	P	F	C	Na
	0	0	72	17	3	1	13	23

VEGETABLE ACCOMPANIMENTS

Quick Microwave Tips: Use your microwave for cooking fresh vegetables tender-crisp in minutes. Wash and prepare vegetables as desired. Prick whole carrots and potatoes with a fork. Place vegetables in plastic bag or covered dish. Consult your owner's manual for cooking times.

Seasoned Veggie Combo Tray

Try this tasty combination and vary it with the season. It adds a rainbow of color to any meal.

1 small zucchini, sliced thin (optional)
2 cups cauliflower florets
2 cups broccoli florets
2 medium carrots, sliced diagonally
1 medium tomato, cut into 6 wedges
Parmesan cheese
Onion salt

Place zucchini slices in center of oval platter. Arrange a ring of cauliflower florets around the zucchini; a ring of broccoli around the cauliflower and the carrots on the outside ring. Sprinkle with 2 tablespoons water and cover tightly with plastic wrap. Microwave on high for 6-8 minutes or until vegetables are almost tender. Drain. Arrange tomato wedges on top and sprinkle lightly with Parmesan cheese and onion salt. Cook uncovered on high 1-2 minutes and serve immediately.

Microwave: High 6-8 minutes and
High 1-2 minutes   **Yield: 6-8 servings**

Per Serving	RCU	FU	Cal	% Ft	P	F	C	Na
	0	0	33	9	3	0	6	67

Creamed Asparagus

Serve this vegetable over toast, baked potatoes, or in an omelet.

1 10-ounce package frozen asparagus pieces
1/2 teaspoon salt
1 tablespoon cornstarch
1 cup skim milk

Steam asparagus until tender. Drain. Mix cornstarch with milk, and add to hot asparagus. Cook until thick, stirring gently.
Cook: 5-10 min   Yield: 4 servings

Per Serving	RCU	FU	Cal	% Ft	P	F	C	Na
	0	0	48	14	4	1	7	270

Creamed Carrots

Golden chunks of sweet eating.

4 large carrots, peeled and sliced or shredded
2 tablespoons water
1/4 teaspoon salt
1/2 cup skim milk

Place carrots, water, and salt in covered pan; steam until carrots are very tender. Drain liquid. Place milk and carrots in blender, and pulse to make creamy chunks. Carrots may also be lightly mashed with a potato masher.
Cook: 8-12 min   Yield: 4-5 servings

Per Serving	RCU	FU	Cal	% Ft	P	F	C	Na
	0	0	35	5	2	0	7	135

Creamed Peas and Potatoes

These creamy vegetables are a year-round favorite.

2 to 3 medium-size red potatoes
1 10-ounce package frozen petite peas
1/2 teaspoon salt
1 cup skim milk
1 tablespoon cornstarch

Peel and cube potatoes. Cook in small amount of boiling, salted water until barely tender, about 10 to 12 minutes. Drain off excess water. Add frozen peas and salt. Mix milk and cornstarch. Add to vegetables, and cook until thickened to desired consistency.

Cook: 10-15 min   Yield: 4-6 servings

Per Serving	RCU	FU	Cal	% Ft	P	F	C	Na
	0	0	34	5	2	0	7	135

Saucy Beets

These brighten any meal.

1/4 cup vinegar
1 tablespoon sugar or honey
1 tablespoon cornstarch
1/4 teaspoon salt
2 cups diced beets

Drain beets and save 1/2 cup liquid. Set beets aside; combine juice with remaining ingredients. Cook and stir with wire whip until mixture thickens. Add beets; heat through and serve.

Tip: Saucy Beets are especially good with Swedish Hot Dish.

Yield: 6 servings

Per Serving	RCU	FU	Cal	% Ft	P	F	C	Na
	0	0	31	6	1	0	6	243

Perfect Corn on the Cob

This corn won't have that "drowned in water" flavor. If possible, pick and husk the corn just before cooking. For additional flavor, put a few inner husks in the bottom of the pan before adding the water.

6 ears corn, husked

Place corn in just 1 inch of boiling water. Cover and let steam on medium-high heat for just 5 minutes. Don't let pan boil dry.

Cook: 5 min   Yield: 6 servings

Per Serving	RCU	FU	Cal	% Ft	P	F	C	Na
	0	0	75	12	3	1	17	0

Mushroom Green Beans

When you get tired of plain green beans, try these.

2 16-ounce cans green beans
1 10 3/4-ounce can cream of mushroom soup, low fat
1 4-ounce can mushrooms, drained
1 tablespoon grated cheese (optional)

Drain hot beans. Add soup and mushrooms, and simmer until hot. Sprinkle cheese on top, if desired. Serve immediately.

Yield: 6 servings

Per Serving	RCU	FU	Cal	% Ft	P	F	C	Na
	0	0	53	17	2	1	9	576

Baked Winter Squash

Use your microwave - squash is ready to eat in just 10 minutes.

1 large piece of banana squash, sweetmeat, or other winter squash

Peel, remove seeds, and cut squash into small serving-size pieces. Place in a 1 1/2-quart casserole dish, and add 1 to 2 tablespoons of water. Cover with lid or plastic wrap.
Microwave: Use high power for 8 to 10 minutes or until tender. Let stand 2 minutes. To oven bake, cover and place in a 400° oven for about 45 minutes.
Microwave: High 8-10 min
Bake: 400° 40-50 min   Yield: 6 servings

Spaghetti Squash

Cut squash into quarters; remove seeds. Place squash in a large saucepan; add about 2 inches water. Bring to a boil. Reduce heat; cover and simmer until tender, about 20 minutes. Before serving, use a fork to shred and separate the squash pulp into strands. Serve with spaghetti sauce if desired.
Microwave: Prick the squash with a sharp knife. Place the whole squash in a baking dish. Cook uncovered on high 8 to 10 minutes or until squash is tender, turning dish once after 5 minutes. Let stand 5 minutes. Cut the squash in half, scoop out and discard seeds, and shred strands with a fork.
Cook: Simmer 20 min
Microwave: High 8-10 min   Yield: 6-8 servings

Per Serving	RCU	FU	Cal	% Ft	P	F	C	Na
	0	0	87	7	3	1	21	1

Summer Squash

1 teaspoon butter
1 medium onion, diced
3-4 young summer or zucchini squash, sliced
1 tablespoon chopped green chile (optional)
1/4 teaspoon salt
Dash pepper

Melt butter in medium saucepan. Add chopped onion and squash. Cover tightly and let steam on low heat until tender. Squash will make its own liquid, so do not add water unless squash is very dry.

Cook: 10-12 minutes   Yield: 6-8 servings

Per Serving	RCU	FU	Cal	% Ft	P	F	C	Na
	0	0	39	10	2	0	8	68

Carrots 'n Cabbage

1/2 medium head of cabbage
2 carrots

Shred cabbage and carrots using hand grater or medium shred blade on food processor. Place in microwave or heavy pan. Add 2 tablespoons water and cover. Cook until tender-crisp. Season and serve.

Cook: Simmer 10-12 minutes
Microwave: High   4-6 minutes   Yield: 6-8 servings

Per Serving	RCU	FU	Cal	% Ft	P	F	C	Na
	0	0	34	0	1	0	7	32

238 / SET FOR LIFE

Candied Yams or Sweet Potatoes

Holiday yams are so good with turkey.

3-4 medium yams or sweet potatoes, boiled or baked
1 8-ounce can unsweetened crushed pineapple
1 to 2 tablespoons brown sugar or honey
2 to 4 tablespoons orange juice concentrate
1/2 teaspoon salt

   Peel cooked yams or sweet potatoes and cut into thick slices. Whip with electric mixer or mash with potato masher until light and fluffy. Add pineapple, brown sugar, orange juice concentrate and salt. Whip 30 seconds longer or until well-mixed. Pour potatoes into a casserole dish. Cover, and bake in a 375° oven for 25-30 minutes or until hot.
   Microwave: Cover and cook on high for 8 to 10 minutes.
Bake: 375° 25-35 min
Microwave: High 8-10 min   **Yield: 10-12 servings**

Sliced Candied Yams

   Cooked yams or sweet potatoes may be cut into thick slices. Place in a baking dish. Mix pineapple, brown sugar, orange juice concentrate, and salt. Pour over slices. Cover and bake as above. Prepare ahead if desired.

Per Serving	RCU	FU	Cal	% Ft	P	F	C	Na
	0	0	78	5	1	0	18	100

Baked Yams

1 large yam or sweet potato

   Set yam on a cradle of foil to prevent dripping in the oven. Bake in a 400° oven until tender, about 1 hour.
   Microwave: Prick yam with a fork and place on a piece of paper toweling. Cook on high until tender, approximately 9 to 11 minutes for one large yam. Turn over once during cooking. Let stand 5 minutes before serving.
   Tip: Baked yams are a satisfying cold snack when you want something sweet to eat.
Bake: 400° 1 hr
Microwave: High 8-10 min   **Yield: 4 servings**

Per Serving	RCU	FU	Cal	% Ft	P	F	C	Na
	0	0	78	6	1	1	18	7

CHAPTER 10

Special Occasions

Here are some favorite desserts and snacks, plus a few salads for those special occasions which always seem to come along. To guide you in selecting recipes, we have coded them as follows:

+ + + This code indicates that the recipe is *Setpoint*. It is probably high in complex carbohydrates and low in fats and sugars. Eat and enjoy these foods.

+ + These recipes may be used for *Special Occasions*. They use lower amounts of fats and sugars than found in their traditional counterparts and higher amounts of complex carbohydrates: whole wheat flour, oatmeal, and the like. Most families have an occasional dessert, and these are good choices. Active children and many teens have high energy requirements and can use the extra calories. They are better off eating these desserts than those prepared from all refined carbohydrates and fats. Anyone with a sticky Setpoint or health problem will want to avoid them.

+ These recipes are *Forbidden Favorites*. They are high in fat and sugar and should be a very infrequent choice. They are definitely not recommended if you're trying to lose weight or overcome a health problem.

As you include more and more wholesome foods in your diet, you may be surprised to find the forbidden favorites losing their appeal as your food preferences change. Then you will know that you are *making real progress!*

COOKIES

Raisin Bars + +

Everyone loves these spicy, moist bars!

1 cup raisins
1 cup water
2 cups whole wheat flour
2 teaspoons cinnamon
1 teaspoon soda
1/2 teaspoon salt
1/2 cup chopped nuts (optional)
1/4-1/3 cup softened margarine or oil
1/2 cup honey or sugar
1 egg
1 teaspoon vanilla

Glaze:
1 tablespoon warm water
1/2 cup powdered sugar
1/2 teaspoon vanilla

Mix raisins and water in blender for 20 to 30 seconds. Combine dry ingredients and nuts in mixer bowl. Add margarine and liquids, including the water-raisin mix. Mix well. Pour into a lightly greased 10 x 15-inch baking sheet. Bake in a 375° oven for 14-16 minutes.

Remove cookies from oven and let cool slightly while combining glaze ingredients in blender. Pulse until smooth. Pour onto warm cookies and spread with spatula. The thin glaze seals the cookies. Cut into bars after glaze sets.

Bake: 375° 14-16 min   Yield: 24 bars

Per Serving	RCU	FU	Cal	% Ft	P	F	C	Na
	1	0	96	21	2	2	16	102

Butterscotch Squares++

Kids love to make these chewy stir n' pour brownies.

1/3 cup butter	2 teaspoons baking powder
1 cup brown sugar	2 cups whole wheat flour — *try 1 cup w/w flour*
1/2 cup honey	1/8 teaspoon salt *1 cup oatmeal,*
2 eggs	1 teaspoon vanilla

Melt butter in a medium-size saucepan. Remove from heat, and stir in brown sugar and honey. Add remaining ingredients, and stir until well blended. Spread in a greased or nonstick 10 x 15-inch baking sheet. Bake in a 350° oven for 15 to 18 minutes or until lightly browned. Cookies will raise and are done just as they start to fall. *Do not overbake.*

Bake: 350° 15-18 min   Yield: 24 bars   *12 minutes*

Per Serving	RCU	FU	Cal	% Ft	P	F	C	Na
	1	1	96	28	2	3	17	70

Raisin & Nut Cookies

Sometimes called breakfast cookies.

1 1/3 cups water	5 cups whole wheat flour
2 cups raisins	1 teaspoon baking powder
2/3 cup oil	1 teaspoon soda
1 cup brown sugar	1 teaspoon salt
1 cup white sugar	2 teaspoons cinnamon
3 eggs	1/4 teaspoon nutmeg
2 teaspoons vanilla	1 cup nuts, optional

Boil water and raisins for 5 minutes; let cool. Cream oil, sugars, eggs and vanilla in mixer bowl. Blend in cooled raisin mixture. Add dry ingredients and mix well. Add nuts if desired. Drop dough from a spoon onto nonstick baking sheet. Bake in a 400° oven for 10 to 12 minutes or just until set.

Bake: 400° 10-12 min   Yield: 60

Per Serving	RCU	FU	Cal	% Ft	P	F	C	Na
	1	0	90	29	2	3	13	58

Alan's Cookies++

This favorite recipe has several tasty variations.

3/4 cup oil
1 cup brown sugar
1/2 cup sugar
2 eggs
1 teaspoon vanilla
1 1/2 cups whole wheat flour
2 cups rolled oats
1/2 teaspoon salt
1 teaspoon soda
1/2 teaspoon baking powder
1 cup raisins

Cream oil, sugars, eggs, and vanilla. Add remaining ingredients and mix well. For bar cookies, spread batter in a 10 x 15-inch lightly greased baking sheet. For regular cookies, drop by tablespoonfuls onto nonstick baking sheets; or use a small ice cream scoop for uniform size. Bake in a 350° oven 12 to 15 minutes for bar cookies, 8 to 12 minutes for drop cookies.

Time will vary with the weight of the baking sheets used.

Bake: 350°   Bar cookies: 12-15 min
              Drop cookies: 8-12 min   Yield: 36

#2 Sunflower Seed Cookies

Prepare cookies as directed above, omitting the raisins. Add 1/2 cup unsweetened coconut and 1/2 cup sunflower seeds.

#3 Crunchy Chip Cookies

Prepare cookies as directed above, omitting the raisins. Add 1/2 cup carob chips and 1/2 cup chopped nuts.

Per Serving	RCU	FU	Cal	% Ft	P	F	C	Na
	1	1	108	43	2	5	13	58
#2	1	1	117	53	2	7	12	63
#3	1	1	109	51	2	6	12	60

Applesauce Cookies + +

Cookies have a soft, cake-like texture.

1/2 cup oil
3/4 cup honey or 1 cup sugar
1 egg
1 cup applesauce
2 cups whole wheat flour
1 cup quick oats

1 teaspoon soda
1 teaspoon cinnamon
1/2 teaspoon nutmeg
1/2 teaspoon salt
1 cup chopped dates or raisins
1/2 cup chopped nuts (optional)

Mix oil, honey, and egg until fluffy. Blend in applesauce. Add remaining ingredients; mix well. Drop by tablespoonfuls onto nonstick baking sheets. Bake in a 350° oven for 10 to 12 minutes or just until set.

Bake: 350° 10-12 min   Yield: 36

Per Serving	RCU	FU	Cal	% Ft	P	F	C	Na
	1	0	94	33	1	3	15	65

Spiced Oatmeal Drops++

Here's a spicy version of an old favorite.

3/4 cup oil
1 1/2 cups sugar
1/3 cup molasses
2 eggs
3 cups whole wheat flour
1 teaspoon cinnamon
1 teaspoon nutmeg

1 teaspoon cloves
1 teaspoon salt
1 teaspoon soda
1 teaspoon baking powder
1 12-ounce can evaporated skimmed milk
3 cups quick oats
1 cup raisins

Mix oil, sugar, molasses, and eggs. In a separate bowl, combine flour, spices, salt, soda, and baking powder. Alternately add with the milk. Mix well. Blend in oats and raisins. Drop dough from a spoon onto nonstick baking sheet. Tip: One tablespoon apple pie spice may be used in place of the cinnamon, nutmeg, and cloves. Bake in a 350° oven for 10 to 12 minutes or until light brown.

Bake: 350° 10-12 min   Yield: 84 small

Per Serving	RCU	FU	Cal	% Ft	P	F	C	Na
	1	0	62	34	1	2	9	45

Creamy Pumpkin Cookies ++

These moist lowfat cookies taste especially good on Halloween.

3/4 cup nonfat mayonnaise or 1/2 cup oil and 2 eggs
1/2 cup sugar
1 cup brown sugar
2 cups canned pumpkin
3 cups whole wheat flour
2 teaspoons baking powder
1 teaspoon soda
1 teaspoon salt
2 teaspoons cinnamon
1/2 teaspoon nutmeg
1 teaspoon ginger
1 cup raisins or 1/2 cup carob chips or chocolate chips

Cream mayonnaise (or oil and eggs), sugars, and pumpkin. Add dry ingredients and mix well. Stir in raisins or chips. Drop from spoon onto non-stick baking sheet. Bake at 350° for 10 to 12 minutes. Do not overbake.

Bake: 350°   **10 to 12 min**   **Yield: 48 large**

Per Serving	RCU	FU	Cal	% Ft	P	F	C	Na
Mayonnaise	1	0	53	3	1	0	11	90
Oil & Eggs	1	0	79	31	1	3	12	73

Peanut Butter Cookies++

Peanut butter cookies are made even better with the sweet nutty taste of fresh whole wheat flour.

1/4 cup margarine
1/2 cup white sugar
1/2 cup brown sugar
1 egg
1/2 cup peanut butter

1/2 teaspoon vanilla
1 tablespoon water
1 cup whole wheat flour
1 cup quick oats
1 teaspoon soda

Cream margarine, sugars, egg, peanut butter, vanilla, and water. Add dry ingredients, and mix well. Drop by spoonfuls onto ungreased baking sheets. Press thumb or handle of knife into center of each cookie. Bake in a 350° oven for 8 to 10 minutes. Cookies will be set, but not firm. Cool on wire racks.

Bake: 350° 8-10 min   **Yield: 36**

Per Serving	RCU	FU	Cal	% Ft	P	F	C	Na
	1	1	123	48	3	7	14	151

Molasses Crinkles + +

They're thick and chewy with crackled tops.

1/2 cup oil
3/4 cup brown sugar
1 egg
1/4 cup molasses
1 cup unbleached white flour
1 cup whole wheat flour
1/4 teaspoon salt
2 teaspoons soda
1 teaspoon cinnamon
1 teaspoon ginger
1/2 teaspoon cloves
Sugar

Mix oil, sugar, egg, and molasses until fluffy. Add remaining ingredients. Mix well. Chill dough. Shape into walnut-size balls. Dip tops in sugar. Place sugar-side up, 3 inches apart on a nonstick baking sheet.

Sprinkle the top of each cookie with 3 drops of water to get a crackled effect. Bake in a 350° oven 10 to 12 minutes, just until set but not hard.

Bake: 350° 10-12 min   Yield: 48

Per Serving	RCU	FU	Cal	% Ft	P	F	C	Na
	0	0	58	44	1	3	6	70

Pineapple Cookies

A delicate taste-treat.

3/4 cup crushed pineapple, slightly drained
1/4 cup oil
1 egg
1 teaspoon vanilla
1 cup brown sugar, packed

2 cups unbleached white flour
1 teaspoon baking powder
1/2 teaspoon soda
1/2 teaspoon salt

Mix pineapple, oil, egg, vanilla and brown sugar. Add flour, baking powder, soda and salt. Mix well. Drop from teaspoon on nonstick baking sheet. Bake in 350° oven for 9 to 11 minutes or until lightly brown.

Bake: 350°   9 to 11 min   Yield: 36

Per Serving	RCU	FU	Cal	% Ft	P	F	C	Na
	1	0	52	29	1	2	8	52

ator Oatmeal Cookies + +

, Aunt Jean Payne makes a hit with her 4-gallon "Cookie Barrel," a plastic hese yummies.

1 cup packed brown sugar
1/2 cup sugar
3/4 cup shortening
2 eggs
1 teaspoon vanilla
1 1/2 cups whole wheat flour
1 teaspoon soda
1/2 teaspoon baking powder
1/2 teaspoon salt
3 cups oats, quick or old fashioned

Cream sugars, shortening, eggs, and vanilla. Add flour, soda, baking powder, and salt. Mix well. Mix in rolled oats. Form dough into two rolls 2 1/2 inches in diameter. Wrap in waxed paper, and chill until stiff. Dough may also be frozen. Cut in thin slices. Place slices slightly apart on ungreased baking sheets. If using frozen dough, make slices a little thicker and bake 2 to 3 minutes longer. Bake in a 375° oven for 8 to 10 minutes.

Variation: Drop unchilled dough by spoonfuls onto ungreased baking sheet if desired. Bake as directed.

Bake: 375° 8-10 min   **Yield: 5-6 dozen**

Per Serving	RCU	FU	Cal	% Ft	P	F	C	Na
	1	1	67	49	1	4	8	45

Granola Bars + +

These high-energy bars are ideal for back-packing trips.

1/2 cup honey
1/2 cup peanut butter
1 teaspoon vanilla
5 cups granola*

Warm honey and peanut butter over low heat and mix well. Stir in vanilla and granola. Spread on large baking sheet and cut into bars.

Yield: 30 small bars

Sugar Cookies +

Children love decorating these cookies for Christmas or Valentine's Day.

1 cup shortening
1 cup sugar
2 eggs
1/2 teaspoon vanilla
3 cups unbleached white flour
1/2 teaspoon soda
1/2 teaspoon salt
1 teaspoon baking powder
1/2 cup sour cream, plain yogurt, or buttermilk

Cream shortening, sugar, eggs, and vanilla. Add dry ingredients and sour cream. Mix will. Cover bowl, and chill dough at least 30 minutes. On floured surface, roll out to 1/8-inch thickness. Cut into desired shapes. Place on ungreased cookie sheets. Bake in a 375° oven for 8 minutes. Do not overbake.

Bake: 375° 8 min   Yield: 4-5 dozen

Per Serving	RCU	FU	Cal	% Ft	P	F	C	Na
	1	1	69	52	1	4	8	40

Cherry Bars

1 white cake mix, lite
1 20-ounce can cherry pie filling, lite

Glaze:
2 tablespoons warm water
1 cup powdered sugar
1/2 teaspoon vanilla

Prepare cake according to package directions. Spread two-thirds of the batter evenly in a 9 x 13-inch pan that has been sprayed with nonstick cooking spray. Spread cherry pie filling on top of batter. Dot remaining batter close together on top of pie filling. Bake in a 350° oven for about 40 minutes. Cool ten minutes. Combine glaze ingredients and spread over top of bars.

Bake: 350° 40 min   Yield: 15 servings

Per Serving	RCU	FU	Cal	% Ft	P	F	C	Na
	5	0	220	8	3	2	48	282

CAKES AND FROSTINGS

Applesauce Cake ++

This is a quick and easy no-egg cake with tasty variations.

1/2 cup oil
1 cup sugar or 3/4 cup honey
1 cup applesauce or other pureed fruit
2 cups whole wheat flour
1/2 teaspoon salt
1 teaspoon soda
1 teaspoon cinnamon
1/2 teaspoon cloves
1/2 teaspoon nutmeg
1/2 cup raisins

Combine all ingredients in bowl and mix on medium speed for 3 to 4 minutes. Pour into a lightly greased 7 x 12-inch or 9 x 13-inch pan. Bake in a 350° oven for 20 to 25 minutes or until cake springs back when touched in center. Cool slightly, and frost with Broiled Coconut Topping* if desired.

Bake: 350° 20-25 min   Yield: 15 pieces

Per Serving	RCU	FU	Cal	% Ft	P	F	C	Na
	3	1	189	37	2	8	27	148

Zucchini Cake

Replace applesauce with 2 cups shredded zucchini.

Apricot Cake

Replace applesauce with 1 cup drained, pureed apricots.

Broiled Coconut Topping ++

This is a favorite topping for almost any cake.

1 cup brown sugar
1/4 cup skim milk
2 to 4 tablespoons butter or margarine
1 teaspoon vanilla
1 cup granola or 1/2 cup chopped nuts and 1/2 cup coconut

Mix brown sugar, milk, and butter in small saucepan. Bring to a boil. Boil 2 minutes, stirring constantly. Remove from heat, and stir in vanilla and granola. Spread on cake. Place cake under broiler for 1 to 2 minutes, until mixture bubbles and turns golden brown. Watch carefully as frosting burns easily.

Per Serving	RCU	FU	Cal	% Ft	P	F	C	Na
	1	0	45	43	1	2	6	30

Banana Cake ++

It looks and smells as good as it tastes!

1/3 cup oil
1 cup sugar or 3/4 cup honey
1 egg
1 teaspoon vanilla
1 cup mashed bananas (approximately 3)
1 cup buttermilk or sour milk
2 cups whole wheat flour
1/2 teaspoon salt
1 teaspoon soda
1 teaspoon baking powder
1/2 cup chopped nuts (optional)

Beat together oil, honey, eggs, and vanilla. Add remaining ingredients. Mix well. Let stand 5 minutes before using. Bake in a lightly greased and floured 7 x 12 or 9 x 13-inch pan. Bake in a 350° oven for 25 to 30 minutes or until center springs back when touched.

Bake: 350° 25-30 min   Yield: 15 pieces

Per Serving	RCU	FU	Cal	% Ft	P	F	C	Na
	2	1	165	29	3	5	27	164

Velvety Slim Frosting ++

This frosting is delicious on Banana, Applesauce, and Oatmeal Cake. Refrigerate any leftovers.

1 tablespoon margarine
2 tablespoons unbleached white flour
3-4 tablespoons brown sugar or honey
1/2 cup frozen apple juice concentrate, thawed
1/2 cup buttermilk
1 teaspoon vanilla

Melt margarine in a small saucepan. Using a wire whisk, stir in flour and brown sugar. Add juice concentrate, buttermilk, and vanilla. Cook over medium heat, stirring constantly, until thickened, about 5 minutes. Serve over cake while topping is still warm, or frost cake and chill.

Variation: For Carrot, Zucchini or Apricot Cake
Follow above recipe, using white sugar in place of brown sugar, and orange juice concentrate instead of apple juice concentrate.

Per Serving	RCU	FU	Cal	% Ft	P	F	C	Na
	0	0	20	32	0	1	3	20

Carrot Cake Supreme + +

A delectable combination of flavors for a special occasion.

1/2 cup oil
1 cup sugar or honey
3 eggs
1 teaspoon vanilla
2 cups finely grated carrot (about 4 large carrots)
1 cup unsweetened crushed pineapple, undrained
2 cups whole wheat flour
1/2 cup unbleached white flour
1/2 teaspoon salt
2 teaspoons baking powder
1 teaspoon soda
2 teaspoons cinnamon
1/2 cup chopped nuts (optional)
1 cup raisins

Mix oil, sugar, eggs, and vanilla. To creamed mixture add carrots, crushed pineapple, and all dry ingredients. Mix well. Fold in nuts or raisins if desired. Pour into a 9 x 13-inch pan that has been sprayed with nonstick cooking spray. Bake in a 350° oven for 25 minutes.

Bake: 350° 25 min   **Yield: 20 pieces**

Per Serving	RCU	FU	Cal	% Ft	P	F	C	Na
	2	1	177	34	4	7	24	147

Cream Cheese Frosting+

1 8-ounce package nonfat cream cheese, softened
2 tablespoons butter
1 teaspoon vanilla
3 cups powdered sugar

Mix cream cheese, butter, and vanilla. Add powdered sugar and mix. Add a little hot water if needed to achieve desired consistency.

Per Serving	RCU	FU	Cal	% Ft	P	F	C	Na
	2	0	55	18	2	1	10	68

Oatmeal Cake ++

This moist cake is luscious!

1 1/2 cups oatmeal, quick or old-fashioned
1/2 cup margarine or butter
1 1/2 cups boiling water
1 cup sugar or 3/4 cup honey
1 teaspoon vanilla
2 eggs
1 1/2 cups whole wheat flour
1/2 teaspoon salt
1 teaspoon soda
1 teaspoon cinnamon
1/2 teaspoon nutmeg

Stir oatmeal and margarine into boiling water. Set pan aside, and let margarine melt. Mix honey, vanilla, and eggs until creamy. Add flour, oatmeal mixture, soda, salt, and spices and mix well. Pour into a lightly greased 9 x 13-inch pan. Bake in a 350° oven for 25 to 30 minutes or until a toothpick inserted in the center comes out clean.
Bake: 350° 25-30 min   Yield: 15 pieces

Per Serving	RCU	FU	Cal	% Ft	P	F	C	Na
	2	1	163	40	3	7	23	236

Coconut Pecan Frosting +

3/4 cup evaporated skimmed milk
1/2 cup honey or 1 cup sugar
1 egg, slightly beaten
1/4 cup butter or margarine
1 teaspoon vanilla
1 cup coconut
1 cup chopped pecans

Combine milk, honey, egg, butter, and vanilla in a saucepan. Cook and stir over low heat until thickened, about 12 minutes. Beat until cool. Stir in coconut and pecans.

Per Serving	RCU	FU	Cal	% Ft	P	F	C	Na
	2	2	167	65	2	12	12	65

Lemon Bundt Cake +

This cake is a birthday tradition for our three sons.

1 package yellow or lemon cake mix
1 3 1/2-ounce package instant lemon pudding mix
1 cup water
1/2 cup oil
4 eggs

Glaze:
1 cup powdered sugar
1 lemon, juiced (3 tablespoons)
1 orange, juiced (3-4 tablespoons)

Place cake mix, pudding, water, oil and eggs in mixer bowl. Beat 5 to 7 minutes. Pour into a greased and floured bundt pan. Place a shallow pan of water on the bottom oven rack while cake is baking. Bake in a 350° oven for 45 minutes. While cake is baking, combine powdered sugar and juices. Remove cake from oven, and immediately remove from pan. Place on a wire cooling rack and place rack over a large plate. Slowly pour glaze over cake, repeating several times. Serve when cool.

Bake: 350° 45 minutes   **Yield: 20 servings**

Per Serving	RCU	FU	Cal	% Ft	P	F	C	Na
	3	1	209	40	2	9	40	237

White Cake

This makes an elegant white cake.

1/2 cup shortening
3/4 cup honey or 1 cup sugar
1 teaspoon vanilla
2 cups unbleached white flour
1/2 teaspoon salt
1 tablespoon baking powder
1 cup skim milk
2 eggs

Cream shortening, honey, and vanilla. Mix in dry ingredients. Add milk, and beat 2 minutes. Add eggs, and beat another minute. Pour into a lightly greased and floured 9 x 13-inch pan or two 8-inch round cake pans. Bake in a 350° oven for 20 to 25 minutes or until a toothpick inserted in the center comes out clean.

Bake: 350° 20-25 min   **Yield: 15 pieces**

Per Serving	RCU	FU	Cal	% Ft	P	F	C	Na
	3	1	188	41	3	9	25	167

Spice Cake

Prepare White Cake as directed. Add to dry ingredients 1 teaspoon cinnamon, 1/2 teaspoon cloves, 1/2 teaspoon nutmeg, and 1/4 teaspoon allspice.

Butter Frosting +

1/2 cup margarine or shortening
2 egg whites or 1 whole egg
3 1/2 cups powdered sugar
1/2 teaspoon salt
1 teaspoon vanilla

Place all ingredients in bowl. Mix on high speed until fluffy.

Per Serving	RCU	FU	Cal	% Ft	P	F	C	Na
	2	1	109	49	0	6	14	140

Gingerbread ++

Everyone loves this fragrant spicy cake.

1/2 cup oil
1 cup sugar or honey
1 egg, slightly beaten
1/2 cup light molasses
2 cups unbleached flour
1/2 teaspoon salt
1 teaspoon soda
1 teaspoon ginger
1 teaspoon cinnamon
1/2 teaspoon cloves
1 cup hot water

Mix oil, sugar, egg, and molasses. Add dry ingredients and hot water. Mix well. Pour into a 7 x 12-inch baking pan that has been coated with nonstick cooking spray. Bake in a 350° oven for about 30 minutes or until toothpick inserted in center comes out clean.

Bake: 350°   30 min   **Yield: 18 pieces**

Per Serving	RCU	FU	Cal	% Ft	P	F	C	Na
	3	1	167	36	2	7	25	104

Chocolate Banana Cake++

2 cups unbleached flour
1 1/2 cups sugar
1/2 cup cocoa
1 1/2 teaspoons soda
1/2 teaspoon salt
1/2 teaspoon cinnamon

4 egg whites or 2 eggs
1/2 cup oil
1/2 cup water
1 teaspoon vanilla
1 cup buttermilk or yogurt
1 banana, mashed

Combine flour, sugar, cocoa, soda, salt and cinnamon. Add egg whites, oil, water, vanilla, buttermilk, and banana. Mix on medium speed for 3 to 4 minutes. Pour into a 9 x 13-inch baking pan that has been coated with nonstick cooking spray. Bake in a 350° oven for 35 to 40 minutes or until cake springs back when lightly touched. This cake needs no frosting.

Bake: 350° 35-40 min   **Yield: 15 pieces**

Per Serving	RCU	FU	Cal	% Ft	P	F	C	Na
	4	1	216	23	4	6	39	187

Gingerbread Sauce++

1 1/2 cups water
1/2 cup brown sugar
2 tablespoons butter or margarine
2 tablespoons cornstarch
1 teaspoon vanilla

Combine ingredients and cook over medium heat until mixture comes to a boil and thickens, stirring constantly. Spoon over individual servings.

Applesauce Topper++

1 cup applesauce
1/2 teaspoon peppermint extract

Combine applesauce and peppermint extract. Warm slightly and spoon over individual servings.

Fruit Cake +

This makes a very special holiday gift.

3/4 cup sugar
1 cup whole wheat flour
1/2 teaspoon salt
1 tablespoon baking powder
1 pound dates, coarsely chopped

1 pound pecan halves
4 eggs, well-beaten
1 teaspoon vanilla
8 ounces dried cherries, whole or halves
8 ounces dried pineapple pieces

Sift dry ingredients over dates and nuts and mix. Add well-beaten eggs and vanilla. Mix well. Add fruit, and mix just until coated. Pour batter into greased and floured loaf pans. Place shallow pan of water on the bottom oven rack while cake is baking. Bake in a 325⁰ oven for 1 hour. Immediately remove from pans and cool on wire racks. Wrap in foil, and store in cool place or freezer. Slice very thin.

Bake: 325° 1 hour   Yield: 4   3″ x 5 3/4″ loaves

Per Serving	RCU	FU	Cal	% Ft	P	F	C	Na
	1	1	96	35	2	4	14	54

Grandma's Holiday Fruit Cake + +

Watch this dark, moist, cake disappear!

2 1/2 cups applesauce
1 cup shortening
1 1/2 cups brown sugar
1/2 cup molasses
4 cups whole wheat flour
1/2 teaspoon salt
4 teaspoons soda

2 teaspoons cinnamon
1 teaspoon cloves
2 cups raisins
1/2 cup nuts
8 ounces dried cherries (optional)
8 ounces dried pineapple (optional)

Slowly heat applesauce to medium hot, and pour into mixing bowl equipped with the kneading arm. Add shortening, brown sugar and molasses. Mix well. Combine flour, salt, and spices in sifter. Put raisins, nuts, and fruit in small bowl, and sift a small amount of the flour mixture over them. Stir until coated. Set aside. Add remaining flour to the liquids in bowl, and mix thoroughly. Add fruit and nut mixture. Pulse lightly to mix. Pour into well-greased and floured loaf pans and bake immediately. Bake in a 350° oven for 15 minutes. Reduce heat to 325° and bake 1 hour. Immediately remove from pans, and cool on wire racks. Wrap in foil and freeze.

Bake 325° 1 hour 15 min   Yield: 3   4 x 8 1/2″ loaves

Per Serving	RCU	FU	Cal	% Ft	P	F	C	Na
	1	0	82	34	1	3	11	92

DESSERTS

Strawberry Cheesecake Delight ++

A light and delicious dessert!

Crust:
2 cups graham cracker crumbs (about 12 crackers)
1/4 cup butter or margarine, melted

Filling:
1 8-ounce package fat free cream cheese, softened
1/2 cup sugar
2 tablespoons milk
1/2 teaspoon vanilla
1 1 1/2-ounce package whipped topping, whipped (Dream Whip)

Topping:
1 4 3/4-ounce package strawberry Danish Dessert
4 cups fresh berries, sliced or whole

Place graham crackers in blender and pulse to make crumbs, or use large shred on food processor. Mix crumbs with melted butter and press into a 9 x 13-inch pan. Chill while preparing the filling. Mix cream cheese, sugar, milk, and vanilla. Fold in the whipped topping and spread over crumb crust. Chill until set. Prepare Danish dessert as directed on package for pie. Cool slightly and add berries. Pour fruit mixture over cheesecake. Chill well.

Chill: 4-5 hrs   **Yield: 20 servings**

Per Serving	RCU	FU	Cal	% Ft	P	F	C	Na
	2	1	128	23	3	3	21	154

Cherry Cheesecake

Prepare crust and filling as directed above. Omit Danish Dessert and berries. Cover with 1 20-ounce can lite cherry pie filling.

Frosty Strawberry Squares + +

Crust:
1 cup whole wheat flour
1/4 cup brown sugar
1/2 cup chopped nuts (optional)
1/4 cup margarine, softened

Filling:
2 egg whites
2 tablespoons sugar (increase to 1/2 cup if using whipping cream)
2 tablespoons lemon juice
1 10-ounce package frozen strawberries or raspberries
2 1 1/2-ounce envelopes Dream Whip, prepared according to package directions,
   or 1 cup whipping cream, whipped

Mix flour, sugar, nuts, and margarine. Spread in a shallow pan. Bake in a 250° oven for 20 minutes, stirring occasionally. When cooled, crumble and press into a 9 x 13-inch pan. In mixer bowl, combine egg whites, sugar, lemon juice, and frozen berries. Beat on high speed until stiff, about 5 to 6 minutes. Add prepared Dream Whip or whipped cream and mix on low speed just long enough to fold in cream. Pour over crust in pan. Freeze until firm.

Chill: 3-4 hrs   **Yield: 15 servings**

Per Serving	RCU	FU	Cal	% Ft	P	F	C	Na
D. Whip	1	1	150	19	2	3	24	59

Strawberry Dessert ++

1 10-ounce package frozen sliced strawberries, thawed
   or 2 cups sliced strawberries
1 quart vanilla or strawberry nonfat yogurt
1 10-inch tube angel food cake

Drain strawberries and fold gently into yogurt. Slice cake and top individual servings with berry mixture.
Variation: Tear cake into 2-inch pieces and arrange in 9 x 13-inch dish. Pour berry mixture over cake and chill until firm.
Yield: 18 servings

Per Serving	RCU	FU	Cal	% Ft	P	F	C	Na
	4	10	152	6	4	1	33	124

Layered Fruit Parfait + + +

Here's a dessert that's simply beautiful.

2 cups fresh or frozen blueberries
1 cup plain nonfat yogurt
2 to 4 tablespoons frozen unsweetened apple juice concentrate
1/2 teaspoon grated lemon peel
1 16-ounce carton lowfat cottage cheese

Partially thaw and drain frozen fruits. Prepare dressing by mixing yogurt, apple juice concentrate, and lemon peel. Place approximately 3 tablespoons cottage cheese in each of the 6 large parfait glasses. Layer with approximately 1 tablespoon dressing, strawberries, a few melon balls, blueberries, remaining cottage cheese, dressing, and strawberries. Top with remaining melon balls. Serve immediately. Tip: Parfaits can be made with any combination of fresh fruit.
Yield: 6 servings

Per Serving	RCU	FU	Cal	% Ft	P	F	C	Na
	0	0	117	14	9	2	16	242

Fruity Muesli Dessert + + +

Gail Gillette shares this tangy Setpoint refreshment.

1/4 cup raisins
1 cup plain nonfat yogurt
1 cup unsweetened crushed pineapple, drained
1 11-ounce can mandarin oranges, drained
2 apples, cored, unpeeled, and diced
2 bananas, mashed
2 tablespoons quick-cooking oats
1 orange, juiced (1/4 cup)
1 to 2 tablespoons honey or frozen apple juice concentrate
(If yogurt is fresh and mild, honey is unnecessary)

Soak raisins in hot water for 10 minutes. Drain well. Combine with remaining ingredients. Cover and chill.
Chill: 2 hrs   Yield: 6 servings

Per Serving	RCU	FU	Cal	% Ft	P	F	C	Na
	0	0	155	4	3	1	32	25

Fruit 'n Berry Compote +++

This delicious versatile dish can be varied to meet the season. It's a good dessert, dessert topping, or spread for toast.

1 6-ounce can frozen apple juice concentrate
1 1/2 cups apple juice or water
1 teaspoon vanilla
1 12-ounce package frozen strawberries, cherries, or cranberries
   or 2 cups fresh berries or pitted cherries
4 apples, peeled and diced
1 cup crushed unsweetened pineapple, undrained
3 tablespoons cornstarch

Combine apple juice concentrate, juice or water, and vanilla in a saucepan and bring to a boil. Add fruit, stirring gently. Simmer uncovered for 10 minutes. Mix cornstarch with small amount of water and stir into fruit mixture. Stir constantly until thick. Let cool. Cover and refrigerate.

Salad variation: Omit cornstarch. Soften 2 packages unflavored gelatin in 1/2 cup of the juice or water. Add to hot mixture after cooking and stir until dissolved. Pour into salad mold and chill.

Yield: 10   1/2 cup servings

Per Serving	RCU	FU	Cal	% Ft	P	F	C	Na
	0	0	82	4	0	0	20	1

Baked Apples +++

Enjoy autumn's bounty with this wholesome dessert.

6 large baking apples
2 tablespoons Granola*
1/2 cup raisins or chopped dates (optional)
1 6-ounce can frozen unsweetened apple juice concentrate, thawed
1 teaspoon cinnamon
1/2 teaspoon nutmeg

Core apples. Mix granola and raisins. Stuff into center of apples. Combine apple juice concentrate and spices to make syrup. Place apples in a glass baking dish. Pour syrup around apples. Bake uncovered in a 350° oven for 45 to 60 minutes or until apples are tender.

Microwave: Make a shallow cut in skin completely around each apple one inch from the bottom to keep skin from shrinking during cooking. Cook on high 9 to 12 minutes or until fork tender. Turn apples halfway through cooking time. Pour syrup over apples before serving.

Bake: 375° **45-50 min**
Microwave: High 9-12 min   **Yield: 6 servings**

Per Serving	RCU	FU	Cal	% Ft	P	F	C	Na
	1	0	98	0	0	0	24	2

Apple Crisp ++

10 large baking apples
  or 2 16-ounce cans unsweetened apple slices
1 6-ounce can frozen unsweetened apple juice concentrate
1 teaspoon cinnamon
Regular or Spicy Oatmeal Topping (see below)

Peel and thinly slice apples. Place in the bottom of a 9 x 13-inch baking dish. Pour thawed apple juice concentrate over apples, and sprinkle with cinnamon. Spread topping evenly over apples. Bake uncovered in a 350° oven for 30 to 40 minutes or until apples are tender but not soggy.

Tip: Any fresh fruit may be substituted for the apples.
Bake: 350° 30-40 min   Yield: 15 servings

Regular Topping

1 cup whole wheat flour or unbleached flour
1/2 cup sugar
1 teaspoon baking powder
1/8 teaspoon salt
1 egg
1/4 cup margarine or shortening, softened

Combine dry ingredients in mixer bowl. Add egg and softened margarine. Mix on low until mixture is crumbly.

Spicy Oatmeal Topping

1/2 cup brown sugar
1/2 cup whole wheat flour
2 cups quick-cooking oats
1 teaspoon cinnamon
1 teaspoon allspice
1/2 teaspoon cloves
1/4 cup butter or margarine, softened

Combine dry ingredients in mixer bowl. Add softened butter, and mix just until mixture is crumbly.

Per Serving	RCU	FU	Cal	% Ft	P	F	C	Na
	1	1	133	23	1	3	24	40

Apple Dumpling Roll + +

Crust:
2 cups unbleached flour (may use half whole wheat)
1/2 teaspoon salt
2 tablespoons sugar
1 tablespoon baking powder
1 tablespoon oil
1 egg, beaten
1/2 cup skim milk

Apples:
8 to 10 medium cooking apples
1 tablespoon cinnamon or apple pie spice
1/4 cup brown sugar or honey (optional)

Syrup:
1 12-ounce can frozen unsweetened apple juice concentrate
1/2 cup water
Few drops red food coloring

Combine the dry crust ingredients. Add oil, egg, and milk. Mix to make a soft dough. Let dough sit while preparing apples. Peel apples, if desired, and shred using hand grater or medium shred on food processor. On lightly floured surface, roll out dough to a 9 x 15-inch rectangle. Spread shredded apples evenly over dough. Sprinkle with cinnamon. Add brown sugar or honey, if desired. Beginning at the 15-inch side, roll up. Using a piece of thread or fishing line, cut into 15 pieces. Place in a 9 x 13-inch baking dish. Combine syrup ingredients, and pour syrup evenly over rolls. Bake uncovered in a 350° oven for 30 to 35 minutes.

Bake: 350° 30-35 min   **Yield: 15 servings**

Per Serving	RCU	FU	Cal	% Ft	P	F	C	Na
	2	0	132	10	2	2	27	155

ruit Cobbler ++

rust while baking — like magic!

*margarine or butter, melted
3/4 cup skim milk
1/2 cup sugar
1 cup unbleached white flour (may use half whole wheat)
2 teaspoons baking powder
1/4 teaspoon salt
1 teaspoon vanilla
3-4 cups "lite" canned fruit, slightly drained
 or fresh fruit (blueberries, apricots, peaches, etc.)

Melt margarine in oven in a 8 x 12-inch glass baking dish or 1 1/2-quart casserole dish while oven preheats. In blender mix milk, sugar, flour, baking powder, salt, and vanilla. Remove pan from oven. Spread margarine evenly in pan. Pour batter over melted margarine. Do not stir. Pour fruit evenly over batter. Do not stir. Bake uncovered in a 325° oven for 30 to 40 minutes or until crust is brown.
Bake: 325° 30-40 min   Yield: 15 servings

Per Serving	RCU	FU	Cal	% Ft	P	F	C	Na
	2	0	100	15	2	2	20	111

Old-Fashioned Rice Pudding ++

Make a double batch and enjoy the leftovers for breakfast!

**2 large eggs
1/4 cup honey
1 teaspoon vanilla
1/4 teaspoon salt
2 cups skim milk
2 cups cooked brown rice
Nutmeg
1/2 cup raisins (optional)**

Place eggs, honey, vanilla, salt, and milk in blender. Pulse to mix well. Pour over cooked rice in a 9 x 9-inch baking dish. Add raisins, if desired. Stir only until mixed. Sprinkle with nutmeg. Bake in a 325° oven for 30 to 35 minutes or just until pudding is set. Tip: A double recipe fills a 9 x 13-inch pan.
**Bake: 325° 30-35 min   Yield: 6 servings
or Microwave: High 9-11 min**

Per Serving	RCU	FU	Cal	% Ft	P	F	C	Na
	2	0	155	19	6	3	27	211

Pumpkin Cake Roll +

3 eggs
1/2 cup honey
2/3 cup canned pumpkin
1 teaspoon lemon juice
3/4 cup whole wheat flour
2 teaspoons cinnamon
1 teaspoon baking powder
1 teaspoon ginger
1/2 teaspoon salt
1/2 teaspoon nutmeg
1/3 cup powdered sugar
1 8-ounce package cream cheese
2 tablespoons soft margarine
1/2 teaspoon vanilla
1 cup powdered sugar

Whip eggs with mixer until lemon colored. Add honey and mix until slightly thickened. Add pumpkin and lemon juice and mix. Add whole wheat flour, cinnamon, baking powder, ginger, salt, and nutmeg. Mix only until flour is blended in. Do not overmix! Spread batter in a greased and floured 10 x 15-inch pan. Bake in a 350° oven for 15 minutes.

Turn out onto a towel sprinkled with 1/3 cup powdered sugar. Starting at the narrow end, roll up cake and towel together. Cool on rack, seam side down. While cake cools, whip cream cheese, margarine, and vanilla until smooth. Add 1 cup powdered sugar, and mix until smooth.

Unroll cooled cake. Spread with cream cheese mixture, and roll up cake. Wrap in waxed paper or plastic wrap. Chill at least 2 hours. Slice to serve. Roll may be frozen if desired.

Bake: 350° 15 min   **Chill: 2-3 hrs**   **Yield: 12 servings**

Per Serving	RCU	FU	Cal	% Ft	P	F	C	Na
	3	1	31	24	2	4	24	152

PIES AND PIE CRUSTS

Fresh Peach Pie Filling ++

Summer isn't complete without one of Loa Maxwell's famous peach pies. Make this without a crust for lowfat enjoyment. This filling also makes a wonderful cheesecake topping.

3 fresh peaches, mashed
1/2 cup sugar
3 tablespoons cornstarch
1/2 cup water
1/4 teaspoon almond extract
1 tablespoon butter or margarine
4 to 5 peaches, peeled and sliced
1 1 1/2-ounce package Dream Whip, prepared according to directions on package, optional

In a saucepan combine mashed peaches, sugar, cornstarch, and water. Cook until mixture boils, about 5 minutes. Add almond extract and butter. Cool in refrigerator while slicing peaches into pie pan. Pour filling over peaches; chill. Top with Dream Whip if desired.

Chill: 2 hrs   Yield: 1   9" pie

Per Serving	RCU	FU	Cal	% Ft	P	F	C	Na
	2	0	108	15	0	2	25	18

Lemon Meringue Pie Filling +

Marguerite Payne's tangy lemon pie is absolutely the best!

1/3 cup cornstarch
1 cup sugar or 2/3 cup honey
1/4 teaspoon salt
1 1/2 cups boiling water
3 egg yolks, slightly beaten
1/3 cup lemon juice
2 tablespoons butter
1 tablespoon grated lemon rind

Meringue:
3 egg whites
1/4 teaspoon cream of tartar
3 tablespoons sugar
1/2 teaspoon vanilla

Mix cornstarch, honey, and salt in a heavy pan. Gradually add boiling water; stir well. Cook over medium heat, stirring constantly until mixture is thick and clear. Boil 1 minute. Slowly stir half the hot mixture into egg yolks, then beat into the hot mixture in pan. Boil 1 minute longer, stirring constantly. Remove from heat. Continue stirring until smooth. Add lemon juice, butter, and grated lemon rind. Cool slightly, and pour into pie pan or baked pie shell.

Meringue: beat egg whites with cream of tartar until frothy. Gradually add sugar, and whip until egg whites are stiff and peaks form. Add vanilla, and mix. Cover pie with meringue, sealing meringue to crust to prevent weeping. Bake in a 400° oven for 8 minutes or until meringue is a delicate brown. Watch carefully; meringue burns easily.

Bake: 400° 8 min   Yield: 1   9″ pie

Per Serving	RCU	FU	Cal	% Ft	P	F	C	Na
w/o crust	5	1	186	12	3	6	34	133

Cherry Pie Filling +

This filling makes a good cherry cobbler when topped with the Stir-n-Drop Biscuits*

3 cups drained, canned, pitted pie cherries
1 cup juice from cherries
3 tablespoons cornstarch
1/8 teaspoon salt
1/2 to 3/4 cup sugar
1/4 teaspoon almond extract

Drain juice from pie cherries. Add water to fill cup if needed. In a medium saucepan, combine cornstarch, salt, and sugar. Stir in juice. Cook and stir over medium heat until thick and bubbly. Cook 1 minute more, and remove from heat. Stir in cherries and almond extract. Cool while preparing pastry. Pour filling in prepared pastry, and place top crust over filling. Crimp edges. Cover edges of pastry with foil to prevent excess browning. Bake in a 375° oven for 25 minutes. Remove foil and bake for 25 to 30 minutes more or until pie crust is golden brown.

Bake: 375° 50-55 min   Yield: 1   9'' pie

Per Serving	RCU	FU	Cal	% Ft	P	F	C	Na
w/o crust	2	0	115	3	1	0	29	32

Pumpkin Pie Filling +

Try this autumn favorite as a delicious pie, pudding, and in Pumpkin Pie Squares.

2 eggs, slightly beaten
1 16-ounce can solid-pack pumpkin (2 cups)
1/2 cup honey or 3/4 cup sugar
1/2 teaspoon salt
1 teaspoon cinnamon
1/2 teaspoon ginger
1/4 teaspoon cloves
1 12-ounce can evaporated skim milk

Mix all ingredients. Pour mixture into 9-inch pie pans. Bake in a 425° oven for 15 minutes; reduce temperature to 350°. Bake an additional 35 to 40 minutes or until knife inserted into center of each pie comes out clean. Cool.
Tip: Bake as a custard without crust for lowfat eating.
Bake: 425° 15 min and 350° 35-40 min   Yield: 2   9'' pies

Per Serving	RCU	FU	Cal	% Ft	P	F	C	Na
w/o crust	2	0	70	11	2	1	13	100

Pumpkin Pie Squares +

Carla Crane shares this easy-to-make and -to-serve recipe.

Crust:
1 cup whole wheat flour
1/2 cup quick rolled oats
1/4 cup brown sugar
1/3 cup butter or margarine

Combine flour, oats, brown sugar, and butter. Mix until crumbly.
Press into ungreased 9 x 13-inch pan.
Bake: 350° 15 minutes

Make Pumpkin Pie Filling and pour into crust.
Bake: 350° 20 minutes. Remove from oven and add topping.

Topping:
1/4 cup brown sugar
2 tablespoons butter
1/2 cup chopped pecans

Combine brown sugar, butter and pecans. Sprinkle topping over pumpkin filling. Return to oven and bake 15 to 20 minutes or until filling is set. Cool in pan. Cut in squares. Top with a dollop of Dream Whip or whipped cream and a pecan half if desired.
Bake: 350° 15 min and 20 min and 15-20 min   **Yield: 24 squares**

Per Serving	RCU	FU	Cal	% Ft	P	F	C	Na
	1	1	104	34	2	4	15	106

Never-Fail Pie Crust +

3 cups unbleached white flour	1/3 cup plus 1 tablespoon ice water
1 teaspoon salt	1 egg, beaten
1 cup lard or shortening	1 tablespoon vinegar

Place flour and salt in mixer bowl. Cut lard into flour until mixture is the size of peas. Remove 1 cup of mixture, and place in a medium-size bowl. Add water, egg, and vinegar. Stir with a fork. Add to mixture in mixer bowl, and mix just until dough sticks together. Divide dough into three or four equal portions. Place one portion in the center of a 12 x 15-inch piece of waxed paper. Place another piece of waxed paper on top. Roll with rolling pin to 1/4 inch thick. Remove top sheet from dough, and invert dough and waxed paper over a 9-inch pie pan. Pull waxed paper from dough. Crimp edges of crust. For an unfilled pie shell, prick dough with a fork every 1/4 inch. Bake in a 400° oven for 10 to 12 minutes or until golden brown. For a filled single- or double-crust pie, bake as directed on pie recipe. Wrap and freeze unused portions of dough.

Bake: 400° 10-12 min   Yield: 3-4   9" pie shells

Per Serving	RCU	FU	Cal	% Ft	P	F	C	Na
	1	2	137	64	2	10	11	82

Perfect Pie Crust +

It's foolproof—always flaky and tender.

1 1/2 cups butter-flavored shortening	1 teaspoon salt
2 1/2 cups unbleached white flour	1 teaspoon baking powder
1 cup whole wheat flour	3/4 cup water
(may use all white flour)	

Mix shortening, 1 1/2 cups unbleached flour, whole wheat flour, salt, and baking powder with mixer. Add cold water; mix lightly. Mix in most of the remaining 1 cup unbleached flour; dough should be manageably soft. Divide dough into five or six equal portions. Place one portion in the center of a 12 x 15-inch piece of waxed paper. Place another piece of waxed paper on top. Roll with rolling pin to 1/4 inch thick. Remove top sheet from dough, and invert dough on waxed paper over a 9-inch pie pan. Pull waxed paper from dough. Crimp edges of crust. For an unfilled pie shell, prick dough with a fork every 1/4 inch. Bake in a 400° oven for 10 to 12 minutes or until golden brown. For a filled single- or double-crust pie, bake as directed on pie recipe. Wrap and freeze unused portions of dough.

Bake: 400° 10-12 min   Yield: 4-5   9" pie shells

Per Serving	RCU	FU	Cal	% Ft	P	F	C	Na
	0	2	109	70	1	9	7	57

FROZEN DESSERTS

Back in the "olden days" when I was a little girl, Sunday evenings on the farm were a time for socializing. In the summer, our large front lawn was a gathering place for friends and relatives from up and down the beautiful Virden Valley. Under the large male mulberry tree were home-grown watermelon and cantaloupe, covered with a wet gunny sack to keep them cool until we ate. On the back step the teenagers cranked out homemade ice cream, arguing about who got to "lick the dash." You'll enjoy these simple ice creams; they may bring back memories for you, too.

Easy Ice Cream++

2 cups sugar or honey
1 tablespoon lemon juice
1 teaspoon vanilla
2 cups fresh or frozen fruit, blended
2 cups half & half
2 quarts milk

Mix sugar, lemon juice, vanilla, fruit and half & half. Pour into freezer. Add milk to 1-inch from the top. Freeze according to manufacturer's instructions.
Tip: For creamier tasting ice cream, thicken with Rennet or 1/3 cup Instant Clear Jel, following directions on package.
Time: 15-20 min (electric ice cream freezer)   Yield: 1 gallon   32 1/2 cup servings

Per Serving	RCU	FU	Cal	% Ft	P	F	C	Na
	2	1	103	33	3	4	14	46

Peach Ice Cream

Prepare Ice Cream as directed, using 2 cups pureed or crushed peaches. Add 1/4 teaspoon almond extract. For added flavor and color, add 1 3-ounce package peach gelatin dissolved in 1/4 cup boiling water.

Raspberry-Banana Ice Cream

Prepare Easy Ice Cream as directed, using 2 cups mashed raspberries and 2 ripe bananas, mashed or pureed.

Karen's Frozen Yogurt +++

Quick and delicious. Be creative and try a wide variety of combinations.

1 cup lowfat vanilla yogurt
1 banana, frozen in chunks
1/2 cup frozen fruit (berries, peaches, pineapple, etc.)

Put yogurt into blender. Add frozen banana. Blend on high speed, adding frozen fruit until thick. Add additional frozen fruit or ice cubes if needed to thicken to desired consistency.
Tip: Use fresh or canned fruit instead of frozen fruit. Mix as directed. Then pour into paper cups and freeze. OR increase recipe and freeze in ice cream freezer.
Time: 5 min   **Yield: 4 1/2 cup servings**

Per Serving	RCU	FU	Cal	% Ft	P	F	C	Na
	2	0	93	11	2	1	19	33

Bavarian Fruit Ice Cream ++

2 quarts milk
4 bananas, mashed
1 1/2 cups sugar or 1 cup honey
1 lemon, juiced (1/4 cup)
2 oranges, juiced (l/2 cup)
1 8-ounce can crushed pineapple, undrained
1 12-ounce can evaporated milk
Whole milk

Combine 2 cups of the milk, bananas, sugar, and juices in blender. Blend well. Pour into ice cream freezer, and stir in remaining ingredients. Add additional whole milk to 1-inch from top. Mixture should be thick. Freeze according to manufacturer's instructions.
Time: 15-20 min (electric ice cream freezer)   **Yield: 1 gallon**

Per Serving	RCU	FU	Cal	% Ft	P	F	C	Na
	2	1	157	26	5	5	23	67

Blender Ice Cream + +

It's quick, delicious, and lowfat!

2 cups 1% milk (use half nonfat yogurt if desired)
1 to 3 tablespoons sugar or honey
1/2 teaspoon vanilla
1 teaspoon lemon juice
1 large banana, frozen
1 to 2 cups frozen fruit, slightly thawed (use fruits such as berries, peaches, or apricots)

Break banana into pieces. Put ingredients into blender. Pulse, then blend on high speed until thick. Add more fruit if a thicker shake is desired.
   Tip: Use fresh fruit and add ice cubes to desired consistency.
Time: 3 minutes   Yield: 4 servings

Per Serving	RCU	FU	Cal	% Ft	P	F	C	Na
	1	0	111	10	5	1	21	66

Creamy Fruit Freeze + +

This delicious dessert is smooth, creamy and fat-free.

1 envelope unflavored gelatin
1/2 cup milk
4 cups fresh sliced peaches
1/2 to 3/4 cup light corn syrup

In small saucepan, sprinkle gelatin over milk; let stand 1 minute. Cook and stir over low heat until gelatin is dissolved. (Mixture may be placed in small glass container and microwaved for one minute.) Place fruit, corn syrup, and milk mixture in blender. Cover, and blend at high speed for 30 seconds or until thoroughly pureed. Pour into a freezer container. Cover and freeze until soft-set.
   Remove from freezer; let stand at room temperature to soften, if needed. Spoon into mixer bowl. Whip on medium speed until smooth and creamy. Serve immediately or pour into a freezer container, cover, and freeze again until soft-set.
   Tip: Watermelon, cantaloupe, raspberries, strawberries, bananas, or other fresh fruit may be used in place of peaches.
Chill: 1-2 hrs   Yield: 12   1/3 cup servings

Per Serving	RCU	FU	Cal	% Ft	P	F	C	Na
	1	0	62	1	1	0	14	15

Fruitsicles +++

2 cups sliced strawberries or peaches, blended
1 cup nonfat yogurt, vanilla or fruit flavored

Puree all ingredients in blender. If using peaches, add 1/2 teaspoon cinnamon. Freeze in small paper cups with a wooden stick inserted in the center of each.
Yield: 6 1/2 cup servings

Per Serving	RCU	FU	Cal	% Ft	P	F	C	Na
	0	0	50	12	2	1	10	19

Lavender Fruit Ice + + +

Serve Carole Griffith's beautiful summer refreshment in sherbet cups.

1 8-ounce can unsweetened pineapple tidbits
1 10-ounce package frozen blueberries
1 10-ounce package frozen raspberries
2 bananas, cubed
Ice cubes as desired

Drain pineapple, reserving juice. Gently mix fruit in a large bowl. Pour a little pineapple juice over berries to separate. Use the rest of the juice to crush enough ice cubes to yield 2 to 4 cups of finely crushed ice. Add more juice as needed to crush the ice. Fold ice into fruit and serve.
Yield: 10 servings

Per Serving	RCU	FU	Cal	% Ft	P	F	C	Na
	0	0	44	3	1	0	11	1

BEVERAGES

Fruit Smoothie +++

This beverage is easy and refreshing. Try it occasionally for breakfast with whole wheat toast or muffins.

2 cups pineapple or orange juice
1 apple, cored and sliced
1 orange, peeled and sectioned
2 bananas (may be frozen)
1 cup fresh or canned fruit, drained
Ice cubes

Place juice in blender. Add fruits and blend well. Drop in ice cubes one at a time until beverage reaches desired consistency. Frozen bananas, broken into small pieces, may be used to thicken beverage. Add more juice if desired.

Yield: 6 servings

Tip: The apples and oranges may be replaced with any seasonal fruit — berries, apricots, peaches, pears, etc. Always add banana for a mellow texture and taste.

Per Serving	RCU	FU	Cal	% Ft	P	F	C	Na
	0	0	124	1	1	0	30	2

Fruit Shake ++

Fruits blend so smoothly you'll think you're eating ice cream. Vary this basic recipe by using in-season fresh fruits.

1 fresh peach
1 large ripe banana, fresh or frozen in chunks
1 peeled orange (optional)
1 cup apple juice, 1% milk, or yogurt
Ice cubes

Blend fruit and apple juice or milk in blender until pureed. Add a few ice cubes, and blend. Continue adding ice and blend until desired consistency is achieved.

Tip: Frozen or fresh strawberries or other fruits may be used in place of the peach or orange.

Yield: 2 cups

Per Serving	RCU	FU	Cal	% Ft	P	F	C	Na
	0	0	157	0	1	0	39	3

Banana Pineapple Slush +++

Cool and frosty, this slush is ideal for a summer party.

1 3-ounce package apricot or strawberry-banana gelatin (optional)
1 cup boiling water
2 cups water
6 large bananas
1 46-ounce can pineapple juice
1 12-ounce can frozen orange juice concentrate
1 6-ounce can frozen lemonade
1 20-ounce can unsweetened crushed pineapple
Sparkling water

Dissolve gelatin in boiling water. Let cool. Put cold water and bananas in blender, and pulse until blended. Mix all ingredients except sparkling water in a 1-gallon or larger container. Cover and freeze. For easier scooping, let sit at room temperature for 15 to 20 minutes before serving. Fill each glass half full of slush, and pour sparkling water over the top.

Tip: This is delicious without the gelatin.

Freeze: 24 hours   **Yield: 1 gallon**

Per Serving	RCU	FU	Cal	% Ft	P	F	C	Na
	1	0	83	0	1	0	20	3

Tropical Fruit Slush +++

Try this for a refreshing summer cooler.

1 quart unsweetened grape juice
1 12-ounce can frozen lemonade concentrate
1 12-ounce can frozen orange juice concentrate
1 46-ounce can pineapple juice
1 46-ounce can apricot nectar
6 cups water
Sparkling water

Thoroughly mix juices and water. Pour into a large container; cover, and freeze. Before serving, let sit at room temperature for about 20 minutes to soften. To serve, place 2 large scoops of the frozen mixture into a tall glass. Fill glass with sparkling water.

Freeze: 24 hours   **Yield: 1 1/2 gallons**

Per Serving	RCU	FU	Cal	% Ft	P	F	C	Na
	1	0	73	0	0	0	18	1

Strawberry Fruit Punch +++

It's beautiful and delicious!

2 cups strawberries, pureed
1 12-ounce can frozen orange juice concentrate
1 48-ounce can pineapple juice
4 cups water
Sparkling water, chilled
Orange slices
Whole strawberries

Mix strawberries, orange juice concentrate, pineapple juice, and water. Chill well. Just before serving, add sparkling water. Float orange slices and strawberries on top.
Chilling Time: 6 hours   Yield: 1 gallon

Per Serving	RCU	FU	Cal	% Ft	P	F	C	Na
	0	0	51	1	1	0	12	1

Fruit Slurpie +++

Teens and kids love to make these. They're a quick summer treat!

3 to 4 cups ice cubes
1/4 cup frozen lemonade concentrate
1/2 to 1 cup water

Put ice cubes in blender. Add lemonade concentrate and 1/4 cup of the water. Pulse to crush ice. Stop blender to scrape down sides. Add additional water as needed until ice is finely crushed and mixture is slushy.
Tip: Any frozen fruit juice concentrate may be used in place of the lemonade. Vary amounts to suit taste.
Yield: 4 servings

Per Serving	RCU	FU	Cal	% Ft	P	F	C	Na
	0	0	6	0	0	0	2	0

Orange Junius ++

This recipe comes from our favorite teen.

1 6-ounce can frozen orange juice concentrate
1 cup water
1 cup 1% milk
2 tablespoons nonfat dry milk (optional)
Ice cubes

Combine all ingredients except ice in blender. Blend at high speed, adding ice cubes until mixture is thick and slushy. Serve immediately.
Yield: 6 servings

Per Serving	RCU	FU	Cal	% Ft	P	F	C	Na
	0	0	105	3	4	0	19	58

Fruit Fizz +++

A refreshing replacement for a soft drink.

1 cup unsweetened fruit juice, any flavor
1 cup sparkling water (no-salt variety)
Ice cubes

Mix fruit juice and sparkling water. For a lighter drink, add more sparkling water. For a heavier drink, add additional fruit juice. Serve over ice.
Yield: cups

Per Serving	RCU	FU	Cal	% Ft	P	F	C	Na
	0	0	55	8	0	0	14	1

Fruit Refresher +++

This beverage makes a good breakfast drink.

1 quart unsweetened apple juice
1 quart unsweetened grape juice

Mix juices and add ice to chill well.
Chill: 4 hours   Yield: 2 quarts

Per Serving	RCU	FU	Cal	% Ft	P	F	C	Na
	0	0	130	3	0	0	33	2

Eggnog +

Wanda Stimpson serves this delicious eggnog on New Year's Eve.

2 quarts 1% milk
1/2 scant teaspoon salt
1/2 cup honey or 3/4 cup sugar
4 to 6 egg yolks
4 to 6 egg whites
1/4 cup sugar
2 teaspoons vanilla
Nutmeg

Heat milk over medium heat in a large 5- to 6-quart pan. While milk is heating, beat salt and sugar into egg yolks. Using a wire whisk, slowly add yolk mixture to milk, mixing well. Cook over medium heat, stirring constantly, until mixture coats a spoon. Do not cook over high heat or let boil; mixture will curdle and separate. Cool.

Beat egg whites until frothy. Slowly add sugar and whip until egg whites peak. Fold egg whites and vanilla into custard. Sprinkle with nutmeg. Chill thoroughly, 5 to 6 hours or overnight.

Cook: 25-30 min   Chill: 5-6 hours   Yield: 16 servings

Per Serving	RCU	FU	Cal	% Ft	P	F	C	Na
	2	0	114	20	6	3	18	158

Hot Wassail + + +

It's perfect for cold weather entertaining. Use a slow cooker to keep it warm. Delicious hot or cold.

1 12-ounce can frozen orange juice concentrate
1 6-ounce can frozen lemonade concentrate
2 quarts water
1 gallon apple juice or cider
5 cinnamon sticks
5 whole cloves

Combine all ingredients in a large pan. Simmer 10 minutes. Remove spices. Serve hot.

Cook: 10 min   Yield: 2 gallons

Per Serving	RCU	FU	Cal	% Ft	P	F	C	Na
	0	0	44	0	0	0	11	1

SWEET TREATS

Karamel Korn +

Uncle Al fixes this treat for company on Sunday evenings.

2 cups brown sugar
1/2 cup margarine
1/2 cup light corn syrup
1 teaspoon vanilla
5 to 6 quarts popped corn

Heat all ingredients except corn in a heavy pan. Bring to a boil, and cook 3 to 4 minutes, stirring constantly. Remove any unpopped kernels from popcorn. Pour syrup over popcorn, and mix well. Cool and break into pieces.

Cook: 5 min   Yield: 24   1 cup servings

Per Serving	RCU	FU	Cal	% Ft	P	F	C	Na
	2	1	139	30	2	5	24	56

Smackies

Prepare syrup as directed for Karamel Korn. Pour syrup over 1 16-ounce package puffed wheat and 1 cup salted peanuts. Mix well. Put in 9 x 13-inch pan and let cool. Cut into 15 squares.

Popcorn Balls +

Linda Haskell shares this quick recipe.

1/2 cup margarine or butter
1 10-ounce package marshmallows
1/4 teaspoon salt
1/2 teaspoon vanilla
Few drops green food coloring
6 quarts popped corn

Melt margarine over low heat. Stir in marshmallows until all are melted. Add salt, vanilla, and food coloring. Remove any unpopped kernels from popped corn by shaking the popped corn in a large bowl. Unpopped kernels will fall to the bottom. Carefully transfer corn into another bowl, and pour syrup over corn. Mix well and shape into small balls. Cool on waxed paper.

Cook: 5 min   Yield: 16-20 small balls

Per Serving	RCU	FU	Cal	% Ft	P	F	C	Na
	2	1	140	35	3	5	23	91

Spudnuts + +

Try these topped with Velvety Slim Frosting

7 cups unbleached white flour
1 tablespoon yeast
2 cups warm milk (125°)
1/2 cup oil or shortening
1/2 cup sugar
2 teaspoons salt
2 eggs, beaten
1 cup mashed potatoes

Mix together 2 cups of flour and yeast in bowl. Add warm milk, and mix for 1 minute. Let sponge 5 to 10 minutes. Stir down. Add oil, sugar, salt, eggs, and potatoes. Add remaining flour, 1 cup at a time, to form a soft dough. Let rise in bowl until double, about 20 minutes. Roll out dough on a lightly greased countertop to 1/2 inch thickness. Cut with a doughnut cutter. Place on lightly greased cookie sheets. Let raise 10 to 15 minutes. Bake in a 425° oven for 8 to 10 minutes or until golden brown. Watch closely.

Bake: 425° 8-10 min   Yield: 4 dozen

Per Serving	RCU	FU	Cal	% Ft	P	F	C	Na
	1	0	95	26	2	3	15	97

MISCELLANEOUS

Hawaiian Fantasy ++

This is a nice do-ahead fruit salad.

1 cup mandarin oranges, drained
2 cups unsweetened crushed pineapple, drained
1/2 cup unsweetened coconut
1 cup miniature marshmallows
1 cup sour cream, fat free
1 cup cooked whole wheat (optional)
2 bananas, sliced (optional

Mix all ingredients together and refrigerate overnight. Add bananas just before serving if desired.

Chill: 8 hours   **Yield: 10 servings**

Per Serving	RCU	FU	Cal	% Ft	P	F	C	Na
	1	0	90	30	3	3	13	20

Cheese Ball ++

This is nice for New Year's Eve entertaining.

2 8-ounce packages nonfat cream cheese, room temperature
1 8-ounce can crushed pineapple, well drained
2 tablespoons finely chopped onion
1/4 cup finely chopped green pepper
1 teaspoon seasoned salt
1 to 2 cups chopped pecans

Mix all ingredients except pecans. Chill 2 to 3 hours. Shape into a ball. Roll in finely chopped pecans.

Chill: 3 hours   **Yield: 1 large cheese ball**   **32 servings**

Per Serving	RCU	FU	Cal	% Ft	P	F	C	Na
	0	0	38	51	2	2	2	97

Frosted Lemon Gelatin Salad ++

This can also serve as dessert!

Salad:
1 20-ounce can crushed pineapple
2 3-ounce packages lemon gelatin
2 cups boiling water
2 cups water
1 cup miniature marshmallows
2 large bananas, sliced

Topping:
1/4 cup sugar
2 tablespoons flour
1 cup pineapple juice
1 egg, slightly beaten
1 cup whipping cream, whipped, or Dream Whip
1 tablespoon Parmesan cheese

Drain pineapple and save juice for topping. Dissolve gelatin in boiling water. Add water. Fold in pineapple, marshmallows, and bananas. Pour into a 9 x 13-inch pan, and chill until firm. To make topping, combine sugar, flour, juice, and egg. Cook until thick; cool. Fold in Dream Whip or whipped cream. Spread on salad, and sprinkle with cheese.

Chill: 3 hrs   Yield: 10-12 servings

Per Serving	RCU	FU	Cal	% Ft	P	F	C	Na
	1	0	84	5	1	0	17	24

Apricot Salad

Substitute orange gelatin for lemon gelatin. Use 2 cups drained and pureed apricots in place of the water.

Ribbon Salad++

Margaret Merrill serves this beautiful salad at Christmas time.

1 3-ounce package lime gelatin
3 cups boiling water
2 cups cold water
1 3-ounce package lemon gelatin
1 10 1/2-ounce package miniature marshmallows
1 8-ounce package cream cheese, fat free
1 8-ounce can crushed pineapple, undrained
1 cup whipping cream, whipped
1 3-ounce package raspberry or cherry gelatin

   Dissolve lime gelatin in 1 cup of the boiling water. Add 1 cup cold water. Pour into 9 x 13-inch pan. Chill until set. Dissolve lemon gelatin in 1 cup boiling water. Add marshamllows, and stir over low heat to melt. Remove from heat and add cream cheese. Stir until melted. Fold in pineapple. Cool. Fold in whipped cream. Pour over lime gelatin, and chill until set. Dissolve red gelatin in 1 cup boiling water. Add 1 cup cold water. Chill until syrupy, and pour over lemon layer. Chill until set. Cut in squares to serve.

Chill: 6 hours   Yield: 20 servings

Per Serving	RCU	FU	Cal	% Ft	P	F	C	Na
	3	0	135	15	4	2	26	98

CHAPTER 11

Off to a Good Start

Healthy babies are not a matter of luck. Having healthy children starts with a healthy mother and the process begins *before conception*. Ideally, a woman should start preparing her body for pregnancy a year before she actually gets pregnant.

Good nutrition during pregnancy is as important to the mother as it is to the unborn child. Many pregnancy related problems such as miscarriage, spotting, nausea, and vomiting can be avoided with proper nutrition. If a nutritional deficiency is suspected, take the responsibility to educate yourself on good nutritional practices by studying the many excellent books now available. Use common sense as you apply what you learn. It's also wise to consult a nutrition-oriented doctor.

It's As Easy As 1, 2, 3

The following guidelines are helpful for a woman before *and* after conception.

1. Eat three well-balanced meals every day. Try to eat at about the same time each day.

2. Avoid refined carbohydrates which include anything made with white flour, sugars of any kind, and white rice. This includes macaroni products made with white flour. The recipes in this book offer hundreds of delicious alternatives to the refined foods many people are accustomed to eating. After eating the *Setpoint* way for a month or two, you will notice an increase in energy and general health.

3. Drink a minimum of six to eight glasses of water a day. If you are retaining water, drink up! Drinking water helps relieve fluid retention. It stimulates the kidneys and helps rid the body of waste and bacteria that can cause disease.

4. Those who strictly follow the *Setpoint* principles will probably gain between twenty and thirty pounds during pregnancy. A suggested guide is one to three pounds or less per month for the first three or four months. If you are gaining at a more rapid rate, analyze your eating habits. Cut down on breads and crackers for snacks, and eat fruits and vegetables instead. Drink extra water, and make sure you are truly hungry before eating.

5. Avoid soft drinks — even diet soft drinks. These beverages affect the insulin level of the body, often increasing hunger and the desire to snack on high-fat and high-sugar foods. In addition, the carbonated water puts undue stress on the kidneys.

6. Many obstetricians recommend that pregnant and nursing women avoid products with aspartame. If a substance is unsafe for a pregnant woman or nursing mother, why should anyone else consume it?[8]

7. Exercise is very important during pregnancy. A daily walk of 30 to 40 minutes is an excellent way to exercise. Walking also helps lessen the effects of morning sickness. Consult your doctor before starting any exercise program.

8. Try a good natural prenatal vitamin. Read the label to make sure it meets the RDA for folic acid and iron. A high amount of synthetic iron can cause constipation and rob the body of vitamin E.

9. Avoid eating after 6 p.m. You will probably sleep better if your stomach is not full at bedtime.

10. Get adequate rest. Sleep a minimum of eight hours at night and take a short nap during the day if needed.

These simple suggestions for a healthy pregnancy really work!

Morning Sickness?

If a woman lives the *Setpoint* way, she is much less likely to suffer from morning sickness. If she does, it is usually less severe. A diet high in fats tends to aggravate this condition. Studies have shown that morning sickness can be greatly relieved by taking 50 to 100 milligrams of vitamin B6 three to four times per day. If you need additional relief, try taking 50 to 100 milligrams of magnesium gluconate along with the B6.

If you are troubled with heartburn, indigestion, or nausea, try drinking a little water mixed with 1/2 to 1 teaspoon of ginger. You will feel a burning sensation for a minute or two, but the symptoms should be relieved almost immediately.

Take My Word For It!

During my last pregnancy I faithfully adhered to the *Setpoint* guidelines. My weight gain was 21 pounds, which was ideal for me. I enjoyed all the nutritious foods my body desired but I didn't overeat. Whenever I was truly hungry, I ate. The first trimester, I ate four to five small meals a day. The second trimester, I went back to three meals a day with a mid-morning and afternoon snack. The last trimester I ate three meals and an occasional snack. I also drank eight to ten glasses of water daily. My labor was short and our fifth child, a beautiful baby girl, was delivered naturally.

If you learn to listen to your body and feed it the right foods at the right times, you should not gain excess weight during pregnancy. Being pregnant may give you an excuse to indulge yourself momentarily, but you will probably pay for it later. Excess fat tends to complicate delivery. Besides, it's much easier to shed a *few* extra pounds after delivery than a *lot* of extra pounds. Two excellent books on prenatal nutrition are *Feed Yourself Right* and *Jane Brody's Nutrition Book.* [9]

BREAST-FEEDING: BABY'S BEST SOURCE OF NUTRITION

Breast-feeding is the best way to nourish a new baby. Your own milk is custom designed with all the necessary nutrients for your own baby. Recent studies have shown that totally breast-fed infants have fewer intestinal upsets, ear infections, and respiratory problems than infants fed formula supplements. [10] In addition to the physical benefits of breast-feeding, mother and baby develop a close relationship through this special bonding.

An excellent resource for more information on breast-feeding is the La Leche League International. They have a chapter in most larger cities across the United States. The national headquarters are located at 9616 Minneapolis Avenue, Franklin Park, Illinois 60131. La Leche publishes a book called *The Womanly Art of Breast-Feeding*[11] which contains complete information on successfully nursing your baby. Another excellent resource book is *Nursing Your Baby*[12], available in many libraries or in paperback at most bookstores.

While nursing, continue to follow the ten eating guidelines for pregnant women. Drink ten to twelve glasses of water every day. A mother's inadequate water intake can cause an inadequate milk supply for her baby. Drink two glasses of water with every meal, plus a full glass each time you nurse.

What's Next Best to Mom?

If you are unable to nurse, don't feel guilty. Choose a formula made from a whole-milk base and one that is not highly sweetened. Make sure the formula doesn't contain added oils, such as coconut or palm oil, which are high in saturated fats.

A good alternative to breast-feeding is goat's milk. The fat globules in goat's milk are similar in size to the ones contained in human milk, and the protein content is much lower than cow's milk. Make sure this milk is from a certified goat dairy, and check with your doctor.

To prepare a custom-made formula from goat's milk, mix 1 quart certified raw goat's milk with 1 to 2 tablespoons lactose powder. If the baby's stools are too soft, reduce the lactose.

It is possible to make a good formula from cow's milk. Two good recipes can be found in *The Parent's Guide To Better Nutrition For Tots To Teens.* [13]

Coping With Stress Days

Some days are more stressful than others, especially when you are dealing with the demands of other children. You may need an additional nutrition boost to help maintain your milk supply. A nutritional yeast powder works well. It supplies B vitamins as well as protein. A suggested amount is 1 teaspoon three times a day in vegetable or fruit juice. Over a two-week time period, gradually increase the amount to 1 tablespoon three times a day. If you are drinking ten to twelve glasses of water daily and are eating well, you should not need this yeast supplement all the time unless you have an unusually high amount of stress.

Be Aware of Growth Spurts

Babies grow rapidly. At the end of two weeks, around six weeks, and between three and four months of age, you may find that your baby demands to be fed more often. In fact, you may feel that all you do is nurse. The baby could be experiencing a growth spurt. To help increase your milk supply during the growth phase, relax, take a nap, and faithfully drink ten to twelve glasses of water each day. Make sure you are eating three well-balanced meals. The nutritional yeast supplement mentioned above helps increase the milk supply. Baby should settle down in three to five days.

At four to five months, your baby may go through another phase which usually lasts five to seven days. You may again find your milk supply inadequate. This time, the deficiency could be due to two factors:

First, nursing babies often begin noticing objects or people in the room. Their attention may wander so they don't nurse as well. They take less milk at a feeding and therefore demand more frequent feedings. Because of the frustration this causes for both mom and baby, many women give up nursing at this time. Don't despair. The following suggestions will get you through with flying colors. If your baby gets distracted easily, use a quiet, darkened room for nursing. Sit on a comfortable chair or lie on the bed so you can both relax and enjoy being together.

Second, you have probably changed. Up until now your activity has been somewhat limited by a newborn baby. Now that the baby is a little older and you feel better, you may find yourself overdoing and not getting enough rest. Vigorous activity can cause your milk supply to dwindle. Slow down and try to catch a daily nap for a week or two. As my mother's rural doctor told her when I was a baby, "You can't run a cow around the pasture all day and expect it to give milk at night."

A big temptation during an early growth phase is to think that the baby needs solid food because he isn't satisfied after nursing. Don't add solids until baby is five or six months old. Instead, follow the suggestions above, including the nutritional yeast supplement, to increase your milk supply.

Another temptation is to supplement your milk with formula. Instead, nurse your baby more often to build up your milk. Nurse every two to three hours for a couple of days if necessary. The stimulation of more frequent nursing tells your body it needs to produce more milk. When a baby becomes accustomed to a bottle, he quickly loses interest in nursing because it is more difficult to suck from the breast than from a bottle.

Don't Overfeed and Undernourish

Anemia and obesity are two of the most common problems with infants. Both are usually attributed to baby formulas which are much higher in sugar and fat than mother's milk. Many babies are overfed and undernourished. If you are bottle feeding your baby, remember not to overfeed! Give your baby a good start and keep the following tips in mind. They are adapted from Weight Watcher's excellent recommendations.

1. Don't insist that your baby finish every bottle. Breast-fed babies drink varying amounts of milk at each feeding. Bottle-fed babies should be allowed the same freedom. If a baby shows disinterest in eating, don't force the issue.

2. Don't worry if your baby refuses to eat at a set time and then sleeps through the scheduled feeding time. Babies have different patterns each day. As they get older the time between feedings will increase. Babies should eat only when they are hungry, not when Mom thinks it's time for them to eat.

3. Don't push a bottle in your baby's mouth every time a cry is heard. Babies cry for many reasons other than hunger. It's their only way of communicating their needs. Crying might signal a need for a diaper change, a burping, or merely a desire for cuddling and attention. Try a pacifier first, and then try a bottle of water, especially if it has only been one or two hours since the last feeding. Most bottle-fed babies aren't given enough water, especially in hot weather.

4. Don't feed a baby fruit-flavored soft drink mixes or flavored gelatin water in a bottle or a cup! These drinks have no nutritional value and take away baby's desire for good food. In addition, they can cause tooth decay and damage forming tooth buds.

Later is Better

Many parents give in to the social pressure of introducing solid foods at an early age. You may hear a parent brag, "My son ate his first spoonful of cereal when he was only two weeks old."

Many nutritionists and doctors have indicated that infants are healthier if solid foods are introduced between six and eight months. The American Pediatric Association makes the same recommendation. The reason for a later introduction to solids is simple: a baby's digestive system is not fully developed at birth and it is designed to handle only milk, preferably mother's milk. Studies now show that solids introduced when the digestive system is immature frequently cause allergies, asthma, and ear infections. [14]

A baby's weight and size have nothing to do with his body's ability to handle solid foods. This ability comes with a more mature digestive system. Foods given before the age of six months don't contribute needed nutrients or energy. Why risk an allergic reaction or infant obesity? Cereal, fruit, and other foods contain more calories than the same amount of milk or formula. These excess calories from solids go to fat, which is not healthy. This may start baby on the road to a life-long weight problem. The squeeze test will tell. If your baby's arms and legs have a marshmallow feel, that's fat!

Introduce Solids Slowly

A baby's body doesn't start producing the digestive enzymes needed to handle a more complex diet until he is around six to eight months of age. [15] This is the logical time to begin the *gradual* introduction of solid foods over a two to three month period. Remember, your baby has been accustomed to only milk. Don't offer all the solid foods at once.

Introducing solids too rapidly may also cause allergies and respiratory problems. Observe the baby's reaction to solids. If he develops diarrhea, an upset stomach, diaper rash, gets a cold, or gets an ear infection within one to two weeks after starting a food, he may be having an allergic reaction. Stop using that food for a week or two. See if the condition improves. Try the food again and see what happens. Babies often outgrow these allergies as their digestive systems mature.

At six to seven months, baby may lean forward and open his mouth or reach for food while you eat. This is a good indication he wants to try a little solid food. The first time you introduce solid food, your baby may eat only one to two teaspoonful. Solid food is a new experience, and the taste and textures are different than the milk a baby is accustomed to.

The following chart gives some suggested guidelines for introducing solid foods.

Birth					Months
0 1 2 3 4 5 6	7	8	9	10 11	12
Breast Milk, Goat's Milk or a Formula with whole milk as a base.		. . . . . Plus			
	Cereals	Vege-tables	Fruits & Other	Eggs Legumes	Finger Foods
NO SOLID FOODS	Brown Rice Millet Oatmeal Barley Pln. Yogurt	Squash Carrots Potatoes Grn. Beans Peas Beets Broccoli Cauliflower	Applesauce Bananas Peaches Pears Fresh Fruit Plain Yogurt	Eggs Legumes	Lean Meats Combination Foods - Whole Wheat Bread

Start with Cereal

Baby needs solid foods only once a day at first. Try starting with the evening meal. Cereal is usually the first solid food suggested for baby. It's easy to make your own cereal by putting the dry whole grain in a blender until it's of a fine meal consistency. This cereal cooks in minutes using about one tablespoon of the grain to one-third cup water. The grocery store varieties for baby cereals are convenient, but some are very refined, and many contain starch and fillers. Be selective.

When starting out, use the same cereal for a week. Babies don't mind having the same food every day and this way baby will get used to the taste and texture. Also, you will be able to detect any reactions to a certain food. Try oatmeal, barley, millet and brown rice cereal. If rice cereal tends to constipate your baby, serve it only once or twice a week and use another grain such as oatmeal on alternate days. Cereal can be sweetened with a little mashed fruit, but sweetening isn't necessary. Don't get baby used to a highly fruit-sweetened cereal.

Introduce the Veggies!

By the time a baby is seven to eight months old, he will probably eat solid foods twice a day. Try cereal for one meal and a vegetable for another. Cooked fresh vegetables are best, but aren't always available. Your next best choice is to use frozen vegetables. As a third choice, serve canned vegetables with reduced or no salt or rinse them with water to remove excess salt. A blender produces a fine puree which baby needs at first. A baby food grinder, available in most health food stores, is inexpensive to buy and easy to use. It makes a slightly coarser texture than a blender and is ideal for baby until he gets a mouthful of teeth and is ready for mashed or regular food. Commercial baby food is convenient to use on busy days and when traveling. There are a wide variety of baby foods to choose from and they are a better choice for meals than giving baby a bottle of milk.

When fixing baby food from canned vegetables such as beets and green beans, you'll always have more than baby needs. If you won't be using it up within a day or two, freeze the extra in ice cube trays. Put the food cubes in freezer bags for future use. They can easily be warmed in a microwave oven.

When your baby is ready for fruits, keep in mind that fruits should be completely ripe. Bananas should have a solid yellow peel with a few brown spots. If using canned fruit, choose the "lite" fruits and drain well, avoiding the syrup.

Eat With the Family

As baby reaches eight to nine months, you can usually feed him the meal you are eating. Make sure his food is ground or finely mashed. These servings may not be very large and the amount he eats will vary daily according to the energy needs of your child. If you are feeding your family correctly, it's easy for baby to get the nutrients he needs.

By the age of nine to ten months, a baby should be eating three to five meals each day. At this age, *formula or milk should no longer be the mainstay of a baby's diet.* This milk lacks many of the important vitamins, minerals (iron), and bulk baby now needs for healthy growth, and can be the cause of infant anemia. It's easy to give a crying baby a bottle because he's hungry instead of taking the time to feed him a good meal. A bottle before breakfast and at mid-morning diminishes a baby's appetite. Reduce the number of bottle feedings and see how quickly your baby's appetite increases for the cereal and vegetables he's been missing. His general health and disposition will improve dramatically. Take baby completely off the bottle between nine to twelve months of age. Make sure he gets adequate milk from a cup.

Daily Menu Suggestions

Two to three servings whole grains (usually cereal until the baby is able to eat bread)
One to two dark green vegetables
One or two orange vegetables or beets (avoid corn)
Two fruit servings
Whole or 2% milk

Breakfast: Homemade cereal, fruit, bread, glass of milk

Tip: Most cereals need longer cooking for a baby. Cook enough for several meals if desired. Run oatmeal or other cereal through the baby food grinder with half a peach, pear, or some other fruit. Thin with milk as needed.

Lunch: Potato, carrots, spinach, bread, milk, fruit

Tip: Cook a potato in the microwave four to five minutes. Puree in a blender with a little milk, or run through the baby food grinder. Cut a carrot in chunks, microwave one to two minutes in a plastic bag, and then puree.

Dinner: Chicken and brown rice, beets, green beans, bread, milk

Tip: Serve baby the Chicken 'n Rice Bake or Swedish Hot Dish you fix for your family. Puree enough for tonight plus lunch tomorrow. Cover and refrigerate the extra immediately. Cooked whole-grain cereals make a good emergency dinner meal, but don't make a habit of using them in preference to vegetables.

Portions will vary according to the age and appetite of your child. Let him tell you when he is full. Don't force him to eat when he doesn't want any more.

Don't expect baby to feed himself at first. As babies start eating solids, they will eat much better if they are fed by someone using a spoon until about 13 to 15 months of age. At that time, they can gradually learn to feed themselves.

When children get teeth and begin eating finger foods, offer them a variety of slightly cooked vegetables (diced beets, green beans, and broccoli are just the right size for little fingers to pick up), small fruit pieces, whole-grain unsweetened prepared cereals, and 100% whole wheat bread. Avoid the typical supermarket diet of graham and soda crackers, chips, hot dogs, cheese, candy, marshmallows, and pre-sweetened cereals. These foods are high in fats and sugars. Sweets diminish a child's natural appetite for the nutritious foods he needs in order to grow into a healthy adult.

Use a Cup

A baby can be weaned from the bottle or breast directly to a cup anytime between nine months and one year. Bottle-fed babies should be weaned by one year. Begin offering baby a drink of water from a cup between three and four months. He will quickly catch on. Continue offering water and occasionally milk from a cup so that when he is ready to be weaned, he will gave grown accustomed to drinking from a cup.

When weaning baby from the breast or formula, use whole milk unless there is a weight problem. If there is a weight problem and you need to decrease their fat intake, use 2% milk, not skim milk. Babies and young children need the fat from whole or 2% milk to allow maximum absorption of the fat-soluble vitamins A, D, E, and K. Check with your doctor for recommendations.

TV Can Undermine Your Efforts

As children grow, they are often influenced by television. During a child's television program, you see many commercials for breakfast cereal. The next time you go to the store your children may yell and scream until you buy the newest brand. Learn to read the labels. Look at the nutritional information on the side of the cereal box. One gram of sugar equals 1/4 teaspoon. Avoid cereals that have more than 3 grams of sugar per serving.

Don't be fooled by artificially sweetened cereals. Just because the cereal doesn't contain sugar, it isn't automatically okay for kids. Avoid artificial sweeteners. Choose unsweetened whole-grain cereals and sweeten with fresh or dried fruit. For more information on the effects of artificial sweeteners on children's health see the Boston Children's Hospitals Parent's Guide to Nutrition. [16]

Skip the Soft Drinks

Another culprit is soft drinks, especially cola drinks and other soft drinks containing caffeine. The U. S. Senate published a report entitled "Dietary Goals for the United States."[17] It states, "There is a suspected connection between caffeine and ulcers, heart disease, and bladder cancer." It also states that not only is the caffeine in cola drinks harmful, but cola syrup contains a substance which has been linked to stomach disorders — evidence that even decaffeinated cola drinks should be avoided.

The October 1981 issue of *Consumer Reports*[18] also reviews the effects of caffeine. It points out that children get too much caffeine for their body weight by drinking soft drinks containing caffeine. Children who habitually consume several soft drinks daily containing caffeine experience jumpiness, insomnia, and other effects seen in adult coffee drinkers.

Limit High-Fat and High-Sugar Foods

Chips—including potato, corn, and cheese puffs—and pastries such as doughnuts, cream-filled snack cakes, and cookies are a big part of the typical American diet for both children and adults. These foods are high in fats and sugars and start to cause cholesterol buildup in children as early as three years of age, as proven by doctors performing autopsies on young children. [19] Oddly enough, many children who are too thin or underweight for their age are high consumers of fats and sugars. Their appetite for good foods has been suppressed, and their sugar addiction makes them crave these empty-calorie foods.

Feed Children Back to Health

If your child gets sick easily, wholesome foods, adequate rest (ten to twelve hours), and daily exercise will help restore health. Refined foods high in sugar and fats weaken the body and make it more susceptible to infections. Start today to implement the *Setpoint* guidelines. You'll be pleased at how quickly positive changes can occur in your family as you adopt a more nutritious and healthful lifestyle.

A child's behavior is often diet-related. Cries and misbehavior are often cries for the nutrients a child's growing body desperately needs. A well-balanced diet of whole grains, lots of fresh vegetables and fruits, lean meats, milk, and eggs will provide these nutrients and improve a child's disposition.

A child's nutritional intake from birth to age five largely determines what type of body he will have—one prone to infections, allergies, and other illnesses or one with only a few minor illnesses. The decision is up to you—the parent.

Educate yourself on the importance of good nutrition. With knowledge you can make proper food choices for your children and assist them in choosing wisely as they grow older. Study and learn about foods which contain the nutrients your children are lacking. Two excellent books which give this information are *Feed Your Kids Right* and *Foods for Healthy Kids* both by Dr. Lendon Smith, M.D. [20]

As you make these changes, don't let your family feel deprived, or they may rebel. Replace their favorite poor food choices (high fats or sugars) with tasty good food choices, such as those found in this book. It takes time to make the transition to wholesome foods. Don't try to change all your eating habits at once.

Snacks Are Okay

Snacking is not all bad! It's the kind of food people snack on that gives snacking a bad name. Children often need snacks because their energy requirements are very high while they are growing. Give them nutritious snacks, not those full of empty calories.

Healthy Snack Suggestions:

> Slice of whole wheat bread with a skiff of butter or jam
> Fresh in-season fruits
> Lowfat unsweetened yogurt with fresh fruit
> Air-popped popcorn with minimal butter and salt
> Homemade muffins (a wonderful and tasty alternative
> to high-fat, high-sugar cookies)
> Fresh vegetables: carrot and celery sticks, green pepper slices, broccoli and
> cauliflower pieces, etc.
> Homemade nutritious cookies and milk
> Homemade granola or trail mix
> Whole-grain prepared cereal with milk
> Raw nuts (serve in the shell, and they won't overeat)

What is Junk Food?

Junk food is any food that provides short-term energy and does not provide essential vitamins and minerals. Junk food may give you a temporary high but soon leaves you more hungry and tired than you were before eating it. Avoid high-sugar, high-salt, and high-fat snack choices such as chips, pop, pastries, ice cream, candy, and other types of junk food. If you and your family are out of the house around meal time and need something to tide you over until you get home, stop at a grocery store. Buy a banana, apple, raw almonds, or peanuts. Even better, plan ahead and take a nutritious snack with you such as a slice of whole wheat bread or some fruit.

Improve Family Eating Habits

1. Follow the *Setpoint Guidelines* but don't try to change everything all at once. Introduce new foods and recipes gradually. If possible, introduce them in familiar foods. Example: when serving brown rice for the first time, use it in rice pudding or a casserole rather than alone.

2. As parents, Mom and Dad should display an enthusiastic united front when introducing new foods.

3. Make sure everyone eats a good breakfast. Remember, cars don't run on fumes. They need a full tank, and so do we. A whole grain cooked cereal is the best way to start the day. Breakfast needn't be elaborate, just nourishing.

4. Feed children when they are hungry. If children seem to be constantly hungry, feed them four to five smaller meals a day instead of three large ones. Feed them a meal instead of offering sweets to momentarily satisfy them.

5. Discourage any snacks one hour before meals. Even sweet fruits may decrease a child's hunger for nutritious meals. If children are hungry at mealtime, they are more likely to eat what is served. Fruit snacks are okay if children have already eaten a good meal.

6. Mealtime should be approximately the same time each day. Children (and adults) thrive on routine. Sit down at the table and eat together as a family instead of everyone grabbing their own food. Make it a relaxed, happy time of day.

7. Don't be a short-order cook, fixing two to three different menus in order to please everyone. Everyone should eat the same meal! Make it nutritious and delicious.

8. If children don't like what's on the menu, encourage them to try a small portion. Don't allow them to fill up later with a peanut butter and jelly sandwich or other preferred food. They will soon learn to like what's being served.

9. Don't use food as a reward for good behavior or deny it as punishment for bad behavior, such as: "If you're good while Mommy is gone, I'll bring you a treat." Food should not be used as a bribe or as an incentive to behave.

10. Teach children to eat an orange instead of drinking a glass of orange juice; to eat an apple instead of drinking apple juice. The whole fruit is much more satisfying because of the fiber and chewing involved.

11. Encourage children to drink at least four to five glasses of water daily.

12. Avoid stocking such foods as fruit-flavored soft drink mixes, soft drinks, fruit juice soft drinks (those with 10 percent fruit juice), powdered chocolate drink mixes, hot dogs, cold cuts, pre-sweetened cereals, soda and graham crackers, pastries, cookies, and white bread.

13. Satisfy sweet tooth cravings with natural sweets such as fresh fruit, dried fruits, raisins, dates, or homemade granola. Cut out high-sugar, high-fat snack items. Keep plenty of wholesome snacks readily available.

14. Use old-fashioned peanut butter. Most name-brand peanut butters have added hydrogenated shortening and sugar. Peanut butter is high in fat and should be used moderately, perhaps once or twice a week, and should not be the mainstay of a child's diet.

15. Teach children why good foods are important to their growth. Children are usually very interested in the whys. Teach them about the vitamins and minerals contained in different food groups and why they need to eat a variety of foods.

16. Involve children in grocery shopping, and teach them how to read labels. Shopping provides a good opportunity to teach children why you buy certain foods and not others.

17. Teach children to make wise food choices if possible when they're away from home. Instead of purchasing a soft drink, suggest they choose a can of unsweetened fruit or vegetable juice, which is about the same price. Remind them that most fast-food restaurants will provide ice water if you ask.

18. Don't forbid certain foods. Children will want them even more. Let children have cake at a friend's party. Even school lunch may not always be up to your standards. Occasional "junk food" is okay if children regularly eat good basic foods at home. The less you make an issue of food, the easier the transition to better family eating habits.

We owe our children the right to healthy minds and bodies. Good health is best attained through regular exercise, adequate rest, and nutritious foods. We love our children. Let's feed them right!

CHAPTER 12

Potpourri

This chapter incorporates a mishmash of guidelines and recipes that may be helpful—either now or later. You will find that living this Setpoint lifestyle, and using the easy-to-store, high-energy foods found in the tasty, wholesome recipes, will help you become much more self-reliant. *Set For Life* will help you achieve good health and weight control naturally, and should not dominate your life; this is a lifetime plan, not a diet. The menu planning and food preparation may take more time initially, but will pay for themselves later in better health, more energy, and a lower food bill. Three weeks of menus and the correlated shopping lists are included here to help get you started. The amounts given in the shopping lists correspond with the recipes; they can be varied to fit your family. Refer to Chapter 5 for complete information, and remember that balance—in every facet of this lifestyle—is your key to success.

Use the *Set For Life Daily Guide* for a few weeks, following the guidelines on pages 37-39. Color or check the open boxes when completed each day so you can identify at a glance the areas that need improvement. This sheet is for your benefit, so be totally honest with yourself. *If it is to be, it is up to me.*

Daily Guide Scoring: Score one point in the small shadowed scoring box (upper right hand corner) for each completed group.

Breakfast . . . . 1 point	Fruit . . . . 1 point
Lunch. . . . . 1 point	Meat Group . . . . 1 point
Dinner . . . . 1 point	Dairy . . . . 1 point
Whole Grains . . . . 1 point	Water . . . . 1 point
Vegetables. . . . . 1 point	Exercise . . . . 1 point

10 points possible per day   70 points possible per week
Goal: 8-10 points daily   56-70 points weekly

You will be successful; this is the way! Have the vision to see, the faith to believe, and the courage to do.

GROCERY LIST — WEEK #1

FRESH VEGETABLES
1 head cabbage
2 heads lettuce
1 bunch celery
1 bunch green onions
5 lb. carrots
2 green peppers
3 tomatoes
1 bunch broccoli
1 head cauliflower
4 dry onions
1 garlic head
1 piece banana squash
10 lb. potatoes

CANNED VEGETABLES
1 - 28 oz. tomatoes
1 - 8 oz. tomato sauce
1 - 17 oz. whole kernal corn
2 - 15 oz. chili beans (red or
    pinto)
1 - 31 oz. pork and beans
1 - 16 oz. pork and beans
1 - 15 oz. kidney beans
1 - 10 oz. enchilada sauce
1 - 16 oz. salsa or mild taco
    sauce

FRESH FRUIT
apples
oranges
bananas
1 lemon

CANNED FRUIT
2 - 16 oz. lite peaches
1 - 29 oz. lite pear halves
1 - 2 oz. jar maraschino
    cherries
1 - 16 oz. unsweetened apple
    juice

MISC.
1 - 16 oz. apple cider vinegar
1 - 28 oz. catsup
1 - 16 oz. dill pickles

1 - 8 oz. fat-free ranch
    dressing
1 - 16 oz. salad dressing or
    mayonnaise, fat-free
1 - 16 oz. low-sugar jam
1 can evaporated skim milk
1 can lowfat vegetable soup
2 cans chicken gumbo soup
2 cans tomato soup
1 can cream of mushroom
    soup, lowfat
1 can tuna, water-packed
1 - 3 oz. low-sodium instant
    chicken bouillon
1 - 3 oz. low-sodium instant
    beef bouillon
1 pkg. dry onion soup mix

BAKING SUPPLIES
2 lb. honey
1 - 24 oz. vegetable oil
1 box cornstarch
1 baking powder
1 baking soda
1 lb. brown sugar
10 lb. sugar
10 lbs. unbleached white flour
5 lbs. whole wheat flour
1 vanilla extract
1 - 16 oz. pkg. raisins
dried basil leaves
paprika
dry mustard
seasoned salt
chili powder
parmesan cheese
cinnamon
allspice
ginger
salt
minced onion
dried thyme leaves
dried parsley flakes
1 pkg. taco seasoning mix

CEREALS & GRAINS
1 box old fashioned rolled oats
1 box Shredded Wheat
1 box Bran Flakes
1 lb. whole wheat berries
2 lb. long grain brown rice
8 oz. whole wheat spaghetti
    noodles

FROZEN
1 pkg. frozen petite peas

BAKERY
3 loaves 100% whole wheat
    bread
8 whole grain hamburger buns
6 whole wheat bread sticks

DAIRY
1 lb. margarine
1-3 gallons 1% or skim milk
2 - 16 oz. cartons lowfat
    cottage cheese
3 dozen eggs
1/2 lb. cheese

MEAT
2 lb. sole (fresh or frozen) or
    other preferred fish
2 lb. extra lean ground beef
3 chicken breasts or 6 thighs
1 - 2-1/2 - 3 lb. chicken,
    cut up
1 dozen corn tortillas
1 small pkg. lean bacon
2-1/2 oz. pkg thin sliced lean
    ham
4 oz. thinly sliced chicken
    breast
4 oz. thinly sliced turkey ham

MENU — WEEK #1

SUNDAY

Breakfast	**Lunch**	**Dinner**
Bran flakes	Chicken and Rice Bake, p. 161	Canned tomato soup
Whole wheat toast	Baked Beans, p. 229	Turkey ham sandwiches
Fruit	Green salad w/fat free	Lettuce and tomato
1% milk	dressing	Fruit
	Frozen petite peas	Water
	Feather rolls, p. 80 or buy	
	Magic Cobbler, p. 264	
	Water	

MONDAY

Breakfast	**Lunch**	**Dinner**
Oatmeal, p. 97	Tuna salad spread, p. 130	Fiesta Bake, pg. 216 (freeze half)
Apple raisin muffins, p. 90	on whole grain bread	Shredded lettuce
(double & freeze half)	Canned lowfat vegetable soup	Raw vegetable plate
OR Whole wheat toast	Fruit	Whole wheat bread
Fruit	Water	Water
1% milk		

TUESDAY

Breakfast	**Lunch**	**Dinner**
Shredded wheat	Chicken and Rice leftovers	Baked fish fillets, p. 175
Whole wheat toast	Peas	Oven fries, p. 226
Fruit (snack)	Baked beans	Steamed broccoli
1% milk	Green salad	Creamy cole slaw, p. 139
	Whole wheat bread	Whole wheat rolls
	Fruit	Water
	Water	

WEDNESDAY

Breakfast	**Lunch**	**Dinner**
Cracked wheat cereal, p. 99	Baked fish leftovers	Quick Fix Chicken, p. 157
Apple raisin muffins (leftovers)	Broccoli	Steamed brown rice, p. 226
OR Whole wheat toast	Coleslaw	Baked squash, p. 236
Fruit (snack)	Fruit	Green salad w/fat free dressing
1% milk	Water	Whole wheat bread
		water

THURSDAY

Breakfast	**Lunch**	**Dinner**
Oatmeal, p. 97	Chicken breast sandwich	Minestrone soup, p. 123
3-minute boiled eggs	Whole wheat bread	Whole wheat bread sticks, p. 86
Whole wheat toast	Lowfat vegetable soup	or buy
Fruit (snack)	Fruit	Water
1% milk	Water	

FRIDAY

Breakfast	**Lunch**	**Dinner**
Rice 'n Apple breakfast, p. 100	Tuna spread sandwich (leftover)	Fiesta Bake (from freezer)
Whole wheat toast	Whole grain bread	Green salad
1% milk	Raw vegetables	Whole wheat bread
	Fruit	Water
	Water	

SATURDAY

Breakfast	**Lunch**	**Dinner**
Blender Pancakes, p. 107	Minestrone Soup over baked potatoes	Sloppy Joes, p. 202
Pancake Topping, p. 114	Whole wheat bread	Whole grain buns
Scrambled eggs	Fruit	Pork and beans
1% milk	Water	Raw vegetables
		Pear Salad, p. 134
		Water

GROCERY LIST — WEEK #2

FRESH VEGETABLES
3 green peppers
1 bunch green onions
6 tomatoes
10 lb. potatoes
3 medium red potatoes
5 lb. carrots
5 large dry onions
3 cloves garlic
2 heads cabbage
2 heads lettuce
1 bunch celery
8 oz. mushrooms

CANNED VEGETABLES
2 - 4 oz. cans mushrooms
1 - 16 oz. can diced beets
1 - 17 oz. can whole kernal
corn
6 oz. tomato paste
1 jar salsa or mild taco sauce
2 - 16 oz. cans pinto beans
    (if not using own Ranchero
    beans)

FRESH FRUITS
apples
oranges
bananas

CANNED FRUITS
16 oz. unsweetened applesauce
20 oz. can lite cherry pie
    filling

MISC.
Soy sauce
3 cans lowfat vegetable soup
1 - 15 oz. can salmon
1 - 2-1/2 oz. sliced olives
16 oz. lite tortilla chips
1 - 16 oz. box graham crackers
1 box Dream Whip
1 fat free Catalina Salad
    Dressing
16 oz. Salsa

BAKING SUPPLIES
yellow cornmeal
3 lb. whole wheat flour
cooking oil
raisins 2 lb.
baking soda
seasoned salt
garlic salt
garlic powder
vanilla extract
1 pkg. pizza seasoning mix
1 pkg. taco seasoning mix

CEREALS & GRAINS
1 box whole grain cold cereal
1 box old fashioned rolled oats
16 oz. pkg. white (navy) beans
1 lb. pkg. pinto beans
3 lb. long grain brown rice
2 - 3 oz. pkg. whole wheat
    or brown rice ramen
    noodles
1 lb. whole wheat kernals

FROZEN
1 pkg. mixed vegetables
1 pkg. petite peas
1 pkg. corn
lemon juice concentrate

BAKERY
3 loaves 100% whole wheat
bread

DAIRY
1-3 gallons 1% or skim milk
16 oz. lowfat cottage cheese
8 oz. cream cheese, fat free
1 lb. margarine
8 oz. skim mozzarella cheese
8 oz. cheddar cheese
3 dozen eggs

MEAT
1 - lean ham hock, ham bone,
      or 8 oz. lean ham
1 - 2 1/2 oz. pkg. thinly
      sliced ham
4 oz. thinly sliced chicken
      breast
3-4 lb. lean beef pot roast
1 1/2 lb. extra lean ground
      beef
1 lb. boneless chicken breast,
      uncooked

MENU — WEEK #2

SUNDAY

Breakfast	**Lunch**	**Dinner**
Whole grain cold cereal	Canned vegetable soup	Roast Beef Dinner, p. 189
Whole wheat toast	Chicken breast sandwiches	Frozen corn
Fruit	Whole wheat bread	Creamy Coleslaw, p. 139
1% milk	Fruit	Feather Rolls, p. 80 or buy
	Water	Cherry Cheesecake Delight, p. 257
		Water

MONDAY

Breakfast	**Lunch**	**Dinner**
Brown rice cereal, p. 100	Roast beef & vegetables (leftover)	Juicy Salmon Loaf, p. 177
Whole wheat toast	Whole wheat rolls	Creamed Peas and Potatoes, p. 234
Fruit	Fruit	Coleslaw
1% milk	Water	Favorite Muffins, p. 89
		(double & freeze half)
		Water

TUESDAY

Breakfast	**Lunch**	**Dinner**
Poached fried eggs, p. 102	Salmon Loaf Sandwiches (leftover)	Favorite Pizza, p. 206
or Boiled eggs	Lowfat vegetable soup or green salad	Green salad w/fat free dressing
Whole wheat toast	Fruit	Water
Fruit	Water	*Cook Ranchero Beans (p. 210) all
1% milk		night for tomorrow's Taco
		Sundaes

WEDNESDAY

Breakfast	**Lunch**	**Dinner**
Cracked wheat cereal, p. 99	Baked Potato, p. 221-222	Taco Sundaes, p. 212
Whole wheat toast	w/frozen mixed vegetables	*Cook extra rice for fried rice and
Fruit	Lowfat cottage cheese	leftovers on Saturday
1% milk	Whole wheat bread	Water
	Fruit	
	Water	

THURSDAY

Breakfast	**Lunch**	**Dinner**
Whole grain cold cereal	Ranchero Beans	Chow Mein, p. 186
Whole wheat toast	Lowfat cottage cheese	Fried Rice, p. 188
Fruit	Raw vegetables	Favorite Muffins (frozen from
1% milk	Whole wheat bread	Monday)
	Fruit	Water
	Water	

FRIDAY

Breakfast	**Lunch**	**Dinner**
Oatmeal, p. 97	Chow mein leftovers	Bean Soup, p. 125
Whole wheat toast	Whole grain bread	Golden Cornbread, p. 92
Fruit	Fruit	Water
1% milk	Water	

SATURDAY

Breakfast	**Lunch**	**Dinner**
Egg Souffle Breakfast Casserole,	Bean soup leftovers	Taco Sundae leftovers
p. 104	Cornbread	Water
Apple Raisin Muffins, p. 90	Raw vegetables	
Fruit	Water	
1% milk		

GROCERY LIST — WEEK #3

FRESH VEGETABLES
1 head cabbage
2 heads lettuce
5 lb. carrots
1 bunch celery
1 bunch green onions
2 dry onions
1 green pepper
2 cloves garlic
2 bunches broccoli
1 head cauliflower
2 yams
10 lb. potatoes

CANNED VEGETABLES
2 - 16 oz. cans tomatoes
1 - 28 oz. can tomatoes
1 - 16 oz. can tomato sauce
2 - 17 oz. whole kernal corn
2 - 4 oz. can mushrooms

FRESH FRUIT
apples
oranges
bananas
other as desired

CANNED FRUIT
8 oz. unsweetened crushed
    pineapple
16 oz. unsweetened apple
    juice
16 oz. fruit cocktail

MISC.
1 can cream of chicken soup,
    lowfat
3 cans tomato soup
3 cans water packed tuna
1 can evaporated skim milk
2 fat-free salad dressings of
    choice
Salad dressing or mayonnaise,
    fat free
1 can lowfat vegetable soup

BAKING SUPPLIES
3 lb. honey
1 box Dream Whip
Small box Knox unflavored
    gelatin
5 lb. whole wheat flour
1 lb. brown sugar
poultry seasoning
bay leaves
minced onion, dry
nutmeg
2 pkgs. spaghetti sauce mix
nonfat dry milk powder
4 oz. slivered almonds

CEREALS AND GRAINS
Shredded wheat
bran flakes
1 lb. whole wheat kernals
2 lb. long grain brown rice
12 oz. whole wheat spaghetti
    noodles
8 oz. pkg. egg noodles
1/2 lb. unprocessed wheat
    bran

FROZEN
2 - 10 oz. frozen broccoli
12 oz. unsweetened apple
    juice concentrate
10 oz. frozen strawberries
1 pkg. frozen green beans
1 pkg. corn
1 pkg. chopped spinach

BAKERY
4 loaves 100% whole wheat
    bread
1 dozen whole wheat rolls
1 loaf french bread

DAIRY
1 lb. margarine
2 dozen eggs
1-3 gallons 1% or skim milk
1 quart buttermilk
8 oz. sour cream, fat free

MEAT
1 lb. chicken breast
1 - 3 lb. chicken, cut up
1-1/2 lb. extra lean ground
    beef
1 pkg. thinly sliced chicken or
    turkey

MENU — WEEK #3

SUNDAY

Breakfast
Shredded wheat
Whole wheat toast
Fruit
1% milk

Lunch
Chicken Divan, p. 164
Baked Yams, p. 238
Green salad w/fat free dressing
Fruit Set Salad, p. 145
Frosty Strawberry Squares, p. 258
Whole wheat bread
Water

Dinner
Chicken breast sandwiches
Whole grain bread
Lettuce
Fruit set salad
Water

MONDAY

Breakfast
Rice Pudding, p. 264
　(rice from Sun.) prepare
　in microwave
Whole wheat toast
Fruit
1% milk

Lunch
Chicken Divan leftovers
Yams
Salad
Fruit
Whole wheat bread
Water

Dinner
Hamburger Soup, p. 126
Whole wheat rolls
Water

TUESDAY

Breakfast
Whole wheat cereal, p. 99
Whole wheat toast
Fruit
1% milk

Lunch
Hamburger soup (leftovers)
Whole wheat bread
Fruit
Water

Dinner
Spaghetti, p. 202 & 203
Frozen green beans
Green salad w/fat free dressing
French bread
Water

WEDNESDAY

Breakfast
French Toast, p. 110
Spicy Apple Syrup, p. 111
Fruit
1% milk

Lunch
Tuna Sandwich, p. 130
Whole grain bread
Green salad or lowfat soup
Fruit
Water

Dinner
Crispy Chicken, p. 158 (can roll in
　unprocessed wheat bran)
Western Potato Strips, p. 224
Steamed broccoli and cauliflower
Whole wheat bread
Water

THURSDAY

Breakfast
Bran flakes
3-minute boiled egg
Whole wheat toast
Fruit
1% milk

Lunch
Spaghetti leftovers
Green beans
Green salad
Fruit
Water

Dinner
Broccoli with Tuna Sauce, p. 179
Frozen corn
Coleslaw, p. 139
Whole wheat bread
Water

FRIDAY

Breakfast
Oatmeal, p. 97
Whole wheat toast
Fruit
1% milk

Lunch
Broccoli w/tuna (leftovers)
Corn
Coleslaw
Whole wheat bread
Fruit
Water

Dinner
Taglarinni, p. 199
Frozen chopped spinach
Raw vegetable
Water

SATURDAY

Breakfast
Pancake Master Mix, p. 108
Poached Fried Eggs, p. 102
Hashbrowns, pg. 105
Fruit

Lunch
Canned tomato soup
Turkey ham sandwiches
Raw vegetables
Fruit
Water

Dinner
Smorgasbord (leftovers from
　the week)
Water

DAILY GUIDE SCORING: Score one point in the small shadowed scoring box (upper right hand corner) for each completed group.
Follow Daily Guide for Menu Planning on page 39.

Breakfast . . . . .1 point
Lunch . . . . .1 point
Dinner . . . . .1 point

Set for Life — Daily Guide   NAME:

		SUNDAY	MONDAY	TUESDAY
B R E A K F A S T		☐	☐	☐
SNACK				
L U N C H		☐	☐	☐
SNACK				
D I N N E R		☐	☐	☐
TOTAL FAT GRAMS				

COMPLEX CARBOHYDRATES		SUNDAY	MONDAY	TUESDAY
	WHOLE GRAINS	☐	☐	☐
	VEGETABLES	☐	☐	☐
	POTATOES, BEANS OR BROWN RICE			
	FRUITS	☐	☐	☐
	MEAT GROUP	☐	☐	☐
	DAIRY	☐	☐	☐
	WATER	☐	☐	☐
	EXERCISE	20 MIN. / 20 MIN. / 20 MIN. ☐	20 MIN. / 20 MIN. / 20 MIN. ☐	20 MIN. / 20 MIN. / 20 MIN. ☐
	DAILY TOTALS			

© 1995 Set for Life   10 points possible per day   Goal: 8–10 points daily

Whole Grains . . . . .1 point   Meat Group . . . . . .1 point
Vegetables . . . . . . .1 point   Dairy . . . . .1 point
Fruit . . . . .1 point   Water . . . . .1 point
                                       Exercise . . . . .1 point

DATE: *WEEKLY TOTAL:*

WEDNESDAY	THURSDAY	FRIDAY	SATURDAY
❏	❏	❏	❏
❏	❏	❏	❏
❏	❏	❏	❏

				❏					❏					❏					❏
❏	❏	❏	❏
❏	❏	❏	❏
❏	❏	❏	❏
❏	❏	❏	❏
20 MIN.	20 MIN.	20 MIN.		❏	20 MIN.	20 MIN.	20 MIN.		❏	20 MIN.	20 MIN.	20 MIN.		❏	20 MIN.	20 MIN.	20 MIN.		❏

70 points possible per week   56–70 points weekly

Nonfat Yogurt

Making yogurt is easy and economical. Start with 1% or skim milk. Adding nonfat dry milk compensates for the lower solids content of low-fat milk and improves the texture, quality, and food value of the yogurt.

1/2 to 3/4 cup nonfat dry milk
1 quart 1% milk or skim milk
1 package freeze-dried yogurt starter
OR 1/4 cup plain unflavored yogurt

1. Combine nonfat dry milk and 1% milk; use blender if desired. Slowly heat milk to scalding temperature, 180°F or 82°C, stirring often. Maintain this temperature for two minutes. This gives a superior, consistent quality yogurt and is worth the few minutes it takes. Remove milk from heat and cool to lukewarm, 112°F or 44°C. Stir yogurt starter or unflavored yogurt into one cup of the lukewarm milk; pour the mixture back into the container of warm milk and mix well.

2. Immediately put mixture into one of the following containers and let incubate *undisturbed* until firm. A yogurt maker takes about three to five hours, a wide mouth thermos bottle may take overnight or five to eight hours, or use a quart jar. Place jar in a pan of warm water over an electric burner turned to *warm* (don't overheat) for four to five hours; then turn off until yogurt is firm. Refrigerate and yogurt will stay fresh for several weeks.

3. To start a new batch, save one-fourth cup yogurt for a starter. To produce high-quality, mild-flavored yogurt, use a new yogurt starter every three or four batches.

4. Serve with fresh fruit, such as oranges, berries, or bananas; or use in recipes that call for plain nonfat yogurt. Yogurt is a good alternative to high-fat sour cream or mayonnaise and a good source of calcium and protein.

Yield: 4 cups   1/2 cup servings

Per Serving	RCU	FU	Cal	% Ft	P	F	C	Na
	0	0	80	11	7	1	9	109

Yogurt Cheese: Make a cream cheese type product by draining yogurt overnight in a colander lined with cheesecloth or a strong white paper towel. Cheese can be used mixed with chives or fruit for a nonfat spread or in most recipes that call for cream cheese. Stabilize in cooked dishes by adding 1 to 2 tablespoons flour.
One quart yogurt yields 1 1/2 cups cheese.

Grow Your Own Sprouts

Sprouts have been called our most perfect living food because they are fresh, uncontaminated, power-packed with nutrients, and are good for you! Growing sprouts is easy and requires little time, effort or expense. You can have a new crop in three to five days, no matter what the climate or where you live. Sprouts are delicious and a very nutritious, high-energy food.

Alfalfa, mung beans, and wheat are three of the most popular seeds for home sprouting; sprouted sunflower seeds make a tasty addition to any salad. For trouble-free sprouting, invest in a small, inexpensive, plastic sprouter. This will eliminate moldy or sour sprouts, a problem which discourages beginners who try to sprout in a bottle or on a wet towel. Always buy sprouting seeds; these are untreated, have a high germination rate, and should be available at a health food store.

Follow these simple instructions for perfect sprouts:

1. Soak seeds in pure room-temperature water. Small seeds should be soaked for 8 to 12 hours or overnight; soak larger seeds such as wheat 18 to 24 hours. Allow three or four times more water than seeds. Try these amounts to begin with:

Alfalfa and related	2 to 4 tablespoons
Mung beans, lentils and other beans	1/2 to 1 cup
Sunflower seeds	1/2 to 1 cup
Wheat, rye, oats, and related grains	1/2 to 1 cup

2. After soaking, pour seeds into a sprouter and drain well. If you don't have a sprouter, put seeds into a wide-mouth quart or gallon jar and cover the jar mouth with a clean piece of nylon hosiery to facilitate draining the water after rinsing. Lay the bottle on its side for better ventilation during sprouting. Since sprouts grow best in the dark, keep your "garden" covered with a light towel and out of direct sunlight; do keep them in a conspicuous place so you won't forget to rinse often. They can't grow without oxygen, so don't cover with a lid.

4. Rinse and drain the sprouts morning, noon and night if possible. Fill sink with several inches of room temperature water and move the sprouter up and down to thoroughly rinse seeds. Drain well by tilting the sprouter slightly. Extra rinsing keeps alfalfa and ming bean sprouts mild and crisp. You can control the growth of your sprouts to some degree by varying the rinse water temperature. Cold water slows their growth; warm water accelerates it; heavily chlorinated water may kill them.

5. Sprouts will be ready to eat in two to five days. Sample them often to see when they taste best to you. Each seed and grain has its peak of quality. Sunflower seeds are crunchy-tender in just 24 hours. Wheat tastes best when the sprout is the same length as the seed, which takes approximately 48 hours. Mung beans and lentils are at their taste peak when they are from one-fourth to one-inch long; this usually takes two to three days. Alfalfa grows from one to one and one-half inches long in four to five days; uncover alfalfa the last day so it will turn green.

6. When sprouts are ready, rinse with cold water to stop their growth. Eat immediately or store in a covered container in the refrigerator.

Wheatgrass

Dr. Ann Wigmore spent many years proving the value of this vitamin and mineral-rich chlorophyll in rebuilding health. Dr. G. H. Earp-Thomas, a noted scientist and soil expert, isolated more than one hundred elements from fresh wheatgrass and concluded that it is a complete food. Researchers report that every known vitamin has been segregated from wheatgrass, in the amounts and qualities best suited for use in the bodies of human beings.[22]

Some years ago, wheatgrass juice and Zip, in addition to living these principles, helped restore my own (Jane's) shattered health, which stemmed in part from an inherently weak digestive system. They were only part—but a very important part—of my therapy for almost a year. I have learned to appreciate the value of good health, and the price that some of us must pay to enjoy this great blessing. Wheatgrass is not a cure; it simply furnishes vital nourishment which the body needs to regenerate. Hippocrates wisely said, "Let food be thy medicine."

How to Grow Wheatgrass

1 cup wheat
2 cups peat moss
9 x 13-inch glass baking dish or plastic
   greenhouse tray

2 to 3 cups top soil
Water

Put wheat in a quart jar and fill with pure water; let wheat soak at room temperature for 18 to 24 hours. Wheat can be planted immediately after soaking, but for best results, put soaked wheat into a plastic sprouter, or use a wide-mouth jar; turn the jar on its side and roll around to spread the wheat; cover either with a cloth, and let sprout for 24 to 36 hours. Rinse with water at least twice a day and drain well to prevent spoilage.

Spread peat moss evenly in the bottom of a tray and dampen with water. Add top soil and sprinkle with water until damp; soil will be about one-inch deep. Using a spatula, spread the sprouted wheat evenly and thickly on the soil, like icing a cake.

Soak eight layers of black and white newspaper in water; lay this over the wheat. Wrap tray loosely with black plastic and put in a dark place.

In two to three days, depending on room temperature, the sprouts will begin to raise the newspaper; they will be 1/2 to 3/4-inches high and very white. Remove coverings and place tray in full light. Water daily; do not allow wheatgrass to dry out. Wheatgrass will begin to turn green almost immediately and will be seven to eight inches high and ready to cut in eight to ten days.

To harvest wheatgrass, use a good pair of kitchen shears and cut as close to the soil as possible. Ideally, wheatgrass should be used immediately after cutting, but it will keep in a plastic bag in the refrigerator for up to a week.

To assure a continuous supply, start soaking more wheat when the previous tray of wheatgrass is two inches high.

Wheatgrass may be used in several ways:

1. Cut wheatgrass into one-inch lengths with scissors; alternate grass and carrots into a Champion juicer. Drink the juice immediately for maximum benefit; wheatgrass juice is very concentrated so dilute with water if necessary.

2. A Norwalk juicer grinds and presses wheatgrass to extract juice.

3. Special electric and hand wheatgrass juicers are available; check with your local health food store.

4. If you don't have a juicer, cut wheatgrass into one-inch lengths; eat as much as possible in salads and other uncooked dishes.

5. Dr. Earp-Thomas discovered that fruits and vegetables contaminated by sprays were cleansed, and dangerous chemicals neutralized, by placing wheatgrass in the wash water. Dr. Ann Wigmore noted that wheatgrass helps give protection against radiation and fall-out poisons when used in the bath and drinking water.[22 (p. 58)]

ZIP — A Mild Grain Drink

Zip is a mild grain drink made from wheat or barley. Sometimes called a new form of acidophilus, Zip is an excellent digestive aid that benefits most everyone. Those who drink it regularly say they avoid colds and flu and have an increase in energy.

How To Make Zip:
1 cup wheat or barley   **3 cups cold water**

Rinse 1 cup grain; place in a quart bottle and fill with water. Let stand at room temperature for 24 hours. Pour off the water and drink it; if desired, mix this water with juice or use it in cooking. Add more water to the same grain, and let stand another 24 hours. Use the same grain for two or three days; then discard and start with fresh grain.

Mustard Plaster

This good old-fashioned remedy really helps to break up chest congestion.

Prepare a piece of cloth twice the size of the chest area. Mix 4 tablespoons flour and 1 tablespoon dry mustard with enough water to make a very thick paste. (Use 2 tablespoons flour and 1 teaspoon dry mustard for an infant.) Spread this mixture on half the cloth, leaving the edges clear. Fold cloth in half, completely enclosing the mixture. Rub chest area liberally with petroleum jelly (Vaseline) and apply the mustard plaster; cover with a small towel and keep warm and quiet for 20 to 30 minutes. The chest area will get warm and pink but the mustard plaster should never burn the skin. After removing the plaster, keep warm and covered to prevent chilling. This treatment can be used once or twice a day if needed.

Lite Jams

These low-sugar jams and spreads are delicious and inexpensive to make. The recipes can easily be adapted to almost any desired fruit combinations. You'll love the natural fruit flavor.

To thicken jams, use cornstarch, gelatin, or no thickener at all. You can easily adjust the thickness of jam while it is cooking; to thin add a little water or juice. If a thickener jam is desired, mix an additional tablespoon or two of cornstarch into a small quantity of water and slowly stir into the boiling jam. One tablespoon of cornstarch will thicken about two cups of fruit. Remember that the jam will thicken a little more as it cools.

Apple Butter

12 cups thick applesauce, fresh or canned
1 6-ounce can frozen apple juice concentrate
1 to 3 cups sugar or honey
2 teaspoons cinnamon

1/2 teaspoon ground cloves
1/4 teaspoon nutmeg
1/4 teaspoon ginger

Mix applesauce and apple juice concentrate in a heavy pan. Add spices and sugar or honey; don't over-sweeten. Cook slowly and stir often until thick enough to round up in a spoon, about 20 minutes. Pour into hot sterile jars and seal, leaving 1/4-inch head space. Process 10 minutes in water bath.

Cook: 30 min   Process: 10 min   Yield: 6 pints

Per Serving	RCU	FU	Cal	% Ft	P	F	C	Na
1 Tablespoon	0	0	12	0	0	0	3	0

Apricot Jam

12 cups crushed apricots
2 to 3 cups crushed pineapple
4 to 6 cups sugar or 2 to 3 cups honey

1/2 cup cornstarch
1/2 cup cold water

Wash apricots and remove pits. Coarsely grind or chop fruit in blender. Put apricots, undrained pineapple, and sugar in a large, heavy pan. Bring to a boil and cook over medium heat for 15 minutes, stirring often to prevent scorching. Mix cornstarch and water. Stir into fruit and cook another 3 to 5 minutes, stirring constantly. Leave 1/4-inch head space and seal in hot sterile jars. Process in a water bath for 15 minutes.

Cook: 20 min   Process: 15 min   Yield: 7-8 pints

Per Serving	RCU	FU	Cal	% Ft	P	F	C	Na
1 Tablespoon	0	0	10	0	0	0	3	0

Heavenly Pear Jam

8 to 10 cups mashed pears
2 cups crushed pineapple, undrained
1/2 lemon, grated and juiced
1 tablespoon fresh lime juice

4 cups sugar or 2 cups honey
1 4-ounce jar maraschino cherries,
  thinly sliced and undrained
1/2 3-ounce package strawberry gelatin

Peel and core pears. Combine pears, undrained pineapple, lemon rind, lemon and lime juice, and sugar in a heavy pan. Bring to a boil and cook over medium heat for about 15 minutes; stir often as mixture scorches easily. Add cherries and gelatin. Cook 5 to 7 minutes more, stirring constantly. Seal in hot sterile jars. Process 10 minutes in water bath. The strawberry gelatin can be omitted but adds a beautiful color and delicate flavor.

Cook: 20 min   Process: 10 min   Yield: 5 to 6 pints

Peach Jam

12 cups crushed peaches
1/2 cup frozen orange juice concentrate
Juice of 1/2 lemon
4 to 5 cups sugar or 2 cups honey

1 3-ounce package orange gelatin
1/4 cup water
1/4 cup cornstarch

Peel and pit peaches. Combine all ingredients in a heavy pan. Bring to a boil and cook over medium heat for about 15 minutes, stirring often. Stir in orange gelatin. Mix cornstarch and water. Stir into hot jam and cook 3 to 5 minutes more, until thick. Seal in hot sterile jars, leaving 1/4-inch head space. Process 15 minutes in water bath.

Cook: 20 min   Process: 15 min   Yield: 6 pints

Freezer Berry Jam

5 cups stemmed and crushed berries
2 to 2 1/2 cups sugar

1/2 cup light corn syrup
1/4 cup Instant Clear Gel

Mix berries and corn syrup. Mix sugar and Instant Clear Gel*; then stir into fruit, mixing well. Allow 10 minutes for mixture to fully thicken. Put into containers and freeze.

Yield: 6 cups

Per Serving	RCU	FU	Cal	% Ft	P	F	C	Na
1 Tablespoon	1	0	22	0	0	0	6	1

*Instant Clear Gel is a modified tapioca starch that thickens food instantly without cooking and is ideal for low-sugar jams. Check your supermarket, health food store, or restaurant supply for availability.

Canned Salsa

This flavorful salsa is a staple that enhances numerous dishes.

4 to 5 quarts tomatoes, quartered, and
   well drained
1 to 3 medium red beets, fresh or canned
6 to 8 large green bell peppers
   or 10 to 12 Anaheim chilies and
     2 to 3 green peppers
6 large onions, peeled

4 to 6 jalapeno peppers, unseeded
   or 1 to 2 teaspoons crushed, dried
   hot peppers
1 6-ounce can tomato paste
1 teaspoon garlic salt
2 tablespoons salt
1/2 cup apple cider vinegar (5% strength)

Peel tomatoes if desired. After quartering, drain off all available juice, 3 or 4 cups if possible. Pureé the beets, which add natural color and rich flavor. Grind vegetables using a coarse blade; or chop coarsely in blender, using tomatoes for liquid. Pour into a large heavy pan and add remaining ingredients. Simmer about 30 minutes or until salsa reaches desired consistency, stirring often. Fill hot jars, leaving 1/2 inch headspace. Adjust lids and process in a pressure canner for 30 minutes at 12 pounds pressure; adjust for your altitude. Salsa may also be frozen.

Cook: 30 min   Processing Time: 30 min 12 pounds pressure   Yield: 8 to 9 pints
                              (Adjust for your altitude)

End-of-the-Garden Vegetable Soup Mix

This makes a wonderful stew or soup base.

6 quarts tomatoes, peeled and quartered
5 lbs. carrots (about 6 quarts carrots)
6 large onions, peeled and chopped
2 bunches celery, sliced
3 sweet red bell peppers, chopped

3 green bell peppers, chopped
1 head cabbage, sliced
4 quarts water
1/4 to 1/3 cup salt
1 teaspoon pepper (optional)

Chop by hand, or use French-fry blade on food processor for quick cutting of all the vegetables except onions and cabbage. Chop onions in blender, using a small amount of the water. Slice cabbage by hand or use wide slice blade on food processor. Put prepared vegetables and water in a large heavy pan. Add salt and pepper as desired. Simmer over medium heat until carrots are tender but still crisp, about 15-20 minutes. Stir often. Let cool and pour into freezer containers, leaving 1-inch head space. Cover and freeze. Caution: Recipe has not been safely-tested for canning times and temperatures.

Yield: 14 quarts or 28 pints

To Use Soup Mix:

1. Mix 1 quart Garden Vegetable Soup Mix with one large can vegetable beef stew. Add water as desired.

2. Mix 1 quart Vegetable Soup Mix with 1 cup cooked extra-lean ground beef, 1 cup cooked brown rice, 1 cup cooked pinto beans and 1 cup cooked potato cubes (potatoes will microwave in minutes in a plastic bag). Add water as needed.

Bibliography

1. Finn, Susan Calvert RD, Ph.D., Chubby Child—Fat Adult?'' American Baby Magazine, July 1987 pp. 44 & 47.

2. Pritikin, Nathan, Diet For Runners, New York: Simon and Schuster, 1982, ch. 1, p. 16.

3. Diehl, Hans Dr., To Your Health, Redlands, California: The Quiet Hour publishing, 1987, p.108.

4. Remington, Dennis M.D., Back To Health, Provo,Utah: Vitality House International, Inc., 1983.

5. Brody, Jane, Jane Brody's Good Food Book, New York: Bantam Books, 1987, p. 181.

6. Remington, Dennis M.D., Fisher, Garth Ph.D., Parent, Edward Ph.D., How To Lower Your Fat Thermostat, Provo, Utah: Vitality House, 1983.
SyberVision Systems, Inc., The Neuropsychology of Weight Control, Audiocassettes and Study Guide, Newark, California.: SyberVision Systems, Inc., 1985.

7. Wigmore, Ann, Be Your Own Doctor, New York: Hemisphere Press, p. 31, p.54-55.

8. Monte, Woodrow C., Ph.D., R.D., Aspartame: Methanol And The Public Health; Journal of Applied Nutrition Vol. 36, Number 1, 1984, pp. 42-54.
Remington, Dennis M.D., The Bitter Truth About Artificial Sweeteners, Provo: Vitality House International,Inc., 1987.

9. Smith, Lendon M.D., Feed Yourself Right, New York: Dell Publishing Co., Inc., 1983.
Brody, Jane, Jane Brody's Nutrition Book, New York: Bantam Books, 1982.

10. Brody, Jane, Jane Brody's Nutrition Book, New York: Bantam Books, 1982, p. 348.

11. La Lache League, The Womanly Art Of Breastfeeding, Franklin Park: 1958.

12. Pryor, Karen, Nursing Your Baby, New York: Harper and Row, 1963.

13. Thurston, Emory, The Parent's Guide To Better Nutrition For Tots To Teens, Keats Publishing, 1976, pp. 68-74.

14. Brody, Jane, Jane Brody's Nutrition Book, New York: Bantam Books, 1982, pp 349,358,359.

15. Brody, Jane, Jane Brody's Nutrition Book, New York: Bantam Books, 1982, p. 358.

Thurston, Emory, The Parent's Guide To Better Nutrition For Tots To Teens, Keats Publishing, 1976, pp. 9-11.

16. Boston Children's Hospital, Parent's Guide to Nutrition, Boston: Addison Wesley, 1986.

17. Select Committee on Nutrition and Human Needs, Dietary Goals for the United States, United States Senate, Feb. 1977.

18. Consumer Reports, Caffeine: What it Does, Consumers Union, October 1981, pp.595-599.

19. Thurston, Emory, The Parent's Guide To Better Nutrition For Tots To Teens, Keats Publishing, 1976, pp.31,32.

20. Smith, Lendon M.D., Feed Yourself Right, New York: Dell Publishing Co., Inc., 1983.

Smith, Lendon M.D., Foods For Healthy Kids, New York: A Berkely Book, published by arrangement with McGraw-Hill, 1981.

21. Thornock, Dana and Chriscilla, EAT & Be Lean, Clearfield, Utah: Thornock International Productions, 1988.

22. Wigmore, Ann, D.D.N.D., Be Your Own Doctor, New York: Hemisphere Press, Part II.

Index

ORDER INFORMATION

Sunrise Publishers

P.O. Box 112112 • Salt Lake City, UT 84147
Phone (801) 595-8155

NAME
ADDRESS
CITY, STATE, ZIP
PHONE

PLEASE SHIP:

☐ Set For Life   QUAN. _____   @ 18.95

☐ Set For Life (Audio Cassette)   QUAN. _____   @ 9.95

☐ Get Set For Life — Your Guide to Personal Success!   Available Soon

Prices subject to change without notice

**PLEASE ADD FOR
SHIPPING AND HANDLING:**

Up to $10.00 . . . . $2.00
10.01 to 30.00 . . . . 3.00
30.01 to 40.00 . . . . 4.00
40.01 to 50.00 . . . . 5.00
50.01 to 70.00 . . . . 6.00
70.01 to 80.00 . . . . 7.00

For Shipment to Canada
Increase shipping by $1.00

SUBTOTAL	
Utah Orders Add 6% Sales Tax	
◄ Shipping and Handling	
TOTAL ENCLOSED	

☐ CHECK   ☐ MONEY ORDER   ☐ MASTERCARD   ☐ VISA

Card No. _____ Expires _____

Signature _____

SEND ORDERS TO: SUNRISE PUBLISHERS
P.O. Box 112112
Salt Lake City, UT   84147
Phone (801) 595-8155

All Orders Prepaid or COD — FOB Salt Lake City, UT   Please allow 4-6 weeks for delivery.